AF414998

HERBAL SYLLABUS

50 Herbal Medications For Healing Naturally

by

Dr. Earendil M. Spindelilus D.N.M., M.H., C.R., PSc.D

HERBAL SYLLABUS

COPYRIGHT © 2020 BY EARENDIL M. SPINDELILUS

ALL RIGHTS RESERVED.

PUBLISHED BY TREE OF LIFE HOLISTIC WELLNESS CENTER

COVER ART BY EARENDIL AND PEGGY SPINDELILUS

NO PART OF THIS BOOK MAY BE REPRODUCED IN ANY WRITTEN, ELECTRONIC, RECORDING OR PHOTOGRAPHING WITHOUT WRITTEN PERMISSION OF THE PUBLISHER OR AUTHOR.

FIRST EDITION - **ISBN - 9798682621712**

DISCLAIMER

THIS BOOK IS INTENDED TO PROVIDE INFORMATION ON THE SUBJECT OF

HEALING NATURALLY WITH HERBS. THIS INFORMATION PRESENTED IS NOT INTENDED

AS A SUBSTITUTE FOR MEDICAL TRAINING OR ADVICE, BUT EVERY EFFORT HAS BEEN

MADE TO ENSURE ACCURACY.

THE BOOK IS SOLD WITH THE UNDERSTANDING THAT THE PUBLISHER AND AUTHOR

ARE NOT LIABLE FOR ANY MISCONCEPTION OR MISUSE OF THE INFORMATION

PROVIDED AND SHALL HAVE NEITHER LIABILITY NOR

RESPONSIBILITY TO ANY PERSON OR ENTITY WITH RESPECT TO ANY LOSS,

DAMAGE OR INJURY CAUSED OR ALLEGED TO BE CAUSED DIRECTLY OR

INDIRECTLY BY THE SAID INFORMATION.

Table of Contents

DEDICATION

To my wife and best friend Peggy, who has stood beside me and put up with all of my time spent getting one degree or certification after another.

To Waya and Sinde, our furry children who love us unconditionally

I would also like to express my gratitude for all of the patients who have taught me so much about how to be a doctor.

Not all doctors are healers and not all healers are doctors.

CHAPTER 1
Introduction

"Everyone has a doctor in him or her; we just have to help it in its work. The natural healing force within each one of us is the greatest force in getting well."
Hippocrates

One of the greatest gifts we can give our selves is the knowledge to help heal our own bodies and those in our care. With the rising costs of conventional medical care and the increase in illness caused by such medical practices as chemotherapy, radiation, surgery and prescription drugs, it is good to know that Nature can provide for us healing modalities that are safe and proven over thousands of years.

At Tree Of Life Holistic Wellness Center, I have over 20 years of medical practice treating and teaching our patients how to heal their own bodies. Within this book are many of the herbs we have used successfully throughout these years, treating literally thousands of patients.

Using such herbs as Comfrey, Plantain (easily found in most front yards), and Chickweed, we have seen some of the worst wounds heal with little to no scarring. For treating infections, we have found the simple yet graceful Garlic and Goldenseal work wonders when modern antibiotics lost their effectiveness due to overuse.

This book stands as an excellent addition to your holistic library with information on over 50 clinically proven herbs and their scientific and medical properties. The information contained within these pages can be of a benefit to both novice and professional alike. This is book seven in the Healing Naturally book series by Dr. Earendil Spindelilus D.N.M., M.H., C.R., Psc.D.

CHAPTER 2
The Herbs

ALOE VERA

LATIN NAME Aloe vera

Kingdom: Plantae
Clade: Tracheophytes
Clade: Angiosperms
Clade: Monocots
Order: Asparagales
Family: Asphodelaceae
Subfamily: Asphodeloideae
Genus: *Aloe*
Species: **A. vera**

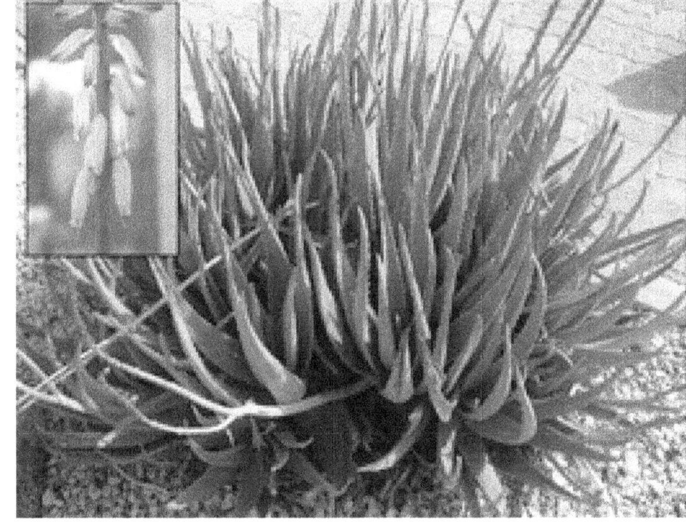

Aloe barbadensis, Aloe capensis
Aloe

Name of Drug

Aloe barbadensis, Curaçao aloe.
Aloe capensis, Cape aloe.

Composition of Drug

Curaçao aloe consists of the dried latex of the leaves of *Aloe barbadensis* Miller [syn.A.vera (L.) N.L.Burm.] [Fam.Liliaceae], as well as its preparations in effective dosage.

Cape aloe consists of the dried latex of the leaves of several species of the genus Aloe, especially *A.ferox* Miller and its hybrids, as well as their preparations in effective dosage.

Aloe contains anthranoids, mainly of the aloe-emodin type.These drugs must conform to the currently valid pharmacopeia.

Pharmacological Properties,

Pharmacokinetics, Toxicology

1,8-dihydroxy-anthracene derivatives have a laxative effect. This effect is primarily caused by the influence on the motility of the colon, an inhibition of stationary and stimulation of propulsive contractions.This results in an accelerated intestinal passage and, because of the shortened contraction time, a reduction in liquid absorption.In addition, stimulation of the active chloride secretion increases the water and electrolyte content.

Systematic studies pertaining to the kinetics of aloe preparations are not available; however, it must be supposed that the aglycones contained in the drug are already absorbed in the upper small intestine.The -glycosides are prodrugs which are neither absorbed nor cleaved in the upper gastrointestinal tract.They are degraded in the colon by bacterial enzymes to aloe-emodin anthrones.Aloe-emodin anthrone is the laxative metabolite. In humans, rhein was demonstrated in the urine after consumption of 86 and 200 mg of aloe powder.

Active metabolites, such as rhein, infiltrate in small amounts into the milk ducts.A laxative effect on nursing infants has not been observed. The placental permeability for rhein is very small.

Drug preparations [i.e., herbal stimulant laxative drugs] have a higher general toxicity than the pure glycosides, presumably due to the content of aglycones. An aloe extract containing 23 percent aloin and less than 0.07 percent aloe-emodin, as well as aloin, produced no mutagenic effects in bacterial and mammalian test systems. For aloe-emodin, emodin and chrysophanol, partially positive results have been obtained. There are no available data regarding carcinogenicity.

Clinical Data

Uses

Constipation.

Contraindications

Intestinal obstruction, acutely inflamed intestinal diseases, e.g., Crohn's disease, ulcerative colitis, appendicitis, abdominal pain of unknown origin. Not to be prescribed to children under 12 years of age or during pregnancy.

Side Effects

In single incidents, cramp-like discomforts of the gastrointestinal tract. These cases require a dosage reduction.

Long-term use/abuse: disturbances of electrolyte balance, especially potassium deficiency, albuminuria and hematuria. Pigment implantation into the intestinal mucosa (*pseudomelanosis coli*), is harmless and usually reverses upon discontinuation of the drug. The potassium deficiency can lead to disorders of heart function and muscular weakness, especially with concurrent use of cardiac glycosides, diuretics and corticosteroids.

Special Caution for Use

Stimulant laxatives must not be used over an extended period of time (1 - 2 weeks) without medical advice.

Use During Pregnancy

Because of insufficient toxicological investigation, this drug should not be used during pregnancy and lactation.

Interactions with Other Drugs

With chronic use/abuse, due to loss in potassium, an increase in effectiveness of cardiac glycosides is possible, as well as an effect on antiarrhythmic agents.Potassium deficiency can be increased by simultaneous application of thiazide diuretics, cortico-adrenal steroids, and licorice root.

Dosage

Aloe powder, aqueous and aqueous-alcoholic extracts in powdered or liquid form, for oral use.

Unless otherwise prescribed:

- 20 - 30 mg hydroxyanthracene derivatives/day, calculated as anhydrous aloin.

The individually correct dosage is the smallest dosage necessary to maintain a soft stool.

Note: The form of administration should be smaller than the normal daily dosage.

Overdosage

Electrolyte and fluid imbalance.

Special Warnings

Usage of a stimulating laxative for longer than the recommended short-term application can cause an increase in intestinal sluggishness.

The preparation should be used only if no effects can be obtained through change of diet or usage of bulk-forming products.

Effects on Operators of Vehicles and Machinery

None known.

Note: During the course of treatment, a harmless red color may occur in the urine.

HISTORY

The generations of past mention the healing methods of Aloe vera plants being handed down through the centuries by word of mouth. We find that the use of Aloe vera appears throughout history with many testimonials of its medicinal values. The earliest record of Aloe vera use comes from the Egyptians. There are records of the Egyptians drawing pictures of Aloe vera plants on the walls of the temples. Many cultures such as the Egyptians would have even elevated the plant to a 'god-like' status. The healing properties of the Aloe vera were utilized for centuries earning the name "Plant of Immortality". One of the common myths about the Aloes was that the two Egyptian queens, Nefertiti and Cleopatra used Aloe vera as part of their beauty treatments. However some sources refute these findings.

The Mahometans of Egypt thought of Aloe vera as a religious symbol, and. they believed that the holy symbol hanging in the doorway would protect them from slanderous and evil influence. The Egyptians used the Aloe vera to make papyrus like scrolls as well as for treatment of tuberculosis. In ancient Egypt when a Pharaoh died, the funeral ceremony was by invitation only with a price tag included: a pound of Aloes. Egyptians used the odorous mixture of Aloe and myrrh for embalming and also placed it with the burial clothes. A man's wealth and esteem for the king were estimated by the number of pounds of Aloes he brought.

The aged people of Mesopotamia, a country located between the Tigris and Euphrates Rivers in present day Iraq used the Aloe vera to hold off the evil spirits from their residences. During the Crusades, the Knights of Templar created a drink of palm wine, Aloe pulp and hemp, which was named 'the Elixir of Jerusalem' and they believed that it added years to their health and life.

The island of Socotra which lies near the Horn of Africa, became known for its Aloe vera plantations as early as 500 BC. The Aloe produced was used for trade to other countries such as Tibet, India and China. Aristotle convinced Alexander the Great to overtake the Isle of Socotra for their Aloe supply containing aloin. The Hindu people thought that Aloe vera grew in the Garden of Eden and named it the 'silent healer'. The Chinese doctors of old thought that Aloe Vera had therapeutic properties so they called it 'harmonic remedy'. In China the juice of Aloes was used to wipe out all rashes. The Russians called Aloe Vera 'the Elixir of Longevity'. The native American Indians used Aloe for its emollient and rejuvenating powers.

Aloe Vera was grown and used by King Solomon (971-931 BC). He highly valued its usage. In Psalm 45:8a it says,"All your garments are fragrant with myrrh and aloes and cassia." Aloes were used on the occasion of a king's wedding, maybe King Solomon's wedding. He most likely grew his own Aloe vera. In Song of Solomon 4:14b it says,"…myrrh and aloes, along with all the finest spices."[10] Aloes were esteemed high with the finest spices. The fleshy leaves contained aloin, a substance which, dissolved in water and added to myrrh, was used in Biblical times for their highly perfected art of embalming. John 19: 38-40 says, "And after these things Joseph of Arimathea, being a disciple of Jesus, but a secret one, for the fear of the Jews, asked Pilate that he might take away the body of Jesus; and Pilate granted permission. He came therefore, and took away His body. And Nicodemus came also, who had first come to Him by night; bringing a mixture of myrrh and aloes, about a hundred pounds weight."

Aloe vera had traveled to Persia and India by 600 BC. by Arab traders. The Arabs called Aloe the 'Desert Lily' for its internal and external uses. They discovered a way to separate the inner gel and the sap from the outer rind. With their bare feet they crushed the leaves, then they put the pulp into the goatskin bags. The bags were then set in the sun to dry and the Aloe would become a powder.

Dioscorides gained most of his knowledge about Aloe vera from traveling with the Roman armies. He first wrote of it in his 'De Materia Medica' in AD 41-68. His commentary uses Aloe vera for boils, healing the foreskin, soothing dry itchy skin, ulcerated genitals, tonsils, gum and throat irritations, bruising, and to stop bleeding wounds. Pliney the Elder, a physician from 23-79 AD, confirmed in his 'Natural History' the discoveries of Dioscorides. Some additional uses that Pliney found for Aloe vera included the healing of leprosy sores and it reduced perspiration as our first anti-perspirant. Two thousand years ago Pliney and Dioscorides saw a difference in the quality of different Aloe vera plants and their processing before use.

Galen (AD 131-201), a physician to a Roman emperor, used Aloe vera as a healing agent. Galen authored over 100 books on herbal and conventional medicine. He gained his knowledge from doctoring the Roman gladiators. Galen followed after the works of Hippocrates and Aristotle.

In the 7th century the Chinese Materia Medicas wrote of using the Aloe vera for sinusitis and other skin conditions. "In the 15th century, a time which heralded a massive explosion in exploration by the then leading maritime powers, namely, Spain, Portugal, Holland, France and Britain, it was the Jesuit priests of Spain who were instrumental in bringing Aloe vera back to the New World as they called it."[16] Many give the Spanish credit for bringing Aloe vera not only to the New World but passing it on to Central America, West Indies, California, Florida, and Texas.

Early Spanish missions had padres that would dispense the healing aids. Some padres would carry an Aloe vera plant up to 50 miles to comfort the sick. Aloes were always found in the mission's yards. During Christopher Columbus' second voyage to America in 1494, a letter was written by his doctor, Dr. Diego Alverez Chanca, said, "A species of Aloes we doctors use are growing in Hispaniola."[18] Christopher Columbus once said, "Four vegetables are indispensable for the well being of man: Wheat, the grape, the olive, and aloe. The first nourishes him, the second raises his spirit, the third brings him harmony, and the fourth cures him."

Aloe Vera lost its potency for healing when it started being imported. The pulp worked best when fresh. This hindered Aloe vera's reputation in the medical community. Europe and North America's medical profession quit using Aloe vera and replaced it with drugs. The scientists determined that the oxidation process hindered the healing properties of Aloe vera. It caused the plant to loose quality and effectiveness, gradually leading to its loss of popularity in areas where it is not grown.

In the 1950's many processing techniques were tried but they failed because of over heating the Aloe can cause it to loose its medicinal value. By the 1970's there was a breakthrough in processing techniques and they successfully; stabilized the leaf gel by using natural ingredients and cold pressing. They also found a way to separate the rind and aloin. These new found processing techniques have created a new market for Aloe vera.

Aloe sales currently supports a multi-billion dollar business world wide. For thousands of years Aloe vera was part of myths and legends but today it plays a role to help improve health and nutrition. Some say that Aloe existed as a predecessor to cortisone on the island of Hawaii in Kona. The Hawiaan people would mash the leaves and stems of Aloe to make a poultice for arthritic conditions. It was quite successful.

Aloe vera maintains being the only thing known to heal atomic burns…the U.S. Government purchased the entire crop from a man in Texas…to make a salve for atomic burns." The invention of the x-ray and atomic bomb brought Aloe vera back into popularity again as it protected against radiation burns. Aloe vera acted as an old natural remedy that is definitely superior to many synthetic drugs and could be called a modern miracle plant.

CHEMICAL CONSTITUENTS

Aloe vera has marvelous medicinal properties. Scientists have discovered over 150 nutritional ingredients in Aloe vera. There seems to be no single magic ingredient. They all work together in a synergistic way to create healing and health giving benefits. The ten main areas of chemical constituents of Aloe vera include: amino acids, anthraquinones, enzymes, minerals, vitamins, lignins, monosaccharide, polysaccharides, salicylic acid, saponins, and sterols.

The amino acids in Aloe vera are the building blocks of protein and influence our brain function. Humans require 22 amino acids and the body will make all of them except for eight essential amino acids which our body gets from the food/drinks that we take in. Every one of the essential amino acids are available in Aloe vera and they include isoleucine, leucine, lysine, methionine, phenylalanine, threonine, valine,and tryptophan. Some of the other non-essential amino acids found in Aloe vera include alanine, arginine, asparagine, cysteine, glutamic acid, glycine, histidine, proline, serine, tyrosine, glutamine, and aspartic acid.

Located in the sap of the leaves you will find twelve anthraquinones, a phenolic compound that has stimulating effects on the bowels and antibiotic properties. In small amounts the anthraquinones do not have a purgative effect. They help with absorption from the gastro intestinal tract and have anti-microbial and pain killing effects. Too many anthraquinones can produce abdominal pain and diarrhea. The most important anthraquinones are aloin and emodin. They are anti-bacterial, anti-viral, and analgesic.[35] The anthraquinones in Aloe vera breakup residue, pus and lifeless cells, bring blood to the region and flush out material from the wounds and ulcers.

Enzymes act as biochemical catalysts that break down the proteins we eat into amino acids. The enzymes turn the food we eat into fuel for every cell in our body, enabling the cells to
function and work efficiently. "The main enzymes found in Aloe vera include Amylase (breaks down sugars and starches), Bradykinase (stimulates immune system, analgesic, anti-inflammatory), Catalase (prevents accumulation of water in the body), Cellulase (aids digestion - cellulose), Lipase (aids digestion - fats), Oxidase, Alkaline Phosphatase, Proteolytiase (hydrolyses proteins into their constituent elements), Creatine Phosphokinase (aids metabolism), and Carboxypeptidase."

The next thing we need to ask ourselves is what fuels the enzymes? The key is the vitamins and minerals we take in. For instance if we lack in zinc and/or Vitamin B6, our body will not be able to break down or use protein. Because of the healing properties of Aloe vera and its synergistic action, the body receives what it needs to work properly. Aloe vera, an anti-oxidant rich plant, contains vitamins such as A, C, and E plus the minerals, zinc, and selenium. Anti-oxidants help boost the immune system and combat free radicals in the body.

It also contains Vitamins B1, B2, B3, B5, B6, and B12 along with choline, calcium (teeth and bone formation, muscle contractions and heart health), magnesium(strengthens teeth and bones, maintains healthy muscles and nervous system, activates enzymes), zinc (speeds up wound healing, mental quickness assists with healthy teeth, bones, skin, immune system, and digestive aid), manganese (activates enzymes, builds healthy bones, nerves and tissues), chromium (assists with protein metabolism and balancing of blood sugars), selenium which all influence our brain performance.

Additional minerals found in Aloe vera include copper (important for red blood cells, skin and hair pigment), iron (involved in oxygen transportation and making of hemoglobin in red blood cells), potassium (helps with fluid balance), phosphorus (helps build bones and teeth, assists with metabolism and body pH), and sodium (regulates body liquids, helps with nerve and muscle performance, and helps deliver nutrients into body cells). Aloe vera also contains the trace minerals of rhodium and iridium used in cancer and tumor research experiments.

Another component of Aloe vera consists of the lignins, a major structural material of cellulose content, that allows for penetrative properties. Aloe vera can soak into the skin up to seven layers deep. Lignins penetrate the toughened areas of the skin being beneficial for skin problems such as eczema and psoriasis.

The next elements of Aloe vera we will discuss include monosaccharides and polysaccharides. Monosaccharides contain the simple sugars which include glucose. The polysaccharides are the more complex long-chain sugars involving glucose and mannose or the gluco-mannans. These sugars are ingested whole from the stomach. They do not get
broken down like other sugars, and appear in the bloodstream in exactly the same form. This process is known as pinocytosis. Once in the blood stream, they exert their healing and immuno-regulating effect. Some of these polysaccharides are not absorbed but stick to certain cells lining the gut and form a barrier preventing absorption of unwanted material so helping to prevent a leaking gut syndrome. The sugars are also used in moisturizing preparations.

One polysaccharide, acemannan, is known for its ability to restore and boost the immune system by stimulating the production of macrophages and improving the activity of T-Lymphocytes by up to 50 %. Acemannan produces immune agents such as interferon and interleukin which help to destroy viruses, bacteria, and tumor cells.[45] Acemannan improves cellular metabolism by normalizing cellular function and regulating the flow of nutrients and wastes in and out of the cells. It knows how to destroy parasites and fungus. In some AIDS patients, it even protected the immune system from the toxic side effects of AZT. Carrington Laboratories in the United States have separated the acemannan from Aloe vera. The product is sold as "Carrisyn" and is being used for treatment of AIDS and Feline leukemia.

Many sources stated that Aloe vera has mucopolysaccharides, nitrogen containing polysaccharides, found in animals and bacteria. A regulation and testing board for Aloe vera products known as the International Aloe Science Council concludes that some people are misinformed and confused on terminology. The Aloe has polysaccharides but not mucopolysaccharides.

Aloe vera contains salicylic acid which is an aspirin-like compound with anti - inflammatory, analgesic, and anti-bacterial properties. It has anti-pyretic properties for reducing fevers. Other constituents of Aloe vera would include prostaglandins, tannins, magnesium lactate, resins, mannins, proteins such as lectins, monosulfonic acid and gibberlin.

Another constituent of Aloe vera includes saponins. These are soapy substances from the gel that is capable of cleansing and having antiseptic properties. The saponins perform strongly as anti-microbial against bacteria, viruses, fungi, and yeasts. The plant sterols or phyto-steroids in Aloe vera include Cholesterol, Campesterol, Lupeol, and B (Beta sign) Sitosterol. The plant steroids have fatty acids in them that have antiseptic, analgesic, and anti-inflammatory properties.

MEDICINAL QUALITIES

The medicinal qualities of Aloe vera are much diversified and adoptogenic. It has the ability to work on different specific problems each person may have. Here lies a plant that can improve the health of the cells throughout the body. Aloe, a therapeutic healing plant, works both externally and internally. When used externally Aloe vera contains properties such as: astringent (causing a contraction of the skin, blood vessels, and other tissues stopping the fluid discharge), emollient (helps to soften and smooth the skin), antifungal (destroys fungi), and cell proliferant (quickly regrows new cells) used to heal wounds and burns.

When we use Aloe vera internally, we get help lowering cholesterol and improving circulation in the lower extremities of the body. Cathartic action of the anthrquinones, emodin and aloin, can be too strong if there contains more than 50 ppm in the Aloe vera juice or gel. Generally it is a good tonic for skin conditions and digestive disorders.[55] The enzymes in Aloe vera will improve digestion and nutrient absorption. It will help bring the body to a pH balance while being beneficial to the whole gastro-intestinal system. Aloe has been known to wash out harmful germs and rebuild with the beneficial flora. Aloe vera sooths indigestion, IBS, colitis and stomach acidity.

Another medicinal property to consider would be anti-bacterial. Aloe-emodin effects the activity of the bacterium <u>Helicobacter pylori</u> as stated in ChungJG Wang HH's research. This bacterium acts as a culprit responsible for causing stomach ulcers. The aloe emodin's antibacterial property also affects four strains of methicillin-resistant <u>Staphylococcus aureus</u> as stated by Hatano's research. In 1964 the Journal of Pharmaceutical Sciences wrote of 'Bacteriostatic Property of Aloe Vera'. They concluded that Aloe vera was a bacteria managing substance that was effective against E.coli, Salmonella, and Streptoccus.

Aloe vera contains another medicinal property known as antiviral. Aloe emodin in Aloe vera makes it so that certain viruses are not able to function. Aloe vera provides a viracudal to <u>herpes simplex virus type 1 and type 2, varicella-zoster virus, pseudorabies virus, and influenza virus</u> according to the research of Sydiskis.

Another important effect that Aloe vera encompasses includes anti-inflammatory. "This effect of Aloe gel may be due to the salicylates, inactivation of bradykinin, and inhibition of histamine formation. It appears that various nonspecified components in the gel reduce the oxidation of arachidonic acid, thereby reducing prostaglandin synthesis and inflammation."[60] The anti-inflammatory occurs naturally in the plant sterols in a synergistic way with the other constituents. It has a steroid like action without the side effects.

In the research of Zhang in 1998, it was discovered that Aloe vera emodin, an anthraquinones, has the ability to suppress or inhibit the growth of malignant cancer cells making it have antineoplastic properties.[62] Aloe vera, a great immune stimulant, contains 90% rhodium and iridium (trace minerals) in the acemannan which is one of the polysaccharides which dramatically increases the white blood cells or macrophages and T cells. It helps enlarge the thymus gland in size by 40%. The thymus is what produces the T cells of the immune system.

Aloe vera has very strong anti-oxidant nutrients. It contains wonderful free radical action in the A, C, and E vitamins. These free radical fighters get rid of the toxins and carcinogenic properties we have in our bodies from the pollution and poor quality foods we eat. We take these free radicals in our bodies through absorption of our skin and through digestion.

Dr. Ivan Danhof, a leading expert on Aloe vera, discovered the rejuvenating ability of Aloe vera, anti-aging. "He believes that one of the main reasons lies in the plant's unique ability to increase production of human fibroblast cells between six and eight times faster than normal cell production. Fibroblast cells are found in the dermis of the skin and are responsible for the fabrication of collagen, the skin's support protein which keeps skin firm, supple, and youthful looking. He found that Aloe vera not only improved fibroblast cell structure but also accelerated the collagen production process. He also believes the clue may lie, once again, with the magic polysaccharides and their moisture binding properties. Aloe vera penetrates the skin with moisture and nutrients up to seven layers deep. The polysaccharides help create a barrier to stop moisture loss from the skin. The fibroblasts will also help protect the skin from damaging rays.

Aloe vera acts as a gentle detoxifier, cleanser, and vermifuge. It is important to use a high quality aloe juice that does not contain more than 50 ppm of aloin in it. Aloin is an anthraquinone that can have purgative actions if too much is used. Aloe will flush out dead skin cells and build new cell growth with healthy tissue, speeding up the healing process of wounds, lesions, and ulcers. It will also help heal skin that is damaged by radiation. Aloe vera will help the body to have better blood flow to the skin because of capillary dilation. The saponins in the aloe have cleansing and antiseptic qualities

DOSAGES

Aloe vera takes time to fix ailments. It may take up to three months for a person to see results. Start your small dosage with a tsp. twice a day an hour before meals. If you feel no adverse reactions, then double your dose until you slowly work up to 4 TBS twice a day. Some people like to take Aloe vera on an empty stomach but taking it before a meal may help with indigestion problems. If your stools get too loose, then cut back on the amount of Aloe vera you are taking.

Aloe vera is a gentle cleanser and purifier of the body causing detoxification to occur. As it carries out toxins and waste, your body may react with aches, pains, rashes, tiredness, nausea, and headaches. Hang in there, this is temporary results. Diarrhea may occur for a day or two. If your symptoms get too bad, cut back on the amount of Aloe vera you are taking and drink plenty of pure water. Start over on a lower dose. Constipation can be helped by taking more Aloe vera daily. Always store your opened bottles of Aloe vera in the refrigerator. It will spoil if left out after opening.

Young children can start with a lower dose such as 1or 2 tsp. a day. You can work up to a comfortable amount that is helping the condition being treated. If a person has a skin condition or allergy, please try a skin patch test first. Aloe vera is non toxic and can be used with other medications without adverse reactions. Be sure to contact your nutritionist if you have questions about using this herb.

Aloe vera can be purchased in gel, juice, or powdered form. Some veterinary practices use Aloe vera for healing epithelial tissues and the immune system. Aloe vera may not be effective on certain tumors or on the nervous system diseases. These aloe treatments are great for animals too. 75% of the time a veterinary is treating a disease that affects the epithelial tissues making Aloe vera a great choice for a healing medium.

ARTICHOKE LEAF

Artichoke leaf

LATIN NAME Cynara scolymus

Kingdom: Plantae
Clade: Tracheophytes
Clade: Angiosperms
Clade: Eudicots
Clade: Asterids
Order: Asterales
Family: Asteraceae
Genus: *Cynara*
Species: *C. cardunculus*
Variety: **C. c. var. *scolymus***

Cynarae folium
Artischockenbltter

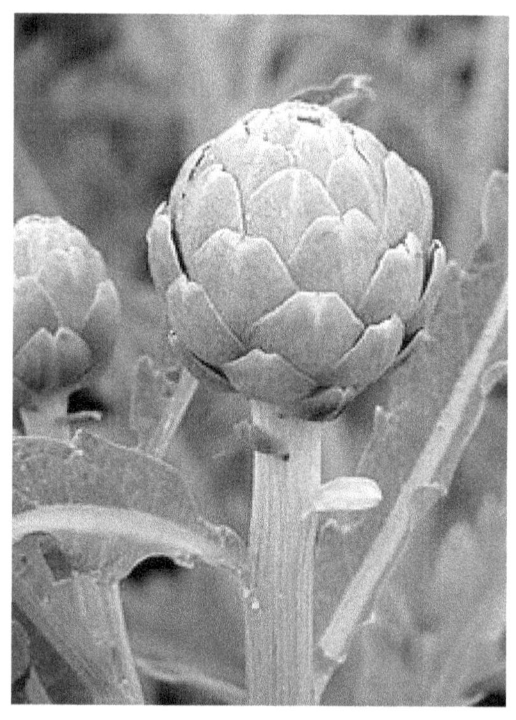

Name of Drug

Cynarae folium, artichoke leaf.

Composition of Drug

Artichoke leaf consists of the fresh or dried leaf of *Cynara scolymus* L. Fam.Asteraceae], and its preparations in effective dosage.

The drug contains caffeoylquinic acid derivatives such as cynarin and bitter principles.

Uses
Dyspeptic problems.

Contraindications
Known allergies to artichokes and other composites.

Obstruction of bile ducts.

In case of gallstones, use only after consultations with a physician.

Side Effects

None known.

Interactions with Other Drugs

None known.

Dosage

Unless otherwise prescribed:
Average daily dosage:

- Drug, 6 g;
- equivalent preparations.

Mode of Administration

Dried, cut leaves, pressed juice of fresh plant, and other galenical preparations for internal use.

Action

Choleretic

1. Loaded With Nutrients

Artichokes are packed with powerful nutrients. A medium artichoke (128 grams raw, 120 grams cooked) contains:

	Raw	Cooked (boiled)
Carbs	13.5 grams	14.3 grams
Fiber	6.9 grams	6.8 grams
Protein	4.2 grams	3.5 grams
Fat	0.2 grams	0.4 grams
Vitamin C	25% of the RDI	15% of the RDI
Vitamin K	24% of the RDI	22% of the RDI
Thiamine	6% of the RDI	5% of the RDI
Riboflavin	5% of the RDI	6% of the RDI
Niacin	7% of the RDI	7% of the RDI
Vitamin B6	11% of the RDI	5% of the RDI
Folate	22% of the RDI	27% of the RDI
Iron	9% of the RDI	4% of the RDI
Magnesium	19% of the RDI	13% of the RDI
Phosphorus	12% of the RDI	9% of the RDI

Potassium   14% of the RDI 10% of the RDI
Calcium   6% of the RDI   3% of the RDI
Zinc   6% of the RDI   3% of the RDI

Artichokes are low in fat while rich in fiber, vitamins, minerals, and antioxidants. Particularly high in folate and vitamins C and K, they also supply important minerals, such as magnesium, phosphorus, potassium, and iron.

One medium artichoke contains almost 7 grams of fiber, which is a whopping 23–28% of the reference daily intake (RDI).

These delicious thistles come with only 60 calories per medium artichoke and around 4 grams of protein — above average for a plant-based food.

To top it off, artichokes rank among the most antioxidant-rich of all vegetables.

Summary Artichokes are low in fat, high in fiber, and loaded with vitamins and minerals like vitamin C, vitamin K, folate, phosphorus, and magnesium. They are also one of the richest sources of antioxidants.

2. May Lower 'Bad' LDL Cholesterol and Increase 'Good' HDL Cholesterol

Artichoke leaf extract may have a positive effect on cholesterol levels.

A large review in over 700 people found that supplementing with artichoke leaf extract daily for 5–13 weeks led to a reduction in total and "bad" LDL cholesterol.

One study in 143 adults with high cholesterol showed that artichoke leaf extract taken daily for six weeks resulted in an 18.5% and 22.9% decrease in total and "bad" LDL cholesterol, respectively.

Additionally, an animal study reported a 30% reduction in "bad" LDL cholesterol and a 22% reduction in triglycerides after regular consumption of artichoke extract.

What's more, regularly consuming artichoke extract may boost "good" HDL cholesterol in adults with high cholesterol.

Artichoke extract affects cholesterol in two primary ways.

First, artichokes contain luteolin, an antioxidant which prevents cholesterol formation.

Second, artichoke leaf extract encourages your body to process cholesterol more efficiently, leading to lower overall levels.

Summary Artichoke extract may reduce total and "bad" LDL cholesterol while increasing "good" HDL cholesterol.

3. May Help Regulate Blood Pressure

Artichoke extract may aid people with high blood pressure.

One study in 98 men with high blood pressure found that consuming artichoke extract daily for 12 weeks reduced diastolic and systolic blood pressure by an average of 2.76 and 2.85 mmHg, respectively.

How artichoke extract reduces blood pressure is not fully understood.

However, test-tube and animal studies indicate that artichoke extract promotes the enzyme eNOS, which plays a role in widening blood vessels.

In addition, artichokes are a good source of potassium, which helps regulate blood pressure.

That said, it is unclear whether consuming whole artichokes provides the same benefits, as the artichoke extract used in these studies is highly concentrated.

Summary Artichoke extract may help lower blood pressure in people with already elevated levels.

4. May Improve Liver Health

Artichoke leaf extract may protect your liver from damage and promote the growth of new tissue.

It also increases the production of bile, which helps remove harmful toxins from your liver.

In one study, artichoke extract given to rats resulted in less liver damage, higher antioxidant levels, and better liver function after an induced drug overdose, compared to rats not given artichoke extract.

Studies in humans also show positive effects on liver health.

For example, one trial in 90 people with non-alcoholic fatty liver disease revealed that consuming 600 mg of artichoke extract daily for two months led to improved liver function.

In another study in obese adults with non-alcoholic fatty liver disease, taking artichoke extract daily for two months resulted in reduced liver inflammation and less fat deposition than not consuming artichoke extract .

Scientists think that certain antioxidants found in artichokes — cynarin and silymarin — are partly responsible for these benefits.

More research is needed to confirm the role of artichoke extract in treating liver disease.

> **Summary** Regular consumption of artichoke extract may help protect your liver from damage and help relieve symptoms of non-alcoholic fatty liver disease. However, more research is needed.

5. May Improve Digestive Health

Artichokes are a great source of fiber, which can help keep your digestive system healthy by promoting friendly gut bacteria, reducing your risk of certain bowel cancers, and alleviating constipation and diarrhea

Artichokes contain inulin, a type of fiber which acts as a prebiotic.

In one study, 12 adults experienced an improvement in gut bacteria when they consumed an artichoke extract containing inulin each day for three weeks .

Artichoke extract may also provide relief from symptoms of indigestion, such as bloating, nausea, and heartburn.

A study in 247 people with indigestion determined that consuming artichoke leaf extract daily for six weeks reduced symptoms, such as flatulence and uncomfortable feelings of fullness, compared to not taking artichoke leaf extract.

Cynarin, a naturally occurring compound in artichokes, may cause these positive effects by stimulating bile production, accelerating gut movement, and improving the digestion of certain fats.

> **Summary** Artichoke leaf extract may maintain digestive health by boosting friendly gut bacteria and alleviating symptoms of indigestion.

6. May Ease Symptoms of Irritable Bowel Syndrome

Irritable bowel syndrome (IBS) is a condition that affects your digestive system and can cause stomach pain, cramping, diarrhea, bloating, constipation, and flatulence.

In one study in people with IBS, consuming artichoke leaf extract daily for six weeks helped ease symptoms. What's more, 96% of participants rated the extract equally as effective as — if not better than — other IBS treatments, such as antidiarrheals and laxatives.

Another study in 208 people with IBS discovered that 1-2 capsules of artichoke leaf extract, consumed daily for two months, reduced symptoms by 26% and improved quality of life by 20%.

Artichoke extract may relieve symptoms in several ways.

Certain compounds in artichokes have antispasmodic properties. This means that they can help stop muscle spasms common in IBS, balance gut bacteria, and reduce inflammation.

While artichoke extract seems promising for treating IBS symptoms, larger human studies are needed.

> **Summary** Artichoke leaf extract may help treat IBS symptoms by reducing muscle spasms, balancing gut bacteria, and reduce inflammation. However, more research is necessary.

7. May Help Lower Blood Sugar

Artichokes and artichoke leaf extract may help lower blood sugar levels.

One study in 39 overweight adults found that consuming kidney bean and artichoke extract daily for two months lowered fasting blood sugar levels compared to not supplementing.

However, it is unclear how much of this effect was due to the artichoke extract itself.

Another small study indicated that consuming boiled artichoke at a meal reduced blood sugar and insulin levels 30 minutes after eating. Notably, this effect was only seen in healthy adults who did not have metabolic syndrome.

How artichoke extract reduces blood sugar isn't fully understood.

That said, artichoke extract has been shown to slow down the activity of alpha-glucosidase, an enzyme that breaks down starch into glucose, potentially impacting blood sugar.

Keep in mind that more research is needed.

> **Summary** Some evidence suggests that artichokes and artichoke leaf extract may lower blood sugar levels. However, more research is needed.

8. May Have Anticancer Effects

Animal and test-tube studies note that artichoke extract impaired cancer growth.

Certain antioxidants — including rutin, quercetin, silymarin, and gallic acid — in artichokes are thought responsible for these anticancer effects.

For example, silymarin was found to help prevent and treat skin cancer in animal and test-tube studies.

Despite these promising results, no human studies exist. More research is needed.

Summary Test-tube and animal studies suggest that artichoke extract may fight the growth of cancer cells. However, no human studies exist, so more research is needed before conclusions can be drawn.

ASTRAGALUS

LATIN NAME Astragalus officinalis

Kingdom: Plantae
Clade: Tracheophytes
Clade: Angiosperms
Clade: Eudicots
Clade: Rosids
Order: Fabales
Family: Fabaceae
Subfamily: Faboideae
Tribe: Galegeae
Subtribe: Astragalinae
Genus: *Astragalus* L.

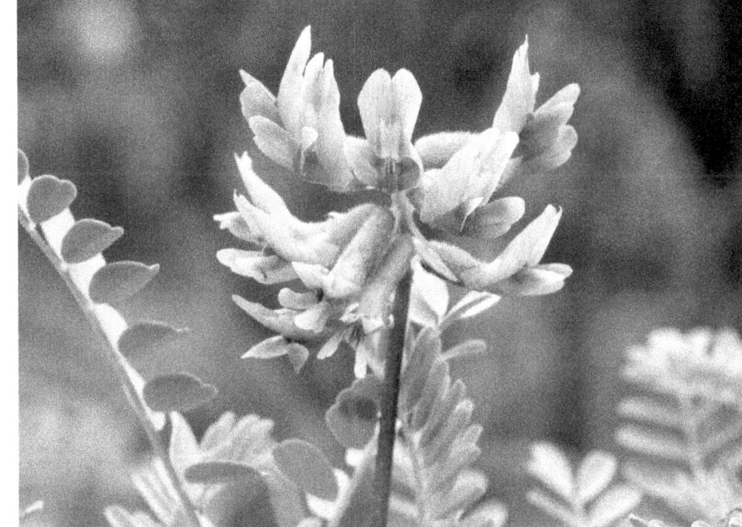

What Is Astragalus?

Astragalus is a plant within the Leguminosae (beans or legumes) family, with a very long history as an immune system booster and disease fighter. Its roots are in Traditional Chinese Medicine, in which it's been used as an adaptogen for thousands of years — meaning it helps the body fight off stress and disease. Today, astragalus medicinal healing and treatment uses span many different illnesses and diseases.

The perennial flowering plant, also called milkvetch root and Huang-qi, grows from 16 to 36 inches tall and is native to the north and eastern regions of China. It's also been traced back to Mongolia and Korea.

Astragalus roots are harvested from 4-year-old plants and are the only part of the plant that's used medicinally. Only two of the over 2,000 species of astragalus, *astragalus membranaceus* and *astragalus mongholicus,* are used medicinally.

Astragalus contains three components that allow the plant to have such a positive impact on human health: saponins, flavonoids and polysaccharides, which are all active compounds contained in certain plants, including some fruits and vegetables. Saponins are known for their ability to lower cholesterol, improve the immune system and prevent cancer.

Flavanoids, also found in astragalus, provide health benefits through cell signaling. They show antioxidative qualities, control and scavenge of free radicals, and can help prevent heart disease, cancer and immunodeficiency viruses. (4) Polysaccharides are known to have antimicrobial, antiviral and anti-inflammatory capabilities, among other health benefits.

Astragalus Benefits

In Traditional Chinese Medicine, the herb was hailed as a protector against stresses, both mental and physical. Astragalus provides health benefits to a number of body systems and ailments. Although more studies in humans are needed to solidify its effectiveness, success in rats, mice and other animals have prompted progressive research on the herb.

Because of the tremendous success of so many research studies and trials, new information about astragalus is coming to light all the time. In general, its greatest strength is preventing and protecting cells against cell death and other harmful elements, such as free radicals and oxidation.

According to continuing research, astragalus health benefits include:

1. Acts as an Anti-Inflammatory

Inflammation is at the root of most diseases. From arthritis to heart disease, it's often the culprit of the damage. Many studies show that thanks to its saponins and polysaccharides, astragalus can reduce inflammatory response in connection to a number of illnesses and conditions, from helping to heal wounds and lesions to reducing inflammation in diabetic kidney disease.

2. Boosts the Immune System

In terms of reputation, boosting the immune system is astragalus' claim to fame. It's been used in this capacity for thousands of years. A study out of Beijing displayed its ability to control t-helper cells 1 and 2, essentially regulating the body's immune responses.

3. Slows or Prevents the Growth of Tumors

Many recent screenings have shown the success of astragalus saponins, flavonoids and polysaccharides in decreasing or eliminating tumors. In instances of chemoresistance treating liver cancer, astragalus has shown potential in reversing multidrug resistance and as an addition to conventional chemotherapy, according to a study published in the *Journal of Pharmacy and Pharmacology*.

4. Protects the Cardiovascular System

The flavonoids present in astragalus are antioxidants that help prevent plaque buildup in arteries and narrowing of vessel walls by protecting the inner wall of the vessel. In addition, a 2014 study published in the *Chinese Journal of Integrative Medicine* suggests injection of astragalus, combined with conventional treatment for viral myocarditis (inflammation of the middle layer of the heart wall), makes treatment more successful in heart conditions.

Other studies have shown its ability to reduce blood pressure and level of **triglycerides**. (10) High levels of triglycerides put individuals at risk for many forms of heart disease, such as stroke, heart attack and hardening of artery walls.

During a heart attack, heart muscle damage occurs when there is a lack of blood supply and oxygen. At that time, calcium overload creates secondary damage. Astragalus may prevent additional heart muscle damage by regulating calcium homeostasis in the heart.

5. Regulates and Prevents Diabetes and Illnesses Related to Diabetes

Astragalus has been studied progressively as an antidiabetic. Studies show its ability to relieve insulin resistance and treat diabetes naturally. The herb's collection of saponins, flavonoids and polysaccharides all are effective in treating and regulating type 1 and 2 diabetes. They're able to increase insulin sensitivity, protect pancreatic beta cells (the cells in the pancreas that produce and release insulin) and also act as anti-inflammatories in areas related to diabetes symptoms.

Kidney disease in diabetics is also a common problem, and astragalus has been used to treat kidney illness for many years. More recent studies in humans and animals have shown astragalus can slow the progress of kidney problems in diabetics and protect the renal system.

6. Contains Antioxidative and Anti-Aging Capabilities

Oxidation due to free radical damage is the main component in disease and aging, and many elements found in astragalus fight free radical damage and prevent of oxidative stress. The herb's polysaccharides have positive effects on the immune system and improvement of the function of the brain, both of which could lengthen life span.

7. Aids in Wound Healing and Minimizes Scarring

Because of its anti-inflammatory qualities, astragalus has a long history of treating wounds. Radix astragali, another name for the dried root of astragalus, has been used in Traditional Chinese Medicine for the repair and regeneration of injured organs and tissues.

In a 2012 study by the Institute of Pharmaceutics at Zhejiang University, wounds treated with astragaloside IV (the active ingredient in dried astragalus root) showed recovery rates increase two- to threefold over 48–96 hours. It was concluded that astragalus is a promising natural product for anti-scarring and healing in wounds.

8. Alleviates Symptoms of Chemotherapy

Astragalus has been shown to help patients receiving chemotherapy to recover more quickly and extend their life spans. In cases of severe chemotherapy symptoms like nausea, vomiting, diarrhea and bone marrow suppression, astragalus has been given intravenously and in combination with other Chinese herbal mixtures. Early research suggests its ability to reduce these symptoms and increase the efficacy of the chemotherapy treatments.

9. Treats Colds and Flu

Because of astragalus' antiviral capabilities, it has long been used to treat common colds and the flu. It's commonly combined with other herbs like ginseng, angelica and licorice. As with many other natural **cold remedies**, it seems to work better when used when healthy individuals use the supplement regularly in order to prevent the illness before it happens. A regimen of astragalus before the colder months of winter may help to prevent or decrease the number of colds and upper respiratory illnesses individuals will have throughout the season.

10. Provides Supplemental Therapy for Chronic Asthma

Astragalus has been used to treat chronic asthma and determined to be a successful supplemental therapy and asthma natural remedy. After being treated, hypersensitivity in airways decreased substantially and mucus production and inflammation were reduced in studies. By preventing or reducing asthma attacks, individuals could be relieved of chronic asthma issues.

There is also evidence to suggest astragalus can successfully:

- prevent collagen degradation
- help heal lung tissue affected by bronchopulmonary dysplasia in newborns

- inhibit herpes simplex virus 1
- prevent the replication of viruses like Coxsackie B-3, a virus that triggers illnesses ranging from mild stomach issues to major heart complications
- treat inflammation in allergic dermatitis (an allergic reaction of the skin)
- help treat hepatitis by inhibiting hepatitis B virus cells in the liver
- treat HIV by protecting t-helper cells fight the virus for much longer
- be used as a mild diuretic

How to Use Astragalus

There are a number of ways to use astragalus root medicinally. Astragalus is currently used as an addition to conventional treatments and should not be used as a replacement for medications unless suggested by a doctor.

According to the University of Maryland Medical Center, astragalus is available at most Chinese markets or health food stores in these forms: (6)

- Tincture (liquid alcohol extract)
- Capsules and tablets
- Injectible forms for use in hospital or clinical settings in Asian countries
- Topically for the skin
- Dried and used in tea

There is not a standardized dosage for astragalus, but you can work with a doctor or specialist to determine how much you should take and how often. There are differences in doses depending on age, health and medical history.

BLACK WALNUT

Walnut leaf

LATIN NAME Juglans nigra

Kingdom: Plantae
Clade: Tracheophytes
Clade: Angiosperms
Clade: Eudicots
Clade: Rosids
Order: Fagales
Family: Juglandaceae
Genus: *Juglans*
Section: *Juglans* sect. *Rhysocaryon*
Species: **J. nigra**

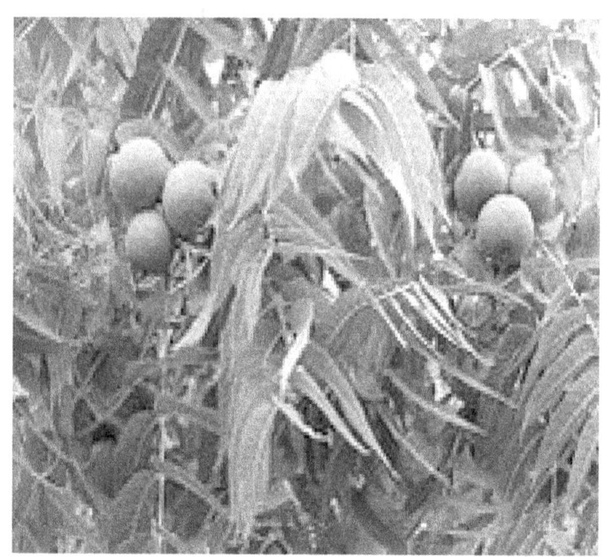

Juglandis folium
Walnubltter

Name of Drug

Juglandis folium, walnut leaf.

Composition of Drug

Walnut leaf consists of the dried leaf of *Juglans regia* L.[Fam.Juglandaceae], as well as its preparations in effective dosage.

The drug contains tannins.

Uses
External:

- Mild, superficial inflammations of the skin; excessive perspiration, e.g., of the hands and feet.

Contraindications
None known.

Side Effects

None known.

Interactions with Other Drugs

None known.

Dosage

Unless otherwise prescribed:

For compresses and partial baths:

- 2 - 3 g herb per 100 ml water;
- equivalent preparations.

Mode of Administration

Comminuted drug for decoctions and other galenical preparations for external use.

Action

Astringent

Walnut hull

Juglandis fructus cortex
Walnufrchtschalen

Name of Drug

Juglandis fructus cortex, walnut hull.

Composition of Drug

Walnut hull consists of the pericarps of *Juglans regia* L. [Fam. Juglandaceae], as well as preparations thereof.

Uses

Walnut hull preparations are used for catarrhs of the gastrointestinal tract, skin diseases, abscesses, inflammation of the eyes, in combinations for diabetes, gastritis, for "blood purification," blood poisoning, and anemia.

The effectiveness for the claimed applications is not documented.

Risks

Fresh walnut hull contains the napthoquinone derivative juglone. The juglone content of the dried walnut hulls has been insufficiently investigated. Juglone acts as a mutagen in various model systems. Application of juglone-containing walnut preparations onto the skin and mucous membranes leads to yellow to brown discoloration. The topical, daily use of juglone-containing preparations of walnut bark is tied to an increased occurrence of cancer of the tongue and leukoplakia of the lips.

THE BENEFITS OF THE USE OF BLACK WALNUT
IN HERBAL PREPARATIONS

MEDICINAL QUALITIES OF BLACK WALNUT
In one region of southern France known as Perigord the long-standing traditional diet is very high in fried foods, rich meats, and fatty patés. Yet, the people suffer fewer heart attacks than Americans. At first medical experts explained this phenomenon by attributing this miracle to the red wine they drink. Red wine is known for its superior antioxidants to protect the heart. Yet, the residents of this region didn't drink any more red wine than those in other parts of Europe. Closer examination revealed that their daily green salads were dressed with walnut oil and chopped walnuts, helping to lower their levels of LDL and overall cholesterol in the bloodstream.

A study published in the American Journal of Clinical Nutrition, May 1994, showed that those whose diets included nuts, either walnuts or almonds, were able to lower their LDL cholesterol by 9 to 10%.

Another study that appeared in the Journal of the American Dietetic Association, July 1995, found that walnuts could also diminish the extent of heart damage after a heart attack.

From ancient times through the nineteenth century herbalists prescribed the walnut, the bark, the roots, and the leaves as an astringent, a laxative, a purgative to induce vomiting, a styptic to stop bleeding, a vermifuge to expel worms or parasites, and a hepatic to tone the liver. The walnut served to induce sweating, cure diarrhea, soothe sore gums and skin diseases, cure herpes, and relieve inflamed tonsils. The nut itself was used to prevent weight gain, calm hysteria, eliminate morning sickness, and to strengthen one's constitution. The hulls were boiled and used to treat head and body lice, herpes, intestinal parasites and worms, skin diseases, and liver ailments. The leaf was decocted to cure boils, eczema, hives, ulcers, and sores.

Even the walnut oil was employed as a medicinal aid. It was first diluted before it was used to treat colic, dandruff, dry hair, gangrene, and open wounds, while the green rind of the walnut was used to treat ringworm.

Alterative; Anodyne; Anti-inflammatory; Astringent; Blood purifier; Blood tonic;//Detergent; Emetic;//Laxative; Pectoral; Vermifuge./
/
The juice from the fruit husk is applied externally as a treatment for ringworm. The husk is chewed in the treatment of colic and applied as a poultice to inflammations.

The bark and leaves are alterative, anodyne, astringent, blood tonic, detergent, emetic, laxative, pectoral and vermifuge. Especially useful in the treatment of skin diseases, black walnut is of the highest value in curing scrofulous diseases, herpes, eczema etc. An infusion of the bark is used to treat diarrhea and also to stop the production of milk, though a strong infusion can be emetic. The bark is chewed to allay the pain of toothache and it is also used as a poultice to reduce the pain of headaches.

A tea made from the leaves is astringent. An infusion has been used to lower high blood pressure. It can be used as a cleansing wash. The pulverized leaves have been rubbed on the affected parts of the body to destroy ringworm. The sap has been used to treat inflammations. Nuts are a highly concentrated form of excellent nutrition; however, it's important to stress that they ought to be eaten in moderation. Because walnuts, like other nuts, are high in fats, it's important to note they are also high in calories.

While one-fourth cup of raw, unsalted walnuts contains 180 calories, be aware they contain 18 grams of fat, 1.5 grams saturated. The fat in walnuts is mostly polyunsaturated. If you are watching the fat, you can calculate your fat intake by dividing the 77% of calories from fat by the 180 calories to learn that a one-fourth cup serving contains 43% fat. That percentage may sound high, but it should not discourage a healthy person from gaining nutritional benefits from eating walnuts in small quantities.

Walnuts are rich in protein, providing 7 grams for that same one-fourth cup, 2 grams of fiber, and only 7 grams of carbohydrates. Walnuts can be considered a super food because they contain a full complement of vitamins, including B1, B2, B3, B5, B6 and folic acid. They also contain a wealth of minerals, such as iron, magnesium, potassium, and zinc.

Walnuts contain Vitamin E-alpha, beta, delta and gamma-tocopherol, making it exceptionally high in antioxidants.

Nutritionists tell us that Omega 3 fatty acids are found in only a few plant food sources, yet are essential to a healthy body. In a 2,000-calorie diet, 3 tablespoons of walnuts will provide our daily requirement of these Omega 3 fatty acids.

THE BENEFITS OF THE USE OF BLACK WALNUT
IN HERBAL PREPARATIONS

**CHEMICAL CONSTITUENTS OF BLACK WALNUT*
The black walnut contains a number of active ingredients, of which the most important are juglone, tannins and iodine. Juglone is a brown constituent of the black walnut hull, leafs, bark and even roots. It is called a phytotoxic allelochemical. Phytotoxic means that it kills plants, and allelochemical means that the black walnut tree produces this chemical to keep other plants from growing around it. You may have noticed that vegetation under black walnut trees is rather scarce, and this is the reason. Since yeast and fungus in humans are also plants, it has been conjectured that it will work against fungus as well and it has been described as an anti-fungal in many herbal reference books.

Chemical Constituent Comparative Scale
*Very Low   Low   Average
            High*
Magnesium (44 mg)   Total Ash (2.9%)   Aluminum (23.1 mg)
Calories (363)
Vit A (s100 IU)   Calcium (309 mg)   Carbohydrates
(82.1%)   Crude Fiber (16.2%
Vit C (0)   Manganese (2.36 gm) Chromium (0.9 mg)
    Fat (5.2%)
Zinc (trace)   Niacin (0.7 mg)   Cobalt (3.6
mg)   Iron (45.5mg)
                Phosphorus (107 mg)   Silicon (2.22
mg)   Potassium (1490 mg)
                Protein (9.8%)   Tin (1.2
mg)   Selenium (2.99 mg)
                Riboflavin (0.1 mg)
                Sodium (13 mg)
                Thiamine (0.2 mg)

THE BENEFITS OF THE USE OF BLACK WALNUT

IN HERBAL PREPARATIONS

**DOSAGES AND APPLICATIONS OF BLACK WALNUT*
The walnut consists of three distinct parts. The edible portion, known
as the kernel or fruit of the nut, is actually the seed of the walnut
tree. It has two lobes. The inner part of the lobe is ivory colored and
is covered by a thin brown skin that is firmly attached.

The shell, called the endocarp, is a very hard material made up of two
distinct halves firmly sealed together. The shell is light brown in
color and has an appearance reminiscent of the convolutions of the human
brain. An inedible, thin, cellulose-like membrane separates the two
lobes of the walnut inside the shell.

The husk, called the pericarp, covers the shell with a soft, fleshy,
green skin that protects the walnut. When fully mature the husk is about
two inches in diameter. Not commonly known, is that the very immature
green husk is edible. At this stage the shell and the nut have not
hardened and both are also edible, though they taste quite sour.
*
Toasting*

To enhance the flavor of walnuts, toast them lightly. Simply put a cup
or two of walnut halves or pieces into a deep, non-stick open skillet
over high heat on the stovetop. Using a wooden spoon, stir constantly
for one to two minutes, taking care not to burn the nuts. Immediately
pour them out onto a dish to cool. If left in the skillet, the residual
heat may burn them.
*
Cracking*

Removing English walnuts from their husks and shells is rarely a
problem. Almost any nutcracker will do. Though they are seldom used
today, a nut pick can be quite handy for pulling the walnut out from its
shell.
*
Chopping*

Chopping nuts can be done in the food processor using the pulse-chop
method. If you only have a few nuts to chop, simply break them up by
hand. If you want coarsely ground walnuts, use a nut mill, an item that
may be available in kitchen shops.
*
Walnut Oil

*

Though the walnut oil was used for many purposes, the first pressing of
the walnut kernel was highly prized by chefs for its lightness and
delicate flavor. High in polyunsaturates, walnut oil is also rich in
gamma-tocopherol, a form of Vitamin E considered nutritionally superior.
Since it is so high in antioxidants, the gamma-tocopherol protects the
oil from becoming rancid quickly.

In France during the eighteenth century, before walnuts were pressed
into oil, they were stored for two to three months to cure. To extract
walnut oil, the nuts were first crushed into a paste. The most highly
valued oils were achieved by heating the paste delicately to bring out
the best flavor of the nuts. Next, the nuts were pressed to extract the
oil. Oil could also be extracted from walnuts without heating, but
heating was preferred, resulting in exceptional flavor. It takes about
four pounds (approximately 2 kilograms) of nuts to press out a scant
quart (a liter) of oil.

Aside from the delicacies of the table, walnut oil served rather diverse
purposes. The ancient Egyptians used the oil in the embalming of their
mummies. Parts of Europe where walnuts were plentiful used a lower
quality of the oil to light their oil lamps. In nineteenth century
France walnut oil was used in the church as holy oil.

European artists favored walnut oil as a paint medium to be mixed with
pigment. In fact, many of the French impressionists preferred it to
poppy and linseed oils that actually surpassed it in quality. The
paintings of Monet, Pissaro, and Cezanne carry traces of walnut oil as
shown by chemical analysis.
*

Using Walnut Oil
*

All vegetable oils are high in calories, and all should be used
sparingly. Walnut oil contains 260 calories per ounce. One tablespoon
contains 120 calories and 14 grams of fat. Use small amounts as a salad
dressing or drizzle delicately over steamed vegetables.

Mode of Administration: Comminuted drug for decoctions and other
galenic preparations for external use.
*

Preparation:* To prepare a decoction, soak 2 teaspoons of herb in 1 cup
of water, boil and strain. An infusion is prepared by using 1.5 g of
finely cut herb, soak in cold water, bring to simmer and strain after
3-5 minutes.

*

Daily Dosage:* The average daily dose for external use 3-6 g of herb.

BLESSED THISTLE HERB

LATIN NAME Cnicus *benedictus*

Kingdom:	Plantae
Clade:	Tracheophytes
Clade:	Angiosperms
Clade:	Eudicots
Clade:	Asterids
Order:	Asterales
Family:	Asteraceae
Subfamily:	Carduoideae
Tribe:	Cynareae
Genus:	*Cnicus* L.
Species:	**C. benedictus**

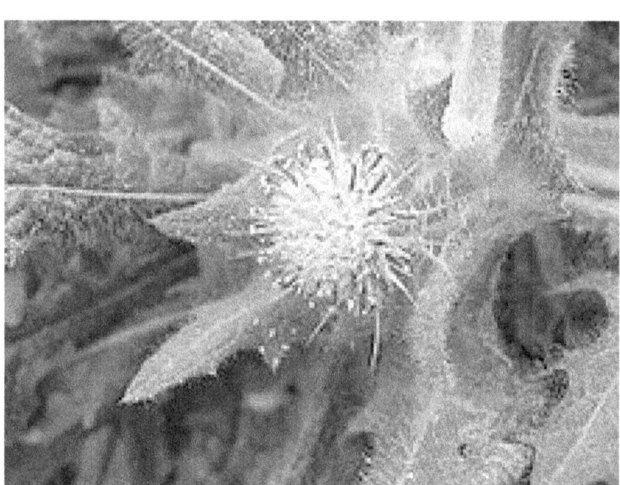

Blessed Thistle herb

Cnici benedicti herba
Benediktenkraut

Name of Drug

Cnici benedicti herba, blessed thistle herb, holy thistle herb.

Composition of Drug

Blessed thistle herb consists of the dried leaves and upper stems, including inflorescence, of *Cnicus benedictus* L.[Fam.Asteraceae], as well as preparations thereof in effective dosage.

The herb contains bitter principles, such as cnicin.

Uses
Loss of appetite, dyspepsia.

Contraindications
Allergies to blessed thistle and other composites.

Side Effects
Allergic reactions are possible.

Interactions with Other Drugs

None known.

Dosage

Unless otherwise prescribed:

Mean daily dosage:

- 4 - 6 g of herb;
- equivalent preparations accordingly.

Mode of Administration

Comminuted herb and dried extracts for teas; bitter-tasting galenical preparations for internal use.

Action

Stimulation of the secretion of saliva and gastric juices

HISTORY

Blessed Thistle has a long and glorious history in herbal medicine. Its history dates back to the Greek and Roman times. It was one of the best known and widely used herbs of the middle ages. Bruno Vonarburg describes the history of Blessed Thistle, "Old folk beliefs states that thistles protect against irritations, restlessness, evil spirits, and witches. It is also known for restlessness and was the witch's herb. The ancient Greeks and Romans used thistles to lite curses, the same as nettles and thorns. People recognized thistles as the seed of evil that grew on graves. Special thorn Gods, from the Greeks such as Hercules, from the Roman Deus, one brought offerings, to protect the fields from thorns and thistles. In the middle ages a healing calendar was chosen to remove thorns from the ground and remove reeds from the ponds." He further states that Martin Luther, a supporter of natural medicine, praised Blessed Thistle for its ability as a tea to soothe pains of the sides and left him symptom free for years. Martin Luther was one of the founders of the religious reformation. The people of that time used herbs from their doctors as well as the common folk. Traditional uses of Blessed Thistle abound and are more fully described in the medicinal uses section of this paper.

It seems that Blessed Thistle has been used, Traditionally in most countries, including England, Russia, China, and Africa, bitters are used to strengthen and tonify the body."

Jacobus Theodorus Tabernaemontanus of the renaissance was a great compiler of works of much old authors and his Kraeuterbuch (herb book), was one of the most in depth and inclusive of all the herbals. The following is his historical description of Blessed Thistle: "…this herb is especially good against the pestilence and all other poisonous weaknesses.

CHEMICAL CONSTITUENTS

Bruno Vonargburg is very thorough in his description of the chemical constituent history of Blessed Thistle: "The research of the chemical substances of Blessed Thistle begin in 1837. There is a high content of bitter principles, the so-called cnicin. The bitterness at 1/1800 is an 1800 dilution where one can still taste the bitterness. Other chemicals are Benedictia, Cnicinolid, Arcticitrol, Arctiing etheric oil with Fenchon, Citral, Cimmonaldehyde and paraffin, further polyencer and oleanol, mucus and tannins, polystyrene, calcium, magnesium, and Vitamin B."

The essential oil of Blessed Thistle is described by R. Vanhoelon-Fastre of the Pharmaceutical Institute of the Free University of Brussels as an antibiotic effect. The essential material influences the stomach secretions, works as an appetite stimulant, and furthers the colon action. It increases the pancreatic secretions, releases cramps of the gallbladder/liver region. It furthers the peristaltic movement of the stomach and strengthens the entire organism.

Bitter herbs keep their importance in medicine as a tonic. There has been 30 different uses of Blessed Thistle as a tonic since the time of Hippocrates.

Its description from the Flora website describes the chemical actions and constituents as follows: "Certain bitter flavonoids found in the leaves, stems, and barks of many plants, particularly the oligomeric proanthocyanidins (OPCs), have indeed been shown to strengthen the walls of blood vessels and capillaries thereby improving overall blood circulation. OPCs have also been shown to bind to collagen and prevent its degradation by enzymes and free radicals and aid in the repair of damaged collagen and elastin. Blessed thistle extracts also have anti-bacterial activity. Research on blessed thistle herb has demonstrated antibiotic properties for: 1) cnicin, 2) the essential oil, and 3) the polyacetylenes contained in the herb. The essential oil has bacteriostatic action against Staphylococcus aureus, S. faecalis, but not E. Coli. Research on blessed thistle has demonstrated that cnicin has considerable activity for stimulating cellular regeneration, detoxification and cleansing. The lignans arctiin and arctigenin, also found in burdock seed, are also noted for this activity and are platelets activating factor (PAF) antagonists and anti-HIV as well. Cnicin also has anti-inflammatory activity."

Continuing with this description: "Active Ingredients: Blessed thistle herb and flowers contain: Bitter substances of the sesquiterpen lactone type, probably occurring in glycosidic form; the principal active ingredient (0.2-0.7%) of the not-too-old dried plant material is a bitter tasting compound called cnicin, a sesquiterpene lactone or germacranolide isolated all the way back in 1837. The seed contains lignan lactones, such as trachelogenin, that also contribute to the bitterness of the drug. Lignans are phyto-estrogen precursors for the key mammalian lignans: enterolactone and enterodiol that are present in humans and animals. The plant also contains: up to 0.3% essential oil which includes n-paraffin (C-9-C13), aromatic aldehydes (cinnamaldehyde, benzaidehyde, cuminaldehyde); phenylpropanes; benzoic acid; monoterpenes (citronellol, fenchone, p-cymene, citral, and others; and flavonoids.

Peter Holmes lists some of the chemical constituents and minerals as follows: "Bitter glycosides (cnicin), alkaloids, flavonoids, essential oil, tannins, sesquiterpone lactone, resin, nicotinic acid, mucilage, minerals (including potassium, calcium, magnesium, iodine)."

MEDICINAL PROPERTIES

Blessed Thistle has an amazing variety of folk history, medicinal uses, and modern applications. One of the first English descriptions of Blessed Thistle medicinal qualities is John Gerard from 1633: "As Carduus Benedictus is bitter, so is it also hot and dry in the second degree, and also withal cleansing and opening. Blessed thistle taken in meat or drink is good for the swimming and giddiness of the head; it strengthens the memory and is a singular remedy against deafness. The same boiled in wine and drunk, heals the griping pains of the belly, kills and expels worms, causes sweat, provokes urine, and drives out gravel, cleanses the stomach; and is very good against the 4 day fever. The juice of the said Carduus is singular good against all poisons, as Heromenous Boeke witnesses, in whatsoever the medicine is taken, and helps the inflammation of the liver, as reported by Joachimus Camerorius of Noremberg. The powder of the leaves ministered in the quantity of half a dram, is very good against the pestilence, if it is received within 24 hours after the taking of the sickness, and the party sweat upon the same: the like virtue has the wine, wherein the herb has been boiled. The green herb pounded and laid to, is good against all hot swellings, as erysipelas, plague, sores and botches, especially those that proceed of the pestilence, and is also good to be laid upon the bites of mad dogs, serpents, spiders, or any venomous beast whatsoever; and so is it likewise if it is taken inwardly. The distilled water thereof is of a less virtue."

Further added is, "It is reported that it likewise cures stubborn and rebellious ulcers, if the decoction is taken for certain days together, and likewise Arnoldus de Villanova reports, that if it is stamped with Barrows grease to the form of an unguent, adding thereto a little wheat flower, it does the same, being applied twice a day. The herb also is good being stamped and applied, so is the juice."

"The extraction of the leaves drawn according to art, is excellent good against the French disease, and quatrain agues, as reported of the aforesaid Camerarius."

"The same author reports, that the distilled water taken with the water of Lovage and Dodder, helps the sauce-flegme face, if it is drunk for certain days together. "

Bruno Vonarburg describes the uses, " …as a tea, it is useful for dyspeptic problems of the gastro-intestinal tract, colon problems, to increase energy, for cramps of the liver-gallbladder area. It is useful for appetite disturbances, hyper and hypo-acidity (too little or too much stomach acidity), and under activity of the pancreas, jaundice, blood problems and sticking pains in the side." (I assume it is the liver or right side.)

The Flora website lists the traditional uses of Blessed Thistle: "Aqueous extract of whole, dried herb and flowers. Traditional usage: Acne, anorexia/appetite loss, anti-inflammatory, antioxidant, cellular regeneration, cleansing, detoxifying, digestive disorders, gastrointestinal disorders, headaches, hormone imbalances, skin disorders. Through its bitter properties, blessed thistle increases the flow of gastric juices relieving dyspepsia, indigestion, and headaches associated with liver congestion. British and German Pharmacopoeias recognize that 'bitters', including blessed thistle, stimulate bile flow and cleanse the liver. In Europe, blessed thistle, as a "bitter vegetable drug" is considered to be a medicinal agent used to stimulate appetite, aid digestion and promote health. Studies confirm that bitters increase gastric juice and bile acid secretions by increasing the flow of saliva through stimulation of specific receptors on the mucus membrane lining of the mouth."

Dr. Fr. Losch talks about the uses of Blessed thistle: "Powdered Blessed thistle of 2 to 4 grams in wine protects against the pestilence, poisons, and removes bad material out of the stomach and kills worms, cleanse the chest and blood, calms colic, promotes sweating, protects against the foul stomach fever, pains of the side, and inner wounds. Blessed thistle taken in food and drink helps dizziness and severe headaches over the eyes."

Earl Mindell lists the folk uses of Blessed Thistle as, "Amenorrhea, stimulates bile production, liver disorders, sluggish appetite, improves circulation, stimulates memory, resolves blood clots, stops bleeding, menstrual problems, and lowers fevers."

Stan Malstrom describes the uses of Blessed Thistle: "For internal parasites; works well for worms. Increases milk while nursing, balances hormones, and helps with cramps and other female problems." Terry Willard, an eminent herbologist describes Blessed thistle, "Tonic, (cold), diaphoretic (hot), emmenagogue and emetic (in double or triple doses)." James Duke describes a newly researched use for Blessed thistle as having anti-HIV activity.

John Tobe describes the action of Blessed thistle as, "Aleipharmic, anthelmintic. From Thomas Green-Universal Herbal "…capable of curing the plague and other malignant feveral disorders…' Useful for ointments externally." E.A. Mueller's book *Die Frau als Hausärztin* (Mother as the home's doctor) is used for "gout, bladder stones, asthma. It is also used for chronic colon disturbances, fever diseases, and seeds are extracted for blood problems."

Schöenenberger describes the traditional Swiss uses: "The inner uses-the entire plant is heart and stomach strengthening, is especially good for mucus congestion. Inflammation and wounds of the stomach and colon. Also from lung mucus, liver problems, jaundice, fevers, cancer like wounds, and weakness from chronic diarrhea,, and constitutional weakness from the tea."

Dieter Podlech recommend Blessed Thistle as "Useful for loss of appetite, colon problems. Useful for liver and gallbladder problems and increase bowel movement." Hugo Hertwig, from pre-world war II Germany from Berlin describes the "…inner and outer uses of Blessed thistle works on the skin. The wound needs to be cleansed with water and then the decoction can be put on. Blessed thistle uses are shown as skin problems over the stomach, liver, kidneys to the lungs areas."

M. Pahlow describes the uses of Blessed thistle: "It stimulates the stomach acid, improves the appetite, protects against colon problems. It stimulates bile production and bile flow. It is useful for chronic stomach problems, and loss of appetite from nervous reasons. Traditional uses include stomach, gallbladder, liver and colon disturbances, appetite loss, bloating, and constipation. It is also used for lung problems, blood poisoning, heart disturbances, and externally for wounds."

Richard Willfort describes internal and external uses of Blessed thistle: "Used for colon problems, gallbladder diseases, liver diseases, jaundice, and gastritis, dyspepsia, gas, and bloating…Also used for constipation, feverish diseases and sluggishness of the gastrointestinal tracts, and weakness of the stomach operations. It also improves and cleanses the blood, anemia. it improves the lung and heart. It is especially good for coughs, catarrh; beginning lung inflammation, lung or heart asthma, heart weakness that are connected with stomach or colon problems. Used externally as a damp warm pack for breast cancer, poor healing wounds, frostbite, and skin lupus of the face. Folk medicine uses include a wound powder, cancer therapy includes a decoction put on breast cancer. It is also useful for cancer-like wounds of the colon and stomach. It regulates excessive menstrual blood flow. It is useful as a nerve calmer. It is also helpful for insomnia, hysteria, and nervous colon tract problems. The seed is used for side pains, purgative, and to induce vomiting." He also discusses the homeopathic uses of Blessed Thistle, known as Carduus Benedictus. In Europe, many natural practitioners use a combination of several therapies to help the body heal. He says, "Homeopathy uses are for glandular diseases, scrofula, wounds, and mucus."

Jacobus Theodorus Tabernaemontanus compiled a very comprehensive list of the uses of Blessed Thistle in various forms, known at that time. The next several paragraphs pertain to his book, and there will only be one foot note to apply to all. Perhaps we have more to learn today. I have translated this from German and this translation is the only known English translation: "The powder (of the herb or the seed), one teaspoon consumed, produces sweating and drives the poison from the heart. It cleanses the blood and kills worms. Used in such a way, is a protection against the pestilence, and doesn't let the poison overrun you. The general person needs this powder against the persistent fever and as prevention against it."

He further states, "The powder consumed in warm wine causes sweating: others boiled the herb in wine and drink therefrom, but it is a bitter drink (If you can't stand the taste make pills.) Taken over a period of time protects against headaches, vertigo, floaters before the eyes, jaundice, edema, and drives the excess dampness from the stomach and uterus, calms the colon, gout, brightens the face, and sharpens the hearing, and cleanses the lungs. This powder taken as one teaspoon, is used for quaternian (four-day) fever, and children's rheumatic complaints…" and again, "This herb is especially good as a liver herb to alleviate constipation. those that have an open wound inside the body should take blessed thistle, boiled in wine or water, and thus drunk, will help him. The new Simplicisten as Matthiolus, Bokius, and others think that this will help migraine headaches that appear above the eyes and sometimes cause vertigo. Use this in food and drink."

"External uses. Matthiolus writes that there is hardly another more precious herb for cancer, and other foul wounds as blessed thistle. He relates that a woman with breast cancer wound open to the bone was healed by the herb (decocted) and it was used to wash the open wound and the dry powder was put in."

Continuing, "The flower of blessed thistle in open wounds heals them up and is often protective. The leaves cut and laid upon, heals the pestilence. The leaves extinguish the burn of the fire (such as the sting or bite of the scorpion or snake). Make a plaster of pork fat and wheat paste with red wine (and blessed thistle powder), lay it on foul wounds."

Also, "You can drive out stones and alleviate women's problems with a steam bath or sweat bath. the leaves mixed with sweet wine, laid on the wound brings good relief."

"Blessed Thistle distilled uses: D. Camerarius says that the distilled water of Blessed Thistle distilled a second time is a special medicinal agent for deafness when it is put in the ears. To treat headaches, soak a linen cloth in the distilled herb water and put on the head. The same water put in the eyes relieves sore, red, itching eyes. One can also remove eye spots by drinking the water and putting it in the corner of the eyes. It is also used for dark and obscured eyes (cataracts). It also takes the pain from burns caused by water or oil; put a cloth soaked with this water. It is also used for old foul wounds also on the face of the female breasts, when washed soothes and furthers wound healing, especially when your put the powder into the wound. This is also for post-birth wounds."

Blessed Thistle in wine: It is useful for all wounds. As with the distilled water, it is useful for the pestilence, poison, headaches, vertigo, dirty blood, and many others. It provokes sweating and menses, as well as urination. It is useful for side aches and sharp pains when associated with wind causes (trapped gas), and drives out the foul stomach fever."

Gaea and Shandar Weiss describe Blessed Thistle, "It is tonic, diaphoretic, emetic, stimulant, and emmenagogic. Considered a tonic for the heart, …it increases circulation. Promotes perspiration, breaks fevers, increases milk in nursing mothers. Blood purifier and a general tonic. In large amounts it induces vomiting, and is a general stomach tonic. In medieval times, … nervous system, treating melancholy, mental agitation, and other nervous disorders with valerian, wood betony, and sage. The name of holy thistle comes from its ability to keep people relaxed, calm peaceful. All thistles are considered tonics for the liver. Blessed thistle is warming, drying, and used for liver problems especially with alcohol. Blessed thistle is a tonic herb for the liver, reproductive system and blood. It is a spleen cleanser.”

Emil Schlegel writes in his book Religion Der Arznei (Religion of the Healer) about the doctrine of signatures. His rendition of the theme is not connected to astrological themes but comes from earlier latin texts. He translates from J.B. Porta in his “Phytognomonica, octo libris contenta; in quibus nova facillimaque affertur methodus, qua plantarum, animalium, metallorum; rerum d enique omnium ex prima extimae faciei inspetione quivis abdiot vires assequatur.” The reader will see an interesting and thorough work where a portion that deals with blessed thistle I translated into English, “Plants that have a similarity with animal parts, have similar powers. The raspberry bush is thorny and works against poisons, for example Carduus Benedictus, not just against snake bites, but against the rabid dog bite, and is effective also for scorpion, spider bites, etc…” (pg 67)

Chapter 5. “Of bitter tastes… Myrrh, aloe, blessed thistle, gentian, wormwood, veronica, etc. It has two wonderful qualities. It keeps the bowel clean and has a balsamic character that prevents fermentation. It prevents and helps septic diseases such as fevers, parasites, and lice.” (pg 91) Chapter 8. “Yellow blooms. They have a sympathy with the gallbladder. It is the bile that removes the toxicity of the joints and body. (In fact the coloring of the stool as well as urine comes from the bile.) Whenever I have a plant, that has a yellow bloom, it removes toxicity from the body...yet a drawing taste, belongs to the spleen and black bile, especially where the root is reddish or gray: Wormwood, yellow iris, tormentil, blessed thistle, potentilla reptans, urginea maritima…”(pg 101)

Chapter 23. “Special Forms of Leaves. All leaves that have thorns, have a pain relieving energy (spiritum), it calms many kinds of puncture wounds of the body, but as the signatur e shows, it is not an opiate, but has a sharp character. Blessed thistle alleviates stabbing pan of the spleen and left side. Frauendistel (Milk Thistle), alleviates stabbing pains of the neck. Eberwurz (Carline Thistle), relieves stabbing pains in pestilent diseases. Mannestreu (Sea Holly), all stabbing pains in the empty spaces (of the body). Wacholderschösslein (Juniper stems), for stabbing pains in the hips. Stechpalmenblätler (Holly leaves), relieve stabbing pains of the joints. All leaves that are long and thin are a sign of the spleen. Spitzwegerich (Plantain), Farnkrauter (Fern herbs), Weidenblatter

(Willow leaves), Blessed thistle. All leaves that have hairy leaves, but are rough, have a power against corrosive inflammations of the arteries…blessed thistle releases the heat of the arteries in the area of the spleen and the quartan (four-day) fevers…" (pg107-108)

Dr. Christopher's therapeutic action of Blessed thistle is, "Tonic (cold), diaphoretic, (hot), emetic (double or triple dosage), emmenagogue, stimulant, febrifuge, antiperiodic, vulnerary. Blessed thistle is wonderful for nursing mothers, stimulating the production of mother's milk. it is very useful in purifying the blood, aiding circulation, and for all liver problems. As a tonic it strengthens the brain, heart, and stomach. Medicinal uses; biliousness, chronic headaches, colds dropsy, dyspepsia, emesis, fractured bones (poultice), heart problems, insanity, intermittent fevers, kidneys, liver, loss of appetite, lungs, strengthens memory, menstrual disorders due to colds, painful menstruation, mother's milk, purification of blood."

Peter Holme puts the use of blessed thistle in Chinese therapeutic terms: "Functions and indications – 1)Stimulates digestion, removes accumulations and relieves appetite loss: reduces liver congestion and resolves mucous damp. Liver and stomach Qi stagnation: appetite loss, painful digestion, depression, constipation, headache. Liver congestion, jaundice. Intestines mucus damp (spleen damp): indigestion, gurgling distended abdomen, alternating constipation and diarrhea. Chronic gastroenteritis. 2) Promotes urination, relieves fluid congestion and relieves edema: resolves toxicosis and promotes lactation. Liver fluid congestion: edema from waist down, nausea. Kidney Qi stagnation: headaches, dry skin, poor appetite, intermittent pains. General toxicosis with rheumatism, arthritis, gout. Poor vision, Scanty or poor quality breast milk. 3) Promotes sweating, dispels wind cold and reduces fever: promotes eruptions. External wind cold: feverishness, fatigue, aching. Cold and flue onset. Eruptive fevers: measles, chickenpox, etc. Remittent fevers (Shao Yang stage) including malaria. Head damp cold: sinus congestion, dizziness, heavy head. 4) Promotes expectoration, resolves viscous phlegm and relieves coughing. Lung phlegm damp: full cough, wheezing, coughing up thick viscous phlegm. Chronic bronchitis, bronchial asthma. 5) Restores the nerves, promotes clear thinking and relieves depression and fatigue. Nerve and brain deficiency: dull thinking memory loss, dizziness, poor hearing, tinnitus, nervous depression. Exhaustion or debility due to overwork, illness, chronic stress. 6) Promotes tissue repair, antidotes poison and reduces tumors. Slow- healing wounds, sores, internal ulcers. Tumors, cancer. Stings, bites, chilblains."

Based upon the previous lists of uses for Blessed thistle from historic, herbal, and folk medicine uses, the top remedy uses are for wounds(15), liver problems (14), fevers, (13), stomach problems (13), colon problems (10), blood problems(10), and appetite disturbances (10).

The next several uses are for headaches (9), lungs (8), heart (7), emetic (6), menstrual problems (6), sweating (6), and parasite problems (6). Other uses of blessed thistle call for pestilence (5), poisons(5), bites (4), cancer (4), constipation (4), deafness (4), depression (4), dizziness (4), dyspeptic problems, jaundice (5), gallbladder problems (4), memory (4), milk production, (4), nervous disorders (4), and side pains (4).

As from the above sources, this next part is a comprehensive list of disorders treated by blessed thistle: Acne, agitation, alexipharmic, amenorrhea, anemia, anorexia, anti-inflammatory, anti-oxidant, anti-periodic, appetite disturbances, bile stimulant, bites, bitter, bladder stones, bleeding, bloating, blood clots, blood problems, botches, bowel movements, brain, breast cancer, bronchitis, burns, cancer, catarrh, cataracts, cellular regeneration, chilblains, chickenpox, circulation, cleansing, colds, colic, colon problems, constipation, coughs, cramps, deafness, depression, detoxification, diarrhea, diaphoretic, edema, emetic, energy, erysipelas, exhaustion, expectoration, eye problems, fatigue, fevers, flu, fractured bones, French disease, frostbite, gallbladder problems, gas, gastritis, hyper-acidity, hypo-acidity, indigestion, inflammation, insanity, jaundice, kidney, lice, liver, lungs, lupus, malaria, measles, memory, menses problems, migraines, milk production, mucus damp, mucus congestion, nausea, nervous system, pancreas, pestilence, plague, poison, purgative, quatrain agues, relaxant, reproductive system, rheumatism, septic diseases, side pains, sinus congestion, skin disorders, sores, spleen, sticking pains, stimulant, stomach problems, stones, stress, sweating, swellings, tonic, toxicity, tumors, ulcers, uterine problems, and urination problems. Thus, Blessed Thistle has a vast array of historical uses.

DOSAGES

The dosage is ½ to 1 teaspoon of the fluid extract. Use ½ teacup 3 times daily. Use 5 to 20 drops of tincture at a time. Bruno Vonarburg related of a French doctor creating a "Vinum Cardui benedicti", or a blessed thistle wine after observing workers, processing the plant having better digestion. A Swiss herb book describes the tincture of blessed thistle as "The tincture can be made in old red wine of the dried herb, left 10 to 14 days in the warm sun or another warm place. Use the tincture 2 to 3 times in a small amount of water or on a sugar cube of 7-10 drops." Dr Fr. Losch uses the distilled water in the ears for deafness.

BUGLEWEED

LATIN NAME Lycopus virginicus

Kingdom: Plantae
Clade: Tracheophytes
Clade: Angiosperms
Clade: Eudicots
Clade: Asterids
Order: Lamiales
Family: Lamiaceae
Subfamily: Nepetoideae
Tribe: Mentheae
Genus: *Lycopus*

Lycopi herba
Wolfstrappkraut

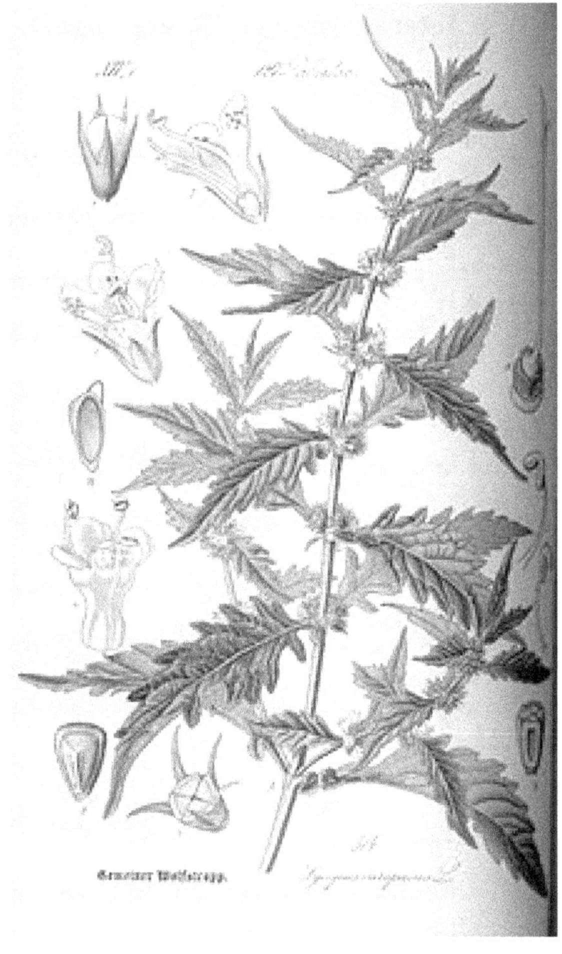

Name of Drug

Lycopi herba, bugleweed, gypsywort.

Composition of Drug

Bugleweed consists of the fresh or dried, above-ground parts of *Lycopus europaeus* L.and/or *L.virginicus* L.Fam.Lamiaceae], as well as their preparations in effective dosage.

The drug contains hydrocinnamic and caffeic acid derivatives, lithospermic acid and flavonoids.

Uses
Mild thyroid hyperfunction with disturbances of the vegetative nervous system.

Tension and pain in the breast (mastodynia).

Contraindications
Thyroid hypofunction, enlargement of the thyroid without functional disorders.

Side Effects

In rare cases, extended therapy and high dosages of bugleweed preparations have resulted in an enlargement of the thyroid.Sudden discontinuation of bugleweed preparations can cause increased symptoms of the disease complex.

Interactions with Other Drugs

None known.

No simultaneous administration of thyroid preparations.

Note: Administration of bugleweed preparations interferes with the administration of diagnostic procedures using radioactive isotopes.

Dosage

The dosage lies between a daily dosage of 1 - 2 g of drug for teas and water-ethanol extracts equivalent of 20 mg of drug.

Note: Each patient has his own individual optimal level of thyroid hormone. Only rough estimations of dosage are possible for thyroid disorders, in which age and weight must be considered.

Mode of Administration

Comminuted herb, freshly pressed juice and other galenical preparations for internal use.

Actions

Antigonadotropic
Antithyrotropic
Inhibition of the peripheral deiodination of T4
Lowering of the prolactin level

Facts About Bugleweed

- Bugleweed is a member of the mint species.
- Its scientific name is **Lycopus virginicus which is very closely related to Lycopus europaeus – its European cousin.**
- Lycopus europaeus is commonly known as gypsywort.
- It was traditionally used by European gypsies for cosmetic purposes hence its common European name.
- Bugleweed is commonly used for respiratory disorders, thyroid issues and anxiety.
- It is also used to normalize the heart rate in people suffering from palpitations.
- Bugleweed can be made into a tea but is also available in supplementary capsule form.

- Few studies into its medicinal effects are available and we are reliant on anecdotal evidence for its medicinal benefits.
- It contains a number of beneficial compounds including tannins, lycopene, lithospermic acid, flavonoid glycosides. ellagic acid, caffeic acid, rosmarinic acid and essential oils.

The Medicinal Properties of Bugleweed

Extracts made from bugleweed contain a good variety of medicinal compounds. These include tannins, flavonoids, phytochemicals and a range of phenolic compounds. In fact the medicinal compounds found in bugleweed are very similar to those found in mint and other members of the mint species such as gypsywort. **In terms of their therapeutic applications, bugleweed and gypsywort have often been regarded as interchangeable.**

Bugleweed is believed to have a respectable range of medicinal properties including antioxidant, anti-inflammatory, astringent, diuretic, nervine and vasoconstrictor properties which give the plant a variety of potential uses when it comes to health and wellness.

The Therapeutic Benefits of Bugleweed

For Respiratory Illnesses

Like so many other herbs, bugleweed contains strong anti-inflammatory compounds which is why **it has traditionally been used to relieve a variety of respiratory complaints**. Bugleweed can be used to relieve many of the symptoms of the cold such as coughs and breathing difficulty. **It is also used to ease the pain of sore throats and relieve sinus and bronchial congestion.**

Bugleweed helps to expel any build up of mucus or phlegm and relieve any inflammation and irritation in the respiratory tracts. With so much going for it, bugleweed seems to be a very attractive natural option especially during those times of the year when people are prone to colds and flu. if you are coming down with a cold, try making a soothing bugleweed tea.

To Relieve Anxiety

As somebody that has experienced their fair share of anxiety and panic disorders, I am always intrigued by the potential of natural remedies. The alternative is not always so attractive. **Pharmaceutical medications are not always as effective as you would hope** and they also come along with the very real risk of serious side effects and dependency.

One of the effects of anxiety that many people suffer are heart palpitations and I have lost count of the times that I thought I was having a heart attack. According to traditional use and proponents of the herb, **bugleweed can help calm the nerves and relieve the irregular heart beats and palpitations associated with anxiety and stress.**

There is no concrete evidence that it will work for you, but giving it a try is a lot less risky than taking a stronger medication.

To Relieve Anxiety

As somebody that has experienced their fair share of anxiety and panic disorders, I am always intrigued by the potential of natural remedies. The alternative is not always so attractive. **Pharmaceutical medications are not always as effective as you would hope** and they also come along with the very real risk of serious side effects and dependency.

One of the effects of anxiety that many people suffer are heart palpitations and I have lost count of the times that I thought I was having a heart attack. According to traditional use and proponents of the herb, **bugleweed can help calm the nerves and relieve the irregular heart beats and palpitations associated with anxiety and stress.**

There is no concrete evidence that it will work for you, but giving it a try is a lot less risky than taking a stronger medication.

For Improved Sleep

Because of its purported ability to calm the nerves, **bugleweed has also been used to overcome sleeping difficulties caused by stress and insomnia.** Millions of people the world over struggle badly to get adequate amounts and quality of sleep and this can have a far reaching impact on their daily lives and ability to function throughout the day.

There is no guarantee that bugleweed will work for you but many people have found use herbal medications as their preferred option and **bugleweed is unlikely to cause any harmful side effects**. If you are one of those many people who suffer from restless nights, it may be worth giving bugleweed a go, especially as part of an overall sleep strategy.

According to proponents of the herb, **it positively interacts with the body's hormones and helps to balance the Circadian rhythms** which can help you achieve a healthy night of rest.

Try a cup of bugleweed tea before bed to relax your mind and hopefully put you in the right state for a good night of sleep.

To Balance the Hormones and Thyroid Health

Undoubtedly the best known reason to use bugleweed is to treat an overactive thyroid. People with hyperthyroidism suffer from numerous uncomfortable symptoms including weakness, fatigue, hair loss and palpitations.

The internet is awash with positive testimonies about the effects of the herb on thyroid levels. **A limited amount of research has demonstrated that bugleweed helps treat elevated thyroid levels by inhibiting T4 output.**

Bugleweed can also play a role in treating other hormonal problems. According to traditional use, it helps to regulate levels of estrogen in women and protects women from breast pain during their menstrual cycle.

For Grave's Disease

Many people also recommend taking bugleweed to treat Grave's disease which is an immune disorder resulting in excessive thyroid hormones being produced. Symptoms of the condition are extremely uncomfortable and include palpitations, tremors, weight loss, lack of libido. It can also cause certain physical changes such as bulging eyes and goiters.

Bugleweed is one of the natural remedies deemed to be an effective remedy for the condition because of its purported **ability to inhibit thyroid production.**

According to anecdotal evidence, **bugleweed helps alleviate many of the symptoms associated with Grave's disease including the elevated heart rate and palpitations** that many sufferers find most difficult to cope with. They do point out however that bugleweed should be taken as part of an overall protocol which includes managing stress. **For thyroid complications, a dose of 5 ml of liquid extract twice a day is generally recommended to start.**

For Heart Health

The ability of bugleweed to steady the heart rate and eliminate palpitations may be significant when it comes to heart health in general. There is no scientific data regarding its efficacy but many people believe that by calming the heart and relieving pressure on the system, **it can help protect against heart attacks, atherosclerosis and stroke.**

It may also help to regulate the heartbeat in people who suffer from palpitations.

For Wound Healing

You can safely apply bugleweed topically to minor wounds, cuts and abrasions to relieve pain and inflammation and to help the wound heal up more quickly. **Bugleweed has excellent antioxidant properties that can promote cell regeneration and reduce inflammation.**

May Help your Complexion

Bugleweed was traditionally used by European gypsies as a topical treatment for the skin. According to traditional use, it helped improve the complexion and was used as a cosmetic remedy in the past. Unfortunately, there is no concrete evidence that it works as a topical skin treatment but it does contain some powerful antioxidants and astringents that can theoretically improve your skin's health.

Antioxidant Benefits

Bugleweed is home to numerous antioxidants which can have an extremely beneficial effect on your body and may protect you from an array of potential diseases in the longer term. The phytochemicals present in the herb can help to neutralize the very damaging effects that free radicals have on your cells and organs and **reduce the risk of disease in the future.**

It is important to get as many natural antioxidants into our system as possible to combat the damage done by free radicals or oxidative stress. Oxidative stress is the root of many diseases including serious illnesses like heart disease and dementia.

How to use Bugleweed

Like most herbs, bugleweed is available in health stores in several different forms. **It can be made into a tea and is also available in tincture or capsule form.** Make sure that you follow the dosage instructions properly and ask an expert if you need any further guidance.

When you stop taking the herb, after long term use, you are advised to **wean yourself off it gradually** as discontinuing the herb abruptly can cause very high thyroid levels.

CATNIP

LATIN NAME Nepata cataria

Kingdom: Plantae
Clade: Tracheophytes
Clade: Angiosperms
Clade: Eudicots
Clade: Asterids
Order: Lamiales
Family: Lamiaceae
Genus: *Nepeta*
Species: **N. cataria**

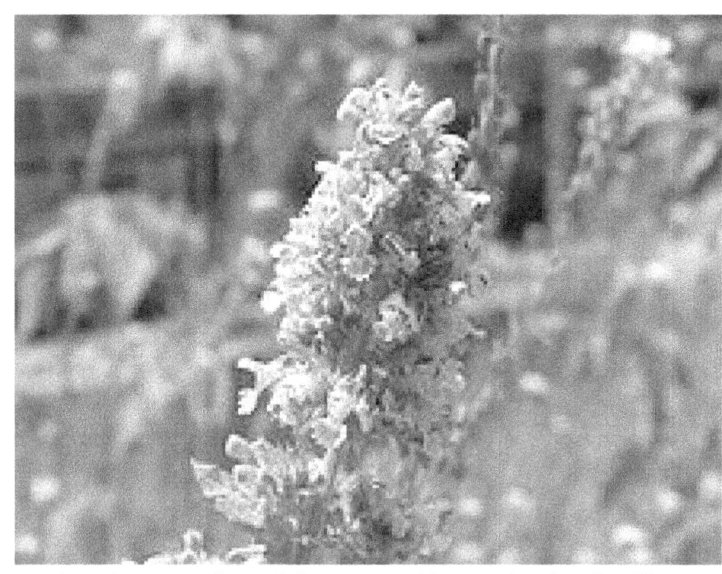

Nepeta cataria, commonly known as **catnip**, **catswort**, **catwort**, and **catmint**, is a species of the genus *Nepeta* in the family Lamiaceae, native to southern and eastern Europe, the Middle East, Central Asia, and parts of China. It is widely naturalized in northern Europe, New Zealand, and North America. The common name catmint can also refer to the genus as a whole.

The names *catnip* and *catmint* are derived from the intense attraction about two-thirds of cats have toward them (alternative plants exist). In addition to its uses with cats, catnip is a popular ingredient in herbal teas (or tisanes), and is valued for its sedative and relaxant properties

Other Common Names: Catmint, catnep, catswort, fieldbalm, Katzenminze (German), hierba gatera (Spanish), katteurt (Danish), cataire (French).

Description

Nepeta cataria is a short-lived perennial, herbaceous plant that grows to be 50–100 cm (20–40 in) tall and wide, which blooms from late spring through autumn. In appearance, *N. cataria* resembles a typical member of the mint family of plants, featuring brown-green foliage with the characteristic square stem of the plant family Lamiaceae. The coarse-toothed leaves are triangular to elliptical in shape. The small, bilabiate flowers of *N. cataria* are pretty and fragrant, and are either pink in color or white with fine spots of pale purple

Scientists have ascertained that the feline reaction to catnip is due to it's content of nepetalactone. The herb is also strongly anti-fungal and a bactericide for Staphylococcus aureus, as well as a close chemical relative to a number of insect repellants that affect mosquitoes and termites… Catnip has also been used as a sedative to help with insomnia, producing similar effects as Valerian.

Plant Parts Used The entire above-the-ground part of the plant is used and can be gathered just after full bloom and then dried for later use. The flowering tops are most commonly used in medicinal applications. (Folklore states that chewing the root may increase aggressiveness and irritability.)

Therapeutic Uses, Benefits

Catnip contains an essential oil (consisting of nepetalactone, carvacrol, citronellol, nerol, geraniol, pulegone, thymol, caryophyllene and nepetalinic acid), iridoids, tannins, and rosmarinic acid.

The soothing effect of catnip is attributed to the substance nepetalactone, not unlike the soothing ingredient found in valerian (*Valeriana officinalis*). Both nepetalactone and nepetalinic acid have been shown to significantly increase sleep duration in mice.

The plant has been cultivated for centuries and has been used both as an herbal medicine and in cooking. It was one of the most important medicinal herbs in medieval monastery gardens.

Catnip has a diaphoretic effect (increasing perspiration without raising body temperature) and antipyretic (anti-fever) effects so it could have uses for treating colds and as an herbal remedy for symptoms of the flu (influenza).

A mild tea made from the flowering tops may be effective in treating colic, restlessness, motion sickness and nervousness in children.

The antispasmodic qualities of this herb help to relieve many gastrointestinal disorders and cramping.

A poultice of the leaves and flowers can be applied to reduce swelling from rheumatism, soft-tissue injuries and other inflammatory conditions.

A mixture of catnip tea and saffron has shown promise in treating scarlet-fever and small-pox.

The Herb Catnip (Nepeta cataria) – ©The Herbal Resource

Catnip is also used as a muscle relaxant and mild sedative, which is why it is often used to relieve the pain of headaches (especially tension headaches) and migraines.

This also explains its use to combat insomnia and other sleep disorders.

Because of the herb's mild sedative effect, it has recently been proposed for use in the treatment of ADHD (hyperactivity) in children.

This plant is also used to bring about the menses in delayed menstruation and increase tone in the uterus.

Nepetalactone, one of the ingredients of the essential oil, is shown to be effective as an insect repellant. It may also work as an external flea treatment on animals.

Catnip has an intoxicating and almost an aphrodisiac effect on many cats. They eat the plants and roll in them with great pleasure. The substance that is most likely responsible for this effect is actinidine, an iridoid glycoside similar to those found in valerian (Valeriana officinalis).

A small cloth bag containing dried leaves can be given to the cat to play with. Most of the time it is a big hit both for the cat and the owner.

Research has shown that approximately one-third of cats do not respond to the plant. It is likely the reaction to it is genetically determined, and is transmitted through a dominant gene. Cats that lack this particular gene do not respond to catnip.

Preparation and Usage

Catnip is used as a herb or seasoning on salads. The oils are extracted and taken in capsule form or used externally. The oils or a potpourri concoction is used for aroma therapy.

The herb can also be steeped as a tea. The tea may be prepared by adding 1 to 2 teaspoons to 1 cup of hot (not boiling) water. Steep it for 10 minutes then strain. It is common to take the capsules or tea three times daily.

CAT'S CLAW

LATIN NAME Uncaria *tomentosa*

Kingdom: Plantae
(unranked):   Angiosperms
(unranked):   Eudicots
(unranked):   Asterids
Order: Gentianales
Family: Rubiaceae
Genus: *Uncaria*
Species: **U. tomentosa**

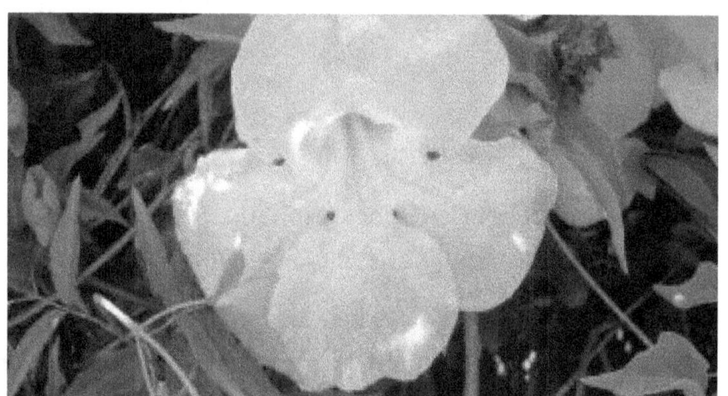

Cat's Claw is a climbing vine indigenous to the Amazon rainforest and other tropical areas of South and Central America, including Peru, Colombia, Ecuador, Guyana, Trinidad, Venezuela, Suriname, Costa Rica, Guatemala, and Panama. The name comes from the claw-like thorns that are used by the vine to climb high into the canopy of the rainforest. There are two main documented species of this plant and they share similar chemical make-ups (U. tomentosa and U. guianensis) Many Native Tribes in the South American Rainforest have used this herb medicinally but the Ashaninka of central Peru are one of the largest commercial producers of Cat's Claw and they as well as many other tribes have made the plant part of their medicinal and spiritual practice for over 2,000 years. Austrian researcher Klaus Keplinger learned about the plant from the Ashaninka, evaluated it in his lab, and then applied for US patents based on the isolation of certain chemicals (oxindole alkaloids) in the plant. The native people's value this plant's spiritual virtues as highly as its medicinal properties.

Since the 1970s, studies and research have been carried out by scientists in Peru, Germany, Austria, England and other countries, to find out more about the powerful healing properties of Cat's Claw. Today, mainly by word of mouth, it has become one of the best selling herbs in the USA. Not since quinine was discovered in the bark of a Peruvian tree during the seventeenth century had any other rainforest plant ever prompted worldwide attention.

The most attention was given to the oxindole alkaloids found in the bark and roots of Cats Claw, which have been documented to stimulate the immune system. It is these seven different alkaloids that are credited with having a variety of different medicinal and healing properties. The most immunologically active alkaloid is believed to be

Isopteropodin (Isomer A), which increases the immune response in the body and act as antioxidants to rid the body of free radicals. Compounds found in Cat's Claw may also work to kill viruses, bacteria, and other microorganisms that cause disease, and they work to inhibit healthy cells from becoming cancerous.

It has been suggested that Cat's claw extracts exert a direct anti-proliferative activity on MCF7 (a breast cancer cell line). This has led to its use as a adjunctive treatment for cancer and AIDS as well as other diseases that negatively impact the immunological system. In addition, the presence of glycosides, proanthocyanidins and beta sitosterol help provide anti-viral and anti-inflammatory support for the body. These alkaloids also exert a beneficial effect on memory. Cat's claw is considered a remarkably potent inhibitor of TNF-alpha production.

This herb's anti-inflammatory properties may help to relieve arthritis, gout, and other inflammatory problems. The primary mechanism for Cat's claw anti-inflammatory actions appears to be immunomodulation via suppression of TNF-alpha synthesis.

Cat's Claw may help create support for the intestinal and immune systems of the body, and may also creates intestinal support with its ability to cleanse the entire intestinal tract. This cleansing helps create support for people experiencing different stomach and bowel disorders, including: colitis, Crohn's disease, irritable bowel syndrome, and leaky bowel syndrome.

In addition, in one study, human volunteers who took Cat's claw for 8 weeks showed improved DNA repair.

Cat's Claw can often be found combined with other 'immune' herbs with similar healing properties such as Echinacea and may:

- reduce pain and inflammation of rheumatism, arthritis and other types of inflammatory problems.
- have anti-tumor and anti-cancer properties that inhibits cancerous cell formation.
- promote the healing of wounds.
- be useful for treatment of gastric ulcers and intestinal complaints
- help to relieve chronic pain.
- enhance immunity by stimulating the immune system.
- help people experiencing stomach and bowel disorders, including colitis, Crohn's disease, irritable bowel syndrome, leaky bowel syndrome, gastritis and duodenal ulcers, intestinal inflammation.
- help fight both viral and fungal infections such as Herpes and Candida

Common Names

Cat's Claw, Una de Gato, paraguayo, garabato, garbato casha, samento, toron, tambor huasca, una huasca, una de gavilan, hawkâ€™s claw

Suggested Properties

Antibacterial, anti-inflammatory, antimutagenic, antioxidant, antitumorous, antiviral, cytostatic, depurative, diuretic, hypotensive, immunostimulant, vermifuge

Indicated for

AIDS, arthritis, balancing intestinal flora, bone pain, bowel disorders, bursitis, cancer, candida, chronic fatigue syndrome, chronic pain, colitis, Crohn's disease, digestive complaints, duodenal ulcers, fungal infections, gastric ulcers, gastritis, gout, herpes, immune system deficiencies, improving DNA repair, inflammatory problems, intestinal complaints, irritable bowel syndrome, kidney cleanser, leaky bowel syndrome, osteoarthritis, parasites, stimulating the immune system, stomach problems, viral infections, urinary tract inflammation, wounds.

CAYENNE

LATIN NAME Capsicum annum

Latin Name: *Capsicum species*
Pharmacopeial Name: capsici fructus, capsici fructus acer
Other Names:
Capsicum annuum L. var. *annuum*: bell pepper, chili pepper, red pepper, sweet pepper, paprika;
Capsicum annuum var. *conoides* Irish: Mexican chili, pimiento;
Capsicum annuum var. *glabriusculum* (Dunal) Heiser & Pickersgill: bird pepper;
Capsicum annuum var. *longum* Sendtner: Louisiana long pepper or hybridized to the Louisiana sport pepper;
Capsicum frutescens L.s.l.: Tabasco pepper, African capsicum, African chili, capsicum, chili pepper, hot pepper.

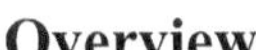

Overview

Capsicum annuum is an annual or biennial plant (Iwu, 1990), while *C. frutescens* is a perennial shrub. Both species are native to tropical America, now cultivated worldwide in tropical and subtropical zones (Leung and Foster, 1996; Whistler, 1992). The degree of pungency, calculated in heat units, of dried *Capsicum* and/or the oleoresin extractive, is what determines its value and end use (Wood, 1987). The material of commerce comes mainly from tropical Africa, China, and India (BHP, 1996).

Chili is the Aztec name for cayenne pepper. It has been used by Native Americans as food and medicine for at least nine thousand years. Based on archeological evidence, its cultivation in Mexico is believed to have begun around seven thousand years ago. It was first introduced to Europe by Dr. Diego Alvarez Chanca, who accompanied explorer Cristoforo Colombo (ca. 1451-1506 C.E.) to the West Indies (Lembeck, 1987; Palevitch and Craker, 1995). From Europe, it was then transported to most tropical, subtropical, and temperate zones around the world (Palevitch and Craker, 1995).

Cayenne was introduced into traditional Indian Ayurvedic medicine as well as traditional Chinese, Japanese, and Korean medicines, respectively. In Ayurvedic medicine, a combination of cayenne, garlic, and liquid amber are used externally in paste or plaster form as a rubefacient (agent which reddens the skin) and local stimulant. It is also combined with mustard seed in a paste form used as a counterirritant (Kapoor, 1990; Nadkarni, 1976). The dried fruit and/or tincture are also used internally to treat flatulent dyspepsia and atony of digestive organs (Karnick, 1994; Nadkarni, 1976). In Chinese medicine, cayenne is considered to have digestive stimulant action and is sometimes used to cause diaphoresis (Shih-Chen et al., 1973). Topically, it is used in China in an ointment form to treat myalgia and frostbite. In Japan, the tincture form is used topically to treat the same conditions (But et al., 1997).

In Germany, cayenne pepper is official in the *German Pharmacopeia* and approved in the Commission E monographs as a topical ointment for the relief of painful muscle spasms in the upper torso (DAB, 1997). In the United States, capsicum tincture and oleoresin were formerly official in the *United States Pharmacopeia* and *National Formulary.* Capsicum USP was used as a carminative, stimulant, and rubefacient (Leung and Foster, 1996; Taber, 1962). Capsaicin, isolated from *Capsicum*, is recognized by the U.S. FDA as a counterirritant for use in OTC topical analgesic drug products (Palevitch and Craker, 1995). It is used as a component in various counterirritant preparations (Leung and Foster, 1996), including ArthriCare (Del Pharmaceuticals, Inc.) arthritis pain relieving rub, which contains *Capsicum* oleoresin (0.025% capsaicin) in combination with menthol USP and *Aloe vera* gel (Arky et al., 1999). *Capsicum* ointments, such as Zostrix cream (GenDerm Corp.), containing 0.025% or 0.075% capsaicin, are used topically to treat shingles (herpes zoster) and post-herpetic neuralgia (Bernstein et al., 1987; Der Marderosian, 1999; Palevitch and Craker, 1995).

Cayenne preparations have demonstrated significant efficacy in the treatment of shingles, trigeminal neuralgia, and reduction of pain following surgical amputation (Tyler, 1993). For topical arthritis relief, capsaicin interferes with the pain of inflammatory joint disease. It may block pain fibers by destroying substance P, which normally would mediate pain signals to the brain (Garrett et al., 1997; Tyler, 1993). It may also interfere with oxygen radical transfers that are intrinsic to pain-producing prostaglandin pathways (Leung and Foster, 1996). While its exact mechanisms are not fully understood, capsaicin is regarded as a neuropathic pain reliever, and has recently been the subject of a phase 3 trial that demonstrated significant reductions in the long-term, postsurgical pain of cancer survivors (Ellison et al., 1997).

Numerous studies on topical preparations containing isolated capsaicin have been documented. Human trials have investigated its use as a treatment for chronic post-herpetic neuralgia (Bernstein et al., 1987; Bernstein et al., 1989; Menke and Heins, 1999; Peikert et al., 1991; Watson et al., 1988; Watson et al., 1993), its effects on normal skin and affected dermatomes in herpes zoster (Westerman et al., 1988), the somesthetic and electrophysiologic effects of topical capsaicin (Walker and Lewis, 1990), its use in the treatment of painful diabetic neuropathy (Basha and Whitehouse, 1991; Tandan et al., 1992), the effect of local capsaicin treatment for chronic rhinopathy (Eberle and Gluck, 1994), its use in the management of surgical neuropathic pain in cancer patients (Ellison et al., 1997), and the effect of topical capsaicin on substance P immunoreactivity (Munn et al., 1997). Additionally, a meta-analysis of trials of topical capsaicin for the treatment of diabetic neuropathy, osteoarthritis, post-herpetic neuralgia, and psoriasis has been published (Zhang and Li Wan Po, 1994).

Other studies on the anti-inflammatory action of capsaicin analogs suggest that the antioxidant nature of the methoxyphenol ring of capsaicin may interfere with the oxygen radical transfer mechanism common to lipoxygenase and cyclo-oxygenase. Cayenne is thought to cause a dose-related (1-100 nM) hemolysis of human red blood cells, and is associated with significant changes in erythrocyte membrane lipid components (decreasing phospholipid and cholesterol content), as well as an acetylcholinesterase activity. There are reported alterations in membranes including calcium homeostasis, lysosomal leakage, and alterations in antioxidant enzyme defense systems (Leung and Foster, 1996).

German pharmacopeial grade cayenne pepper consists of dried, ripe fruit of *C. frutescens* L. sensu latiore., usually removed from the calyx. It must contain not less than 0.4% capsaicinoids with reference to the dried drug. Determination of total capsaicinoids is carried out with liquid chromatography. Botanical identification must be confirmed by thin-layer chromatography (TLC), macroscopic and microscopic examinations, and organoleptic evaluation. Fruit from *C. annuum* L. var. *longum* (de Candolle) Sendtner may not be present (DAB, 1997). The *German Homeopathic Pharmacopoeia,* however, requires the dried ripe fruits of *C. annuum* L. and considers the fruits of *C. frutescens* L. to be foreign constituents (GHP, 1993).

Japanese pharmacopeial grade cayenne pepper consists of the fruit of *C. annuum* L. or its varieties. Identity is confirmed by TLC plus macroscopic and organoleptic evaluations. It must contain not less than 9.0% ether-soluble extractive (JSHM, 1993).

Description

Cayenne consists of the dried fruits of various capsaicin-rich *Capsicum* species [Fam. Solanaceae] and its preparations in effective dosage. Cayenne pepper consists of the dried, ripe, usually removed from the calyx, fruits of *C. frutescens* L., and its preparations in effective dosage. The preparations contain capsaicinoids.

Chemistry and Pharmacology

Cayenne pepper contains up to 1.5% capsaicinoids (pungent principles) including 0.11% capsaicin, 6,7-dihydrocapsaicin, nordihydrocapsaicin, homodihydrocapsaicin, and homocapsaicin; fixed oils (Budavari, 1996; Leung and Foster, 1996; Wood, 1987); carotenoid pigments including capsanthin, capsorubin, alpha- and beta-carotene (Budavari, 1996; But et al., 1997; Leung and Foster, 1996); steroid glycosides, including capsicosides A, B, C, and D (But et al., 1997); 9-17% fats; 12-15% proteins; vitamins A and C; trace of volatile oil (Leung and Foster, 1996; Newall et al., 1996).

The Commission E reported local hyperemic and local nerve-damaging activity.

The *British Herbal Pharmacopoeia* reported rubefacient and vasostimulant actions (BHP, 1996). *The Merck Index* reported the therapeutic category of capsaicin, a pungent principle isolated from cayenne or paprika, as topical analgesic (Budavari, 1996). Cayenne has been shown to have counterirritant, antiseptic, diaphoretic, rubefacient, and gastric stimulating properties (Newall et al., 1996; Stecher, 1968).

Uses

The Commission E approved cayenne for painful muscle spasms in areas of shoulder, arm, and spine of adults and children. Preparations are used to treat arthritis, rheumatism, neuralgia, lumbago, and chilblains. It is also used as a deterrent for thumb sucking or nail biting in children (Leung and Foster, 1996). Human studies on cayenne have found different results in duodenal ulcer patients. One study administered 10 g of red chilies in wheatmeal to the control group and duodenal ulcer sufferers and found no significant effect on acid or pepsin secretion, or on sodium, potassium, and chloride concentrations in the gastric aspirate (Pimparkar et al., 1972). In contrast, a study on capsicum showed that it increased acid concentration and DNA content of gastric aspirates in control subjects as well as in patients with duodenal ulcers (Locock, 1985).

Contraindications

Application on injured skin, allergies to cayenne preparations.

Side Effects

In rare cases hypersensitivity reaction may occur (urticaria).

Use During Pregnancy and Lactation

No restrictions known.

Interactions with Other Drugs

None known.

Note:No additional heat application.

Dosage and Administration

Unless otherwise prescribed: Preparations of cayenne exclusively for external uses.

Liniment: Hot oil emulsion containing dried cayenne powder or alcoholic tincture, applied locally by friction method.

Ointment or cream: Semi-liquid preparation containing 0.02-0.05% capsaicinoids in an emulsion base, applied to affected area.

Poultice: Semi-solid paste or plaster containing 10-40 µg capsaicinoids per cm^2, applied locally.

Tincture 1:10 (g/ml), 90% ethanol: Aqueous-alcoholic preparation containing 0.005-0.01% capsaicinoids, applied locally.

Duration of administration: Not longer than two days; 14 days must pass before a new application can be used in the same location. Longer use on the same area may cause damage to sensitive nerves.

Solanaceae

A farmer used to give Cayenne to his chickens and cows when they were ailing, but never to the children when they were sick. One of the sons said, "We were worth more to him than those animals! He should have given it to us, too." Dr. Christopher assured us that Cayenne is one of the greatest herbs of all time-though it is also one of the most misunderstood and ridiculed. He said that every home should have a good supply of Cayenne   pepper.

When only a young man in his thirties, Dr. Christopher was told by the medical doctors that he could not live past his fortieth year because of arthritis, hardening of arteries, stomach ulcers, and some automobile accidents that had damaged him rather badly. He was so concerned that he started using Cayenne, working up to a teaspoon taken three times a day. By the time he was forty-five years old, he was working in a business wherein the group wanted him to have a $100,000 insurance policy because of the importance of the business deal.

Because it was such a large policy, the company required the examination to be given by two medical doctors, each to examine twice. At the end of one of these physicals, one of the doctors said, "This is astounding! You have the venous structure of a teenage boy, at forty-five years of age !"

The other doctor kept pumping up his blood pressure equipment over and over again, repeating the blood pressure check. Dr. Christopher began to be perturbed, and asked him if the equipment was broken. "It always has worked up till now, but I keep looking at your chart, which says you are forty-five years old, and yet your systolic over your diastolic is absolutely perfect. I cannot comprehend it." Dr. Christopher assured him that it was indeed perfect, and he attributed this clean bill of health to Cayenne.

However, Dr. Christopher needed to be converted to the use of Cayenne. When he was attending the Herbal College in Canada, the teacher announced that they were going to study Cayenne. "Why Cayenne?" asked Dr. Christopher. "It will burn the lining out of the stomach."

"Where did you get your information," asked the teacher, Dr. Nowell. "Oh, my mother told me," answered Dr. Christopher.

Everybody in the class laughed - except the teacher and Dr. Christopher. Dr. Nowell took Dr. Christopher around Vancouver and introduced him to over a dozen people whose lives had been saved with Cayenne: people with heart troubles, ulcers, asthma, and many other ailments. Wherever they went, the people were full of gratitude for being taught about Cayenne, and from then on Dr. Christopher was sold on it.

While Dr. Christopher was working in the business world, he was taking Cayenne, and on one business trip, he was traveling with an athlete, a man who had a black belt in karate and who was, in Dr. Christopher's words, "a husky little guy." Yet he came from a family with a history of high blood pressure, and his uncle had died of varicosity. He was under the care of a doctor at the time. Every morning, Dr. Christopher would take a spoonful of Cayenne in a glassful of water, followed by a few tablespoons of wheat germ oil. The young man wanted to know what Dr. Christopher was taking and wanted to try some. "You're probably too chicken," Dr. Christopher told him! This reverse psychology worked; Dr. Christopher noticed that his Cayenne was disappearing gradually. When they returned from the trip, the man continued taking Cayenne, one teaspoonful three times a day. The doctor was astonished at the young man's next checkup - after a lifetime of high blood pressure, he now had a clean bill of health.

Once a child was shot in the abdomen; a bullet hit the spine, ricocheted, and made a second wound leaving the body. One of Dr. Christopher's herbal students, living next door, heard the shot and raced over, as she knew that the parents were not home and that the children, ages eight and four, would not be shooting guns. There was the eight-year-old gushing blood out both sides. She ran to the cabinet and mixed a tablespoonful of cayenne in a glass of water; she poured it down the boy and immediately called the ambulance, which was eighteen miles away. The emergency room attendant said that the boy would probably bleed to death, being that the distance was so great. The ambulance arrived and rushed the child (who had been playing "Cops and Robbers" with his fathers pistol, which he had found Under the pillow of the bed, to the Primary Children's Hospital eighteen miles away. When he arrived, he was the center of attraction, not because his ease was so dangerous, but because he was chatting a mile a minute - and there was not bleeding. The bleeding had stopped by the time they arrived at the hospital. The chief doctor said to the parents, "I have seen many accident victims in my life, but this is the first time in such an emergency operation that I have opened an abdomen to find no blood, except for a small amount that was there before the bleeding stopped so quickly.   This   has   saved   your   boy's   life."

In that same year, Dr. Christopher treated four other gunshot victims, and each ease responded the same, although sometimes the blood coagulates and comes out in clumps before it stops completely. By the time you count to ten, however, the heavy bleeding should stop completely after administering Cayenne. The Doctor even used tincture of Cayenne on open wounds and, as he put it, "There may be a bit of muttering about it," referring   to   the   burning   feeling   of   the   Cayenne,   but   the   bleeding   stops.

Dr. Christopher related the humorous story of a very fine student of his who had begun teaching herb classes on his own. This young man happened to precede Dr. Christopher's lecture one evening in Arizona. The young man said, "You know, ladies and gentlemen, that Dr. Christopher has always made me gasp. I've seen him drink two or three tablespoons of Cayenne in water - and I'd just shudder. But tonight I'm going to do something that he may have never done himself." With that, he reached down into a container of Cayenne and threw a pinch right into his eye. Dr. Christopher thought that the man must have gone crazy and he was concerned that one of his students would do such a thing in public, although he knew that Cayenne can never hurt the cell structure, no matter how delicate it is. The tears ran down the man's cheek as he continued talking, and when he was finished, he opened his eye and invited everyone to look. The eye just sparkled; it was by far the brighter of the two, although Dr. Christopher said that he never had   seen   this   antic   performed   again   -   and   that   he   never   dared   to   try   it   himself.

A lady who had been attending Dr. Christopher's lectures over the years told the story of her husband who had a severe ease of stomach ulcers. The doctor recommended that part of the stomach be removed, but the man preferred to suffer the pain rather than risk such an operation. But he also ridiculed his wife's recommendations to use Cayenne and other herbs. Whenever he would see Dr. Christopher in town, he'd bellow, "Hello, Doc! Killed anybody with Cayenne today?" Naturally, Dr. Christopher tried to avoid him, but one day he came directly to the Doctor—but this time without any sarcasm, instead being very apologetic, telling this story.

He had come home from work one night, so sick he wanted to die, with stomach ulcers. His wife was not home, but he was in such pain that he decided to commit suicide. When he looked into the medicine cabinet to find some kind of medicine poisonous enough to kill him, he discovered that his wife had discarded all the old bottles of pharmaceutical medicines. All he could find were some bottles of herbs and a large container of Cayenne pepper. He figured that a large dose of that would kill him, so he took a heaping tablespoon in a glass of hot water, gulped it down, rushed into the bedroom, and covered his head with a pillow so that the neighbors couldn't hear his dying screams.

The next thing he knew, his wife was shaking him awake the next morning. He had slept all night, the first time in years, instead of waking every half hour or so for anti-acid tablets. To his amazement, all his pain was gone. He continued using the Cayenne faithfully, three times a day, and never had any more trouble with ulcers.

Once, when traveling with a business partner, Dr. Christopher recommended Cayenne to him, as the man had extremely high blood pressure and such bad hemorrhoids that he had to wear a belt. Dr. Christopher used the same reverse psychology on this man - "I don't think you are brave enough"—and pretty soon the man was taking the Cayenne and the wheat germ oil, too. In a few months, he did not have to wear a belt any longer, and his systolic and diastolic at his blood pressure examination were nearly perfect. He no longer had to go to the doctor—and he lived many long years, for he kept taking his Cayenne.

Early in Dr. Christopher's practice, he was called in the middle of the night by a woman whose husband had just passed out from a heart attack. The Doctor told the woman to heat some water, and he arrived at the house and mixed a teaspoon of Cayenne into the water, propped up the man, and gave him just a little. When he came to, he finished the cup, and within a few minutes felt much stronger. Soon he was well, and became converted to the use of herbs, even buying and running one of the health food stores in Salt Lake City for many years.

One young man had cut his hand deeply, fingers as well as the palm. The blood spurted out in streams. He poured a large amount of Cayenne into the wound, and within seconds the blood flow slowed down, congealed, and stopped. He wrapped with wound, covering it first with a goodly amount of Cayenne. He was so excited about these results that he could hardly wait to attend the next herb lecture to tell about it. But when he unwrapped the bandage to show the audience, instead of a deep, ugly scar, the area was healed and there was no scar at all!

Cayenne can be used on any part of the body and for anybody, Dr. Christopher claimed. He even saved the life of a six-week-old baby who was born with chronic asthma by giving Cayenne tea, from an eyedropper, until the baby was able to breathe again. He said that Cayenne could even be given by enema for chronic constipation (if you are brave!).

At the age of seventy, a few years before he died, Dr. Christopher was asked by a premed student if he could take his blood pressure. The lecture group saw the blood pressure reading of a healthy young man, not the average reading of a seventy-year-old. In addition to a healthy life-style and the mucusless diet, Dr. Christopher attributed this good reading to his thrice-daily dose of Cayenne.

To show what a miracle worker Cayenne really is, Dr. Christopher related the experiment performed by medical doctors in the eastern United States—and printed in the medical journals. They put some live heart tissue in a beaker filled with distilled water, and fed it nothing but Cayenne pepper, cleaning off sediments periodically and adding nothing else but distilled water to replace that which was lost from evaporation. During the experiment, they would have to trim the tissue every few days, because it would grow so rapidly! Having no control glands (pituitary and pineal), the tissue just continued to grow rapidly. They kept this tissue alive for fifteen years. After the doctor doing the experiment died, his associates kept it alive for two more years before destroying it for analysis. This shows the tremendous regenerative and healing power of Cayenne, especially upon the heart.

CEDAR BERRY

LATIN NAME Juniperus monosperma

Kingdom: Plantae
Division: Pinophyta
Class: Pinopsida
Order: Pinales
Family: Cupressaceae
Genus: *Juniperus*
Species: ***J. monosperma***

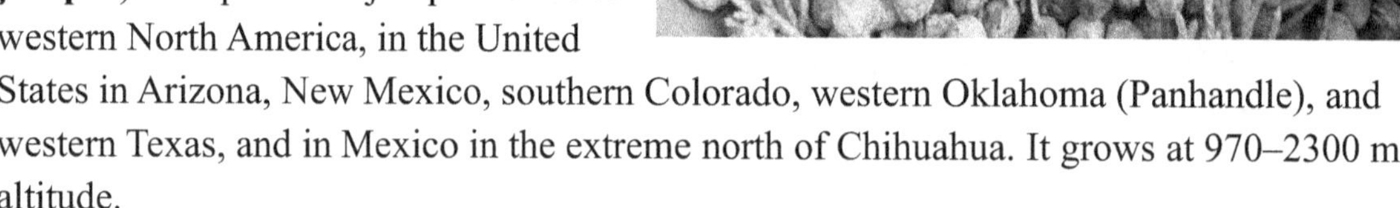

***Juniperus monosperma* (one-seed juniper)** is a species of juniper native to western North America, in the United States in Arizona, New Mexico, southern Colorado, western Oklahoma (Panhandle), and western Texas, and in Mexico in the extreme north of Chihuahua. It grows at 970–2300 m altitude.

It is an evergreen coniferous shrub or small tree growing to 2–7 m (rarely to 12 m) tall, usually multistemmed, and with a dense, rounded crown. The bark is gray-brown, exfoliating in thin longitudinal strips, exposing bright orange brown underneath. The ultimate shoots are 1.2–1.9 mm thick. The leaves are scale-like, 1–2 mm long and 0.6–1.5 mm broad on small shoots, up to 10 mm long on vigorous shoots; they are arranged in alternating whorls of three or opposite pairs. The juvenile leaves, produced on young seedlings only, are needle-like. The cones are berry-like, with soft resinous flesh, subglobose to ovoid, 5–7 mm long, dark blue with a pale blue-white waxy bloom, and contain a single seed (rarely two or three); they mature in about 6–8 months from pollination, and are eaten by birds and mammals. The male cones are 2–4 mm long, and shed their pollen in late winter. It is usually dioecious, with male and female cones on separate plants, but occasional monoecious plants can be found. Its roots have been found to extend to as far as 61m below the surface, making it the plant with the second deepest roots, after *Boscia albitrunca*.

Uses

The Navajo eat the ripened cones in the fall or winter, and make a dye from the bark and cones. They use its wood for various purposes. Among the Zuni people, a poultice of the chewed root is applied to increase the strength of newborns and infants. An infusion of the leaves is also taken for muscle aches and to prevent conception. An infusion of the leaves is also taken postpartum to prevent uterine cramps and stop vaginal bleeding. A simple or compound infusion of twigs is used to promote muscular contractions at birth and used after birth to stop blood flow. The wood is also used as a favorite and ceremonial firewood, and the shredded, fibrous bark is specifically used as tinder to ignite the fire sticks used for the New Year fire.

Nutrient Rich:

Cedar berries are packed full of nutrients that will not only help to maintain your general health, but also tackle a number of other health issues that may be troubling you. This particular berry has been known to help with digestive issues such as IBS, but it can also help with heartburn issues along with a number of other health problems.

Cedar berries are also fantastic at helping to regulate your blood sugar levels and this does mean that they are great for diabetics and you are also boosted by the fact that it helps improve kidney filtration and all of this means it can reduce the chances of you even becoming diabetic at some point in your life.

Studies

Studies have also shown that due to the high levels of vitamin C in the berries they are also very effective at combating fever and colds and of course high levels of nutrients and vitamins will also be fantastic at boosting your immune system in general as well. Finally, it is possible that it will help with rheumatism for some people, but in order to get the full effect you may have to combine these berries with other natural ingredients to get the correct levels of vitamins.

So those are some of the main health benefits of cedar berry and the only thing left for you to do is to buy some and start taking it on a regular basis. You may not feel the difference straight away, but it has certainly helped a number of people and there is no reason to doubt that you should then be any different.

Cedar berry tea benefits are varied and are especially known to many Native American tribes as being potent for respiratory and tumor-related ailments. Even while the therapeutic effects of the cedar berry has yet to be officially and scientifically established, studies already completed on the cedar berry suggest that it may possess antibiotic and antiseptic properties.

The cedar berry comes from the evergreen coniferous shrub that typically abounds in the Western areas of North America, particularly in the U.S. states of Arizona, New Mexico,

Texas and in the northern areas of Mexico.

Bearing the scientific name of juniperus monosperma (one-seed juniper), the cedar berry tree can grow to a height of up to 25 feet. It possesses flat, scale-like leaves.

The cedar berry commonly has a dark bluish-green hue with a dull blue-white waxy bloom. It is actually a modified cone that has a soft resinous flesh, and has a shape that is either subglobose to ovoid. The cedar berry contains a single seed and becomes mature in about 6 to 8 months from pollination.

The cedar berry is typically available commercially in the form of dried herb. It may be used as flavoring agent in cooking and also as a natural food preservative. The cedar berry may also be eaten as food, though it has a strong and unusual flavor that may be an acquired taste.

The active constituents of the cedar berry are the following: alcohols, cadinene, camphene, flavone, flavonoids, glycosides, podophyllotoxin, vitamin C, volatile oils, resin, sabinal, sugar, sulfur, tannins, and terpinene. Podophyllotoxin is the substance that is known to imbue the cedar berry with its anti-tumor properties.

Cedar berry tea can be made either as an infusion or a decoction. As an infusion, the berries are usually steeped in a cup of newly-boiled water for about 3 to 5 minutes. As a decoction, the berries may be soaked in boiling water for up to 15 minutes.

Cedar berry tea may help in the treatment of cough, tuberculosis and other respiratory ailments.

Cedar berry tea may help in the treatment of fever.

Cedar berry tea may aid in alleviating pain from rheumatism and arthritis.

Cedar berry tea may help in lowering risk of developing tumors.

Cedar berry tea may help promote menstruation.

Cedar berry tea may help contribute to strengthening the immune system.

Cedar berry tea may help fight muscle stiffness.

Cedar Berries have an excellent history in treating diabetes.

CHAMOMILE

Chamomile flower, German

LATIN NAME **Matricaria chamomilla**

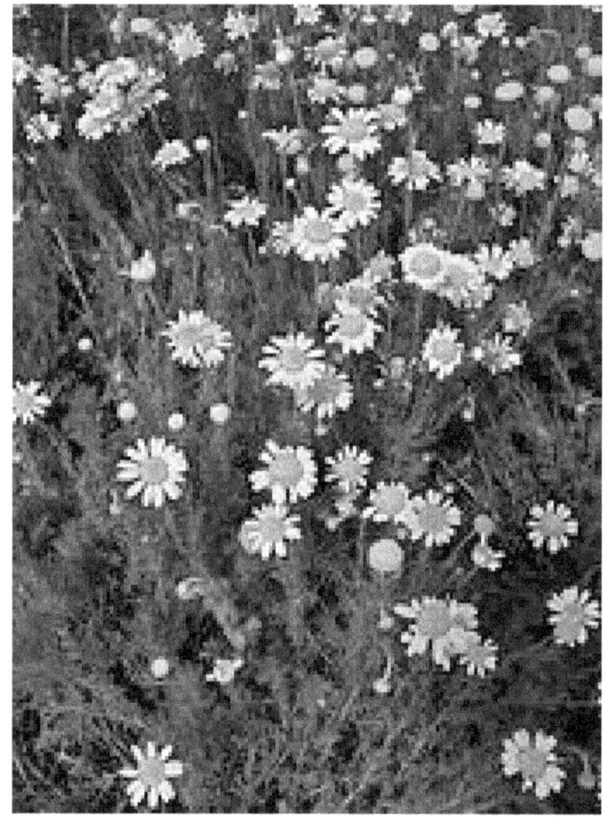

Kingdom:	Plantae
Clade:	Tracheophytes
Clade:	Angiosperms
Clade:	Eudicots
Clade:	Asterids
Order:	Asterales
Family:	Asteraceae
Genus:	*Matricaria*
Species:	**M. chamomilla**

Matricariae flos
Kamillenblten

Name of Drug

Matricariae flos, chamomile.

Composition of Drug

Chamomile, consisting of fresh or dried flower heads of *Matricaria recutita* L.(syn. *Chamomilla recutita* (L.) Rauschert) [Fam.Asteraceae], and preparations thereof at effective dosage.The flowers contain at least 0.4 percent (v/w) essential oil. Main ingredients of the essential oil are a-bisabolol or bisabolol oxide A and B.

The flowers also contain matricin and flavone derivatives such as apigenin and apigenin-7-glucoside.

Uses
External:

- Skin and mucous membrane inflammations, as well as bacterial skin diseases, including those of the oral cavity and gums.Inflammations and irritations of the respiratory tract (inhalations).
  Ano-genital inflammation (baths and irrigation).

Internal:

- Gastrointestinal spasms and inflammatory diseases of the gastrointestinal tract.

Contraindications

None known.

Side Effects

None known.

Interactions with Other Drugs

None known.

Dosage

Boiling water (ca.150 ml) is poured over a heaping tablespoon of chamomile (ca.3 g), covered, and after 5 - 10 minutes passed through a tea strainer.

Unless otherwise prescribed, for gastrointestinal complaints a cup of the freshly prepared tea is drunk three or four times a day between meals.For inflammation of the mucous membranes of the mouth and throat, the freshly prepared tea is used as a wash or gargle.

External:

- For poultices and rinses, 3 - 10 percent infusions;
- As a bath additive, 50 g - 10 liters (approximately 2- gallons) water;
- Semi-solid formulations with preparations corresponding to 3 - 10 percent herb.

Mode of Administration

Liquid and solid preparations for external and internal application.

Actions

Antiphlogistic
Musculotropic
Antispasmodic
Promotes   wound   healing
Deodorant
Antibacterial
Bacteriostatic
Stimulates skin metabolism

CHICKWEED

LATIN NAME Stellaria *media*

Kingdom: Plantae
Clade: Tracheophytes
Clade: Angiosperms
Clade: Eudicots
Order: Caryophyllales
Family: Caryophyllaceae
Genus: *Stellaria*
Species: **S. media**

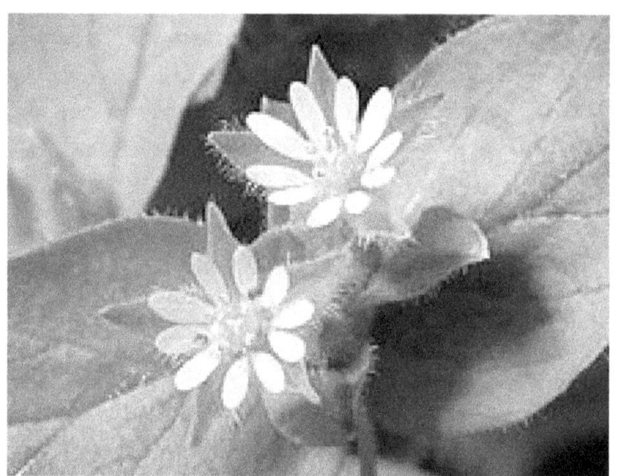

***Stellaria media*, chickweed**, is an annual and perennial flowering plant in the family Caryophyllaceae [1]. It is native to Eurasia and naturalized throughout the world. This species is used as a cooling herbal remedy, and grown as a vegetable crop and ground cover for both human and poultry consumption. It is sometimes called **common chickweed** to distinguish it from other plants called chickweed. Other common names include **chickenwort**, **craches**, **maruns**, and **winterweed**. The plant germinates in autumn or late winter, then forms large mats of foliage.

Description

This species is an annual and perennial with weak slender stems, up through 40 cm long. Plants are sparsely hairy, with hairs in a line along the stem. The leaves are oval and opposite, the lower ones with stalks. Flowers are white and small with 5 very deeply lobed petals. Some plants have no petals. The stamens are usually 3 and the styles 3.[2] The flowers quickly form capsules. Plants have flowers and capsules at the same time.

Herbal Medicine Uses

Chickweed was widely used as an anti-inflammatory herb. For example, chickweed cream was used to soothe eczema, sunburn and insect stings as well as to draw out boils and splinters.

COMFREY

Comfrey root

LATIN NAME Symphytum officinale

Kingdom: Plantae
Clade: Tracheophytes
Clade: Angiosperms
Clade: Eudicots
Clade: Asterids
Order: Boraginales
Family: Boraginaceae
Subfamily: Boraginoideae
Genus: *Symphytum* L.

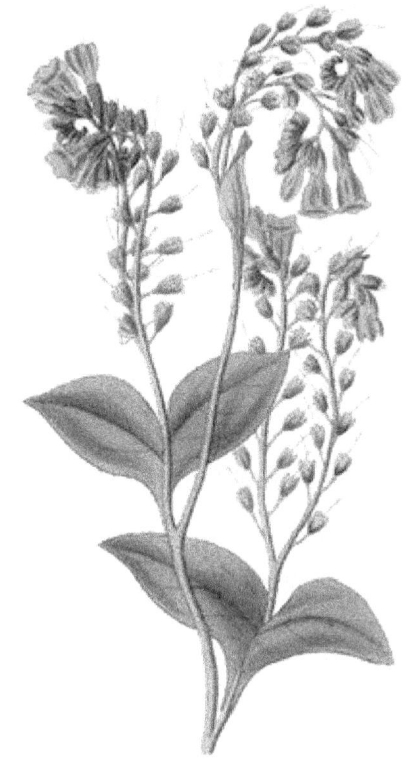

Symphyti radix
Beinwellwurzel

Name of Drug

Symphyti radix; comfrey root.

Composition of Drug

Comfrey, consisting of the fresh or dried root section of *Symphytum officinale* L. [Fam.Boraginaceae], and effective pharmaceutical preparations thereof.

The drug contains allantoin and muco-polysaccharides. Comfrey also contains various amounts of pyrrolizidine (senecio) alkaloids with 1,2-unsaturated necine ring structure and their N-oxides.

Uses
External:

- Bruising, pulled muscles and ligaments, sprains.

Contraindications
None known.

Note: Application should only occur on intact skin; during pregnancy use only after consulting a physician.

Side Effects

None known.

Interaction with Other Drugs

None known.

Dosage

Unless otherwise prescribed:

- Ointments or other preparations for external use are made up with 5 - 20 percent of the drug and prepared accordingly.

The daily dose should not exceed more than 100 mcg pyrrolizidine alkaloids with 1,2-unsaturated necine structure, including its N-oxides.

Mode of Administration

Crushed root, extracts, the pressed juice of the fresh plant for semi-solid preparations and poultices for external use.

Duration of Treatment

Not longer than 4 - 6 weeks per year.

Actions

Antiinflammatory
Furthers the formation of callus
Antimitotic

HISTORY OF COMFREY

Comfrey has enjoyed a long, noble, and quiet existence - until the 1990's. The tea was a common sight on most store shelves, being very popular in the 1970's and 80's as a wonderful healing and tonic herb. It has been part of folk medicine since 400 BC, but Dr. John R. Christopher, noted herbalist, believes that it is an herb that "harkens back to the Garden of Eden." Having common names like knitbone, bruise-wort, wound wort, gum plant, healing herb and slippery root, it is easy to imagine some of its uses. It was famous as a universal salve for the various wounds of war and life in general, specifically in its ability to knit bones. In fact, the very name "symphytum" comes from the Greek meaning "to make grow together." The Latin "officinale" was added when the herb became a part of the official pharmacy list of herbs kept in the apothecary's shop. Our use of the word "comfrey" comes from the Latin "confera", also meaning "knitting together."

Early documents reveal that comfrey was included in the herbal (AD 50) of Dioscorides, an ancient Greek Botanic physician, who traveled with Alexander the Great's army. Comfrey was found growing wild along the way as they went about conquering the known world. During the middle ages, several herbals and material medica of the day described comfrey's medicinal uses, such as treatment of wounds and fractures. The roots were used as a tea for patients that would spit up blood. Most of these references indicate the Russian and, later, European varieties of comfrey. The Turks and Saracens used comfrey to heal wartime wounds. Comfrey was introduced into England and by the mid 1800's was being cultivated by the ton, being used mostly as a crop food for animals. Later, a Quaker by the name of Henry Doubleday (1812-1902) had a hybrid from the Caucasus and European strains of comfrey imported into the US for which he also used mostly as animal fodder. Samuel Thomson, a nineteenth century botanic physician and outspoken herbalist, gave us the earliest recording of the use of comfrey in this country. Later it was included in the U.S. Pharmacopoeia, but toward the end of the century, the medical community relegated it to the list of "trivial" medicines. In the last 25 years, Comfrey has gained attention, but not in a good way. This valuable herb has fallen from grace and is now on the "banned " list, hailed not as a healer, but as a killer.

CHEMICAL CONSTITUENTS OF COMFREY

Comfrey is a complicated herb, containing a large number of constituents. The Pyrrolizidine-type alkaloids (PA) have been the major topic of concern. There are 12 known PA's in comfrey which include: symphytine, symlandine, echimidine, intermidine, lycopsamine, myoscorpine, acetyllycopsamine, acetylintermidine, lasiocarpine, heliosupine, viridiflorine, and echiumine. It also contains carbohydrates e.g. glucose and fructose in the form of Inulin, as well as the gums: arabinose, glucoronic acid, mannose, rhamnose, and xylose. Comfrey contains tannins which are substances that bind up proteins giving them astringent properties; and the Triterpenes: sitosterol, stigmasterol, steroidal saponins and isobauerenol. Other constituents include allantoin, caffeic acid, carotene, chlorogenic acid, choline, lithospermic acid, rosmarinic acid and silicic acid. The therapeutic value of comfrey is attributed to its content of allantoin, a cell proliferant, and rosmarinic acid, an anti-inflammatory agent and inhibitor of microvascular pulmonary injury. The rhizome of comfrey contains a higher percentage of allantoin in the early spring (January to March), decreasing as the plant grows. The allantoin then transfers to the young shoots and buds until the fall. Comfrey also contains an abundance of mucilage, a slimy, moist polysaccharide that works to moisten and soothe tissues.

Nutritionally, comfrey is rich in constituents. It contains sodium, potassium, calcium, chromium, cobalt, copper, magnesium, manganese, boron, zinc and iron. It is high in vegetable protein; in fact, you can get 20 times more protein from an acre of comfrey than you can from the equivalent amount of soybeans. Comfrey is one of the few plants that contain B-12 and is high in vitamin A, plus B-1, B-2, B-3, B-5, B-6, C and E. It has been considered as a potential food source for starving countries due to its protein content and is high in chlorophyll.

Unfortunately, poorly conducted laboratory studies have caused comfrey to garner a rather bad reputation. In 1993, the FDA posted a list of supplements that had associated illness and injuries and included Chaparral, **comfrey**, yohimbe, lobelia, germander, willow bark and Ma huang. The culprit constituent is the PA's in comfrey, which is present in higher concentrations in the root. In 2001, the FDA and the FTC announced its intentions to take action against manufacturers who sold comfrey for internal use and promoted any health giving claims. In fact, Christopher Enterprises,Inc. and Western Botanicals, Inc. were targeted and suits were brought against them. Canada, Germany and the United Kingdom have similar laws restricting the distribution, sale and/or use of comfrey.

So what are pyrrolizidine alkaloids (PA's) and are they as dangerous as the FDA would lead us to believe? Technically, the PA's are not toxic in themselves. They are transformed in the liver to pyrroles which then exert their toxic effect by reacting with the proteins and DNA of the cells. If the liver retains these new toxins, it will result in chronic tissue changes. However, it is possible that the PA's could be detoxified by the liver into a more soluble form and safely excreted by the kidneys. Also there is evidence that other metabolites may play a role in the toxic effects that have been attributed solely to PA's.

These PA compounds are widely present in as many as 6,000 plant species. However, only about ½ of the identified PA's are toxic. There is a great difference in the type and extent of toxicity within the various PA's. Variations may include the stability of the toxic metabolite (pyrrole) that is produced from it, the rate at which the reactive metabolite is produced, the species and sex of the exposed subject, the dose, the route of administration and the healthy/nutritional status of the test subject. Toxicity will also depend on what plant part is being used e.g. the root, leaf, etc., the growth stage of the plant, the individual plant used and how long the plant has been stored. It is important to note that these variations place comfrey PA's in a class with lower toxicity than the PA's implicated in significant human poisonings. In fact, the journal "Science" published data by biochemist Bruce Ames, Ph.D., of the University of California at Berkeley, that indicates that comfrey leaf tea is less carcinogenic than an equivalent amount of beer. Cheers!

MEDICINAL QUALITIES OF COMFREY

The traditional therapeutic actions of comfrey include demulcent (soothes mucous membranes), cell proliferant, pectoral (relieves disorders of the chest and lung), astringent, nutritive, tonic, expectorant, hemostatic, alterative (promotes a beneficial change in the body), vulnerary (heals fresh cuts and wounds), mucilage and styptic (arrests hemorrhage and bleeding). These claims have been backed by thousands of years of successful, albeit anecdotal evidence.

Comfrey's leaves or roots can be applied as a poultice, wash or ointment and are used for bruising, sciatica, boils, rheumatism, neuralgia, varicose veins, bed sores, wounds, ulcers, insect bites, tumours, muscular pain, pulled tendons, gangrene, shingles and dermatological conditions. It can be added to bath water to promote a youthful skin. Its emollient effects are very soothing, inhibiting further damage to tissues, stimulating the production of cartilage, tendons and muscles. It is highly regarded as a blood, bone and flesh builder.

Internally, comfrey has been used for indigestion, stomach and bowel problems, excessive menstrual flow, hoarseness, periodontal diseases, bleeding gums, thyroid disorders, diarrhea, gastro-intestinal ulcers, hernia, glandular fever, coughs, lung conditions, hemorrhaging, cancer, catarrh, anemia, sinusitis, lupus, lowering blood pressure, hiatal hernia, blood purifier and to ease inflammation of the joints and mucous membranes.

In addition to its medicinal use in humans, it has been used to feed animals from horses to zoo animals due to its rich vegetable protein content. Its ability to knit flesh and bones together has been known from the beginning. It will promote healthy cells but not malignant ones. The monks used comfrey for its ability to cure bronchial disorders and injuries. The roots made into a tea were beneficial for those spitting up blood. Nicholas Culpeper, an 18th century herbalist, described the properties of comfrey as being "cold, dry and earthy". He used it to treat fresh wounds, to dry up the fluids from old ulcers and cankers and stopped hemorrhages. He found the root beneficial for blood in the urine, to help patients to expectorate from the lungs and belly, for broken bones, hemorrhoids, and to cool and ease pain.

But in our modern "scientific" age, the thousands years of use and anecdotal evidence is not adequate to recommend this wonderful plant for safe use now. Research and clinical trials/studies are the standards in finding any food, drug or herb safe and therapeutic. There are obvious flaws in this method e.g. political and economic biases. But one of the less obvious flaws is a consistent short-coming that modern scientific methods refuse to overcome. That is their insistence that the sum of the parts should equal the whole, and in dealing with live, biological plants with hundreds of active constituents; this simply doesn't work. Nowhere is this more evident than in the nutritional research done by Dr. T. Colin Campbell. In his ground breaking, 20-year research called *The China Study*, where he studied the health benefits of whole "foods" in the Chinese diet, instead of singling out certain nutritional components e.g. specific vitamins. He was accused of "shotgun" science by his colleagues and they have been trying to deny the validity of his research since his findings were published. But the evidence is overwhelming. Whole foods make a difference where supplementation of isolated "active" constituents do not.

Comfrey has fallen victim to this "reductionist" type of science. Studies were done with rats, using only certain PA's, in differing amounts over differing amounts of time. In all cases where only certain PA constituents were used, the results ranged from liver tumors to death. In one feeding where the rat was fed up to 30% of its diet from the *whole leaf* over 21 days, there were no adverse effects.

There were many things wrong with this study. First, only one species of rat was used which limits the broad applicability of the results and poorly translates to predicting human response. In fact, the characteristics of PA toxicity in animals can differ tremendously between species from that of humans. In rats, the confounding result was tumors/cancer/death whereas humans have never manifested tumors, instead developing veno-occlusive disease of the liver. Secondly, the doses given the rats far exceeded any equivalent human dosing. Humans typically use comfrey as an infusion which extracts only about 1/3 of the alkaloids present in the plant. In one feeding, the rats were given a single dose of the total leaf and they all showed evidence of liver damage. But the dose was the equivalent of a human taking in 4.4 pounds of root or 29 pounds of the leaf in one single dosing. This would be impossible to do. Thirdly, in very few cases do humans take in comfrey consistently over the majority of their life span. The studied rats were given comfrey daily for up to 600 days or until they died, their life spans being only two to three years. The death was then attributed to liver toxicity. And lastly, the route of administration did not mimic traditional and approriate use. In some studies the lab animals were injected with the PA's, thus bypassing the gastrointestinal system when taken internally and the integumentary system when applied externally. These systems are necessary for appropriate absorption. The result was that these animals were exposed to greatly increased levels of PA's. It has never been recorded that humans inject comfrey or any other herb, therefore this does not parallel the normal delivery route.

So, in reality, no research has been done to determine the validity of the traditional uses of comfrey e.g. in the treatment of broken bones, tendon damage, ulcerations in the gastrointestinal tract and lung congestion. However, there have been several studies done documenting the anti-inflammatory, analgesic, wound healing and immune modulating effects which support the use of comfrey as a vulnerary. In the majority of subjects studied, they observed relief or healing over the placebo groups.

DOSAGES & APPLICATIONS OF COMFREY

Traditionally, Comfrey has been taken as an infusion (tea) made from the leaves. If a stronger solution is needed, a decoction can be made from the bark. Both the infusion and the decoction are able to extract the active constituents into distilled water. Decoctions are more suitable for fomentations, enemas or as a base for ointments.

Extracts or tinctures of comfrey can also be made by soaking comfrey leaves or root in a menstruum of 100 proof vodka, pure, undistilled apple cider vinegar or olive oil. For more detailed instructions on making extracts and tinctures, refer to *School of Natural Healing* by Dr. John R. Christopher. These can be purchased and one alternative is Herb Pharm, who produces a pyrrolizidine-free comfrey extract. The herb extracts that contain the PA's are run through an ion exchange bed that removes them. The finished extract contains less than one part-per-million of PA's. Comfrey oil is wonderful when massaged into pregnant bellies to promote elasticity and prevention of stretch marks.

The dried leaves/roots can be powdered and put into vegetable-based or gelatin-based capsules for internal use as well. It is important not to forget the use of Comfrey as a poultice. The fresh leaves are best used for this application. Pick the leaves, rinse and shake them dry, then blend with enough distilled water to create a thick mash. Apply to affected area and wrap with gauze. In an emergency, pick the leaves, bruise them and apply directly to wound. Another application is by suppository.

The following chart is taken from *School of Natural Healing* and is the recommended dosages for comfrey:

Decoction:2 fl.oz. three times/day

Fluid extract:½ - 1 teaspoonful three times/day

Infusion(tea):1 cupful, three times/day

Capsule:2 - "00" capsules three times/day or 1 teaspoonful of the powder

Tincture:½ - 1 teaspoonful three times/day

CRAMP BARK

LATIN NAME Viburnum opulus

Kingdom: Plantae
Clade: Tracheophytes
Clade: Angiosperms
Clade: Eudicots
Clade: Asterids
Order: Dipsacales
Family: Adoxaceae
Genus: *Viburnum*
Species: **V. opulus**

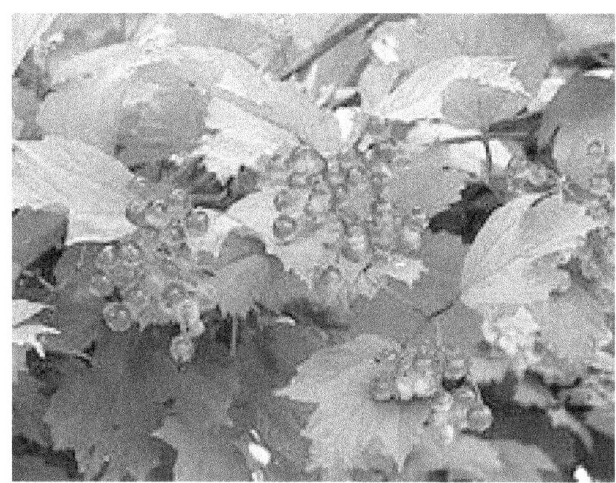

Viburnum opulus (common name: **guelder-rose**[1] or **guelder rose**; /ˈgɛldər/[2]) is a species of flowering plant in the family Adoxaceae (formerly Caprifoliaceae) native to Europe, northern Africa and central Asia

The common name 'guelder rose' relates to the Dutch province of Gelderland, where a popular cultivar, the snowball tree, supposedly originated.[4] Other common names include **water elder**, **cramp bark**, **snowball tree**, **common snowball**[5], and **European cranberrybush**, though this plant is not closely related to the cranberry. Some botanists also include the North American species *Viburnum trilobum* as *V. opulus* var. *americanum* Ait., or as *V. opulus* subsp. *trilobum* (Marshall) Clausen.

Specifically indicated in irregular uterine contractions, [Viburnum opulus] is also used for muscle spasms of all types, including in smooth and skeletal muscles, bronchi (such as in asthma), arteries (contributing to hypertension), and the bladder. Its effect on smooth muscle appears to be greater than on skeletal muscle.

- American Herbal Pharmacopoeia

Cramp bark is the herb that many herbalists reach for to relieve painful menstrual cramps. It seems to work best if taken 1-2 days before cramping starts, but can also be taken as needed.

Cramp bark is considered a uterine decongestant. Signs of uterine congestion include bloating, cramping before menstruation, as well as delayed menses. Uterine congestion can also be a pattern associated with endometriosis, fibroids and ovarian cysts.

I've talked to many women who have had menstrual cramps their whole lives and think that this is "normal." Painful menstruation is not natural! It's a symptom and can be addressed.

My take-home message is that, yes, cramp bark is stellar for relieving painful menstrual cramping. However, if a woman is continually experiencing painful cramps or other PMS symptoms, then it is far better to get to the root cause of the matter and get rid of them once and for all!

The chief therapeutic error made when treating acute severe menstrual cramps is to under dose, both in the size of the dose and its frequency. The German author R.F. Weiss suggests minimum doses of 20-30 drops, and a maximum of a teaspoon (Weiss). Doses may be repeated every several hours. Ellingwood suggests 20 drops every hour.
- Paul Bergner, NAIMH Course Materials

Viburnum Opulus to Relieve Urinary Pain

Urinary tract infections and bladder infections are often associated with frequent and painful urination. Cramp bark can relieve the pain and decrease the urgent frequency as well. Of course, the infection itself will still need to be addressed, but cramp bark will ease a lot of the discomfort.

Cramp bark combines well with bearberry for bladder infections with painful cramping and frequent urination with little passed. - Herbalpedia

Viburnum Opulus to Relieve Abdominal Cramps (Irritable Bowel Syndrome, Diarrhea)

Cramp bark can also relieve the pain of cramping that originates in the bowel. This is especially useful for more chronic conditions like Irritable Bowel Syndrome (IBS).

For acute cases of diarrhea, such as in food poisoning, we don't necessarily want to prematurely stop the diarrhea. However, it is doubtful that cramp bark would have an inhibitory effect.

Viburnum Opulus to Relieve Spasmodic Coughing

Spasmodic coughing can be the worst kind of cough. This is characterized by a dry cough, meaning no mucus is expectorated, and often gets worse at night. It can be spasmodic in nature, resulting in repeated coughing that keeps you from sleep, burns the throat and is all-around unpleasant.

Antispasmodic herbs like cramp barkcan relieve the muscle spasm causing this type of cough and therefore promote restful sleep.

Viburnum Opulus to Relieve High Blood Pressure

There are many causes for high blood pressure and many ways to find solutions for high blood pressure. Cramp bark can relieve tension in the cardiac muscle, arteries and veins, which can contribute to decreased blood pressure. This is especially suited for the person with lots of stress, tension and a type A attitude. Of course, diet, lifestyle and other cardiac herbs will need to be used to make a difference in someone's long-term health.

Viburnum Opulus to Relieve Muscle Cramps, Muscle Spasms, and Muscle Twitches

Have you ever "thrown out your back"? I have, countless times. One minute you're doing a seemingly innocent thing like picking something off the floor (or you're totally overdoing it gardening) and bam! something slips out of place and the pain increases steadily until lifting your pinky finger creates excruciating pain.

After a while the muscles around the area seize up, which immobilizes you even more. This is not necessarily a bad thing! Those seized muscles are protecting this vulnerable area. The holistic approach here is rest! Popping some pills or herbs and then heading back out to the garden is not a good idea and it can injure you further.

I often use cramp bark as a fomentation over cramped muscles when I've thrown out my back AND I rest and stay mostly immobilized. The cramp bark fomentation significantly decreases the discomfort, but I am also not going to push myself too much and increase the risk of further injury.

Another common way that cramp bark can be used is for restless legs. Restless legs are when your legs jump and move involuntarily as you are falling asleep. The underlying cause needs to be addressed, whether it is a nervous system issue or nutrient deficiencies (hint: magnesium deficiency is common). However, while figuring out what is going on, cramp bark tincture or cramp bark tea can relieve the spastic muscles and promote sleep.

Viburnum Opulus for Threatened Miscarriage, Early Labor and Labor

Cramp bark is used by midwives for both a threatened miscarriage, early labor and during labor. Kinda sounds a bit contradictory. That's the beautiful complexity of herbs.

Cramp bark can relax the uterus to stop uterine contractions if they are happening too early, such as in a threatened miscarriage or early labor. However, cramp bark also helps to tone and regulate contractions, which can facilitate a healthy labor.

Even though cramp bark is a uterine relaxant, it does not appear to interfere with labor. Rather, it promotes uterine muscle tone and regulates the rhythm of the contractions, resulting in effective uterine contractions. Cramp bark is also indicated for afterpains and is useful in helping the uterus to regain its normal shape.
- American Herbal Pharmacopeia

Viburnum Opulus for Tension Headaches

Headaches and migraines that are associated with tension respond well to formulas that include cramp bark. Here's an example of such a formula from herbalist Robert Dale Rogers:

For migraines associated with stress, combine with hawthorn, linden, marsh hedge nettle, and skullcap.

DANDELION

LATIN Taraxacum officinale

Kingdom: Plantae
Clade: Tracheophytes
Clade: Angiosperms
Clade: Eudicots
Clade: Asterids
Order: Asterales
Family: Asteraceae
Subfamily: Cichorioideae
Tribe: Cichorieae
Subtribe: Crepidinae
Genus: *Taraxacum*

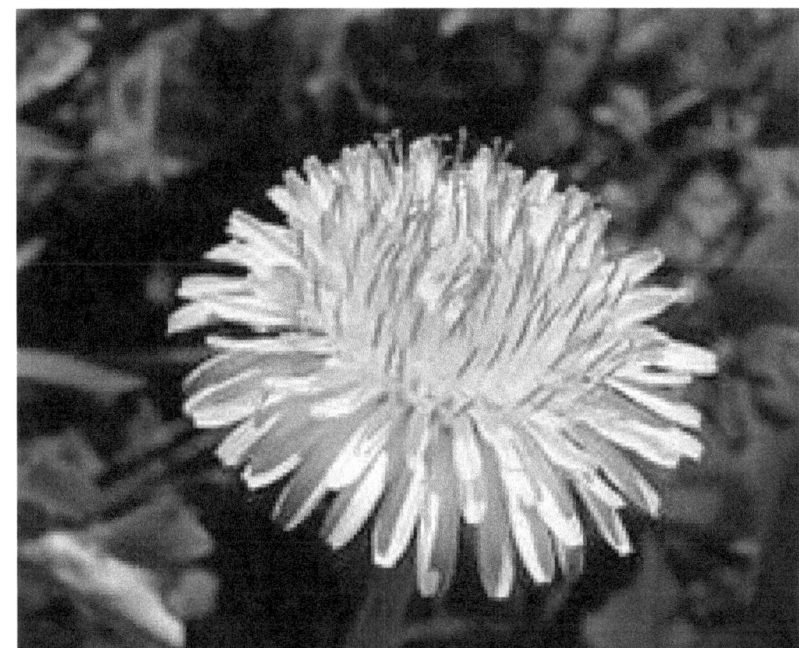

Dandelion root with herb

Taraxaci radix cum herba
Lwenzahnwurzel mit-kraut

Name of Drug

Taraxaci radix cum herba, dandelion root with herb.

Composition of Drug

Dandelion root with herb consists of the entire plant *Taraxacum officinale* G.H.Weber ex Wiggers *s.l.* [Fam. Asteraceae], gathered while flowering, as well as its preparations in effective dosage.

Ingredients include the bitter principles lactucopicrin (taraxacin), triterpenoids, and phytosterol.

Uses
Disturbances in bile flow, stimulation of diuresis, loss of appetite, and dyspepsia.

Contraindications

Obstruction of bile ducts, gall bladder empyema, ileus. In case of gallstones, use only after consultation with a physician.

Side Effects

As with all drugs containing bitter substances, discomfort due to gastric hyperacidity may occur.

Interactions with Other Drugs

None known.

Dosage

Unless otherwise prescribed:

As tea:

- 1 tablespoon of cut drug per cup of water.

As decoction:

- 3 - 4 g of cut or powdered drug per cup of water.

As tincture:

- 10 - 15 drops 3 times daily.

Mode of Administration

Liquid and solid preparations for oral use.

Actions

Choleretic
Diuretic
Appetite-stimulating

HISTORY

The first mention of the Dandelion as a medicine is in the works of the Arabian physicians of the tenth and eleventh centuries, who speak of it as a sort of wild Endive, under the name of *Taraxcacon*. In this country, we find allusion to it in the Welsh medicines of the thirteenth century. Dandelion was much valued as a medicine in the times of Gerard and Parkinson, and is still extensively employed.

Dandelion roots have long been largely used on the Continent, and the plant is cultivated largely in India as a remedy for liver complaints. Dandelion (Indian Name: - Kukraundha or Kanphool) is a hardly perennial herb and a tasty salad vegetable. The flower stems of this plant grows up to a height of 30 cm. The sharply toothed leaves from flat rosettes on the ground. The common name dandelion comes from the French dent de lion, meaning lion's tooth and refers to the dentate leaf edges. A very common plant, dandelion grows wild almost everywhere. Dandelion is a native of Europe. In India it is found through Himalayas. Nutritionally, the dandelion has remarkable value. It contains almost as much iron as spinach, four times Vitamin A content. An analysis of dandelion shows it to consist of protein, fat and carbohydrates. Its mineral and Vitamin contents are calcium, phosphorus, iron, magnesium, sodium, Vitamin A and C.

The root is perennial and tapering, simple or more or less branched, attaining in a good soil a length of a foot or more and 1/2 inch to an inch in diameter. Old roots divide at the crown into several heads. The root is fleshy and brittle, externally of a dark brown, internally white and abounding in an inodorous milky juice of bitter, but not disagreeable taste.

Only large, fleshy and well-formed roots should be collected, from plants two years old, not slender, forked ones. Roots produced in good soil are easier to dig up without breaking, and are thicker and less forked than those growing on waste places and by the roadside. Collectors should, therefore only dig in good, free soil, in moisture and shade, from meadowland. Dig up in wet weather, but not during frost, which materially lessens the activity of the roots. Avoid breaking the roots, using a long trowel or a fork, lifting steadily and carefully. Shake off as much of the earth as possible and then cleanse the roots, the easiest way being to leave them in a basket in a running stream so that the water covers them, for about an hour, or shake them, bunched, in a tank of clean water. Cut off the crowns of leaves, but be careful in so doing not to leave any scales on the top. Do not cut or slice the roots or the valuable milky juice on which their medicinal value depends will be wasted by bleeding.

The Food & Drug Administration (FDA) continues to treat dandelion as a weed. The agency's official position is: "There is no convincing reason for believing it possesses any therapeutic virtues." Many herbalists of today disagree with that. They say that the FDA forgot to read their Ralph Waldo Emerson.

"What is a weed?" Emerson wrote. "A plant whose virtues have not yet been discovered."

Thanks to some modern herbalists the dandelion's virtues have been well documented.

Studies show that the dandelion to be a rich source of vitamins and minerals. The leaves have the highest vitamin A content of all greens. Herbalists say that dandelion root heads the list of excellent foods for the liver because of its relatively high amounts of choline which is an important nutrient for the liver. Dandelion leaves are a diuretic, meaning that they help flush excess water from the body. Dandelion flowers are well endowed with lecithin, a nutrient that has been proven useful in various liver ailments.

CHEMICAL CONSTITUENTS

The chief constituents of Dandelion root are Taraxacin, acrystalline, bitter substance, of which the yield varies in roots collected at different seasons, and Taraxacerin, an acrid resin, with Inulin (a sort of sugar which replaces starch in many of the Dandelion family, *Compositae*), gluten, gum and potash. The root contains no starch, but early in the year contains much uncrystallizable sugar and laevulin, which differ from Inulin in being soluble in cold water. This diminishes in quantity during the summer and becomes Inulin in the autumn. The root may contain as much as 24 per cent. In the fresh root, the Inulin is present in the cell sap, but in the dry root it occurs as an amorphous, transparent solid, which is only slightly soluble in cold water, but soluble in hot water.

There is a difference of opinion as to the best time for collecting the roots. The British Pharmacopoeia considers the autumn dug root more bitter than the spring root, and that as it contains about 25 per cent insoluble Inulin, it is to be preferred on this account to the spring root, and it is, therefore, directed that in England the root should be collected between September and February, it being considered to be in perfection for Extract making in the month of November.
Bentley, on the other hand, contended that it is more bitter in March and most of all in July, but that as in the latter month it would generally be inconvenient for digging it, it should be dug in the spring, when the yield of Taraxacin, the bitter *soluble* principle, is greatest.

On account of the variability of the constituents of the plant according to the time of year when gathered, the yield and composition of the extract are very variable. If gathered from roots collected in autumn, the resulting product yields a turbid solution with water; if from spring-collected roots, the aqueous solution will be clear and yield but very little sediment on standing, because of the conversion of the Inulin into Laevulose and sugar at this active period of the plant's life.

In former days, Dandelion Juice was the favorite preparation both in official and domestic medicine. Provincial druggists sent their collectors for the roots and expressed the juice while these were quite fresh. Many country druggists prided themselves on their Dandelion Juice. The most active preparations of Dandelion, the Juice (*Succus Taraxaci*) and the Extract (*Extractum Taraxaci*), are made from the bruised fresh root. The Extract prepared from the fresh root is sometimes almost devoid of bitterness. The dried root alone was official in the United States Pharmacopoeia. In every 100 gm of fresh dandelion there are plenty of nutrients and minerals, which are as follows:

VITAMINS (MG/100G) fresh leaves
A 14,000
Thiamine .19
Riboflavin .26
Niacin .0
C 35

MINERALS (MG/100G)
Calcium 187
Phosphorus 66
Iron 3.1
Sodium 76
Potassium 397

OTHER NUTRIENTS (MG/100G)
Calories 45
Protein 2.7
Fat 0.7
Carbohydrates 9.2

MEDICINAL QUALITIES

There are so many uses claimed for the plant that it takes place among the herbal cure-alls. Its most frequent use, however, is an herb to heal the liver. In Europe, many scientific experiments have been undertaken which prove the traditional belief that the herb truly does cure hepatic ailments (Lucas: Herbal: 33). The herb acts in two ways for these conditions: it promotes the formation of bile and removes excess water from the body in edematous conditions resulting from liver congestion (Lust: 171). It is thought to be especially useful in cases of enlargement of the liver and for jaundice, even in little children. Dr. Swinburne Clymer wrote: "Dandelion has a beneficial influence upon the biliary organs, removing torpor and engorgement of the liver as well as of the spleen...only the green herb, whether for tincture or infusion should be used...." (Lucas: Common: 12). Grieve suggests that the herb is particularly useful in hepatic conditions of persons long resident in warm climates, taken in a broth with some leaves of sorrel and the yolk of an egg, daily for several months (Grieve: 254).

Dandelion is not only official but is used in many patent medicines. Not being poisonous, quite big doses of its preparations may be taken. Its beneficial action is best obtained when combined with other agents.

The tincture made from the tops may be taken in doses of 10 to 15 drops in a spoonful of water, three times daily.

It is said that its use for liver complaints was assigned to the plant largely on the doctrine of signatures, because of its bright yellow flowers of a bilious hue.

In the hepatic complaints of persons long resident in warm climates, Dandelion is said to afford very marked relief. A broth of Dandelion roots, sliced and stewed in boiling water with some leaves of Sorrel and the yolk of an egg, taken daily for some months, has been known to cure seemingly intractable cases of chronic liver congestion.

A strong decoction is found serviceable in stone and gravel: the decoction may be made by boiling 1 pint of the sliced root in 20 parts of water for 15 minutes, straining this when cold and sweetening with brown sugar or honey. A small teacupful may be taken once or twice a day.
Dandelion is used as a bitter tonic in atonic dyspepsia, and as a mild laxative in habitual constipation. When the stomach is irritated and where active treatment would be injurious, the decoction or extract of Dandelion administered three or four times a day, will often prove a valuable remedy. It has a good effect in increasing the appetite and promoting digestion.

Dandelion combined with other active remedies has been used in cases of dropsy and for induration of the liver, and also on the Continent for phthisis and some cutaneous diseases. A decoction of 2 OZ. of the herb or root in 1 quart of water, boiled down to a pint, is taken in doses of one wineglassful every three hours for scurvy, scrofula, eczema and all eruptions on the surface of the body.

Any herb, which acts beneficially upon the liver, has good effect on the rest of the system. Of particular interest is its action upon the digestion and eliminative systems. Kloss claimed that Dandelion is extremely high in nutritive salts, which purify the blood and destroy the acids in the blood. He said, "Anemia is caused by the deficiency of nutritive salts in the blood and really has nothing to do with the quantity of good blood. Dandelion contains these nutritive salts" (Kloss: 237). It is thought to tremendously benefit the stomach and intestines. Lukewarm Dandelion tea, claims Lust, is recommended for dyspepsia with constipation, fever, insomnia and hypochondria (Lust: 171). It is given in chronic constipation and catarrhal gastritis, of particular use in autointoxication, which result in skin eruptions. In other words, many people who suffer from acne or other skin eruptions due to toxins in the system can benefit from taking a daily cup of tea. Furthermore, it promotes good absorption of nutrients and so is recommended for chronic indigestion. Where the stomach is irritated, it can be given in moderate does several times a day; it increases the natural appetite and promotes good digestion.

According to *Peter Gail* author of The Health Benefits of Dandelions, if you are looking for a miracle remedy, which when eaten as a part of your daily diet or taken as a beverage, could, depending on the peculiarities of your body chemistry:

Prevent or cure liver diseases, such as hepatitis or jaundice; act as a tonic and gentle diuretic to purify your blood, cleanse your system, dissolve kidney stones, and otherwise improve gastro-intestinal health; assist in weight reduction; cleanse your skin and eliminate acne; improve your bowel function, working equally well to relieve both constipation and diarrhea; prevent or lower high blood pressure; prevent or cure anemia; lower your serum cholesterol by as much as half; eliminate or drastically reduce acid indigestion and gas buildup by cutting the heaviness of fatty foods; prevent or cure various forms of cancer; prevent or control diabetes mellitus; and, at the same time, have no negative side effects and selectively act on only what ails you. Then Dandelion is for you.

All the above curative functions, and more, have been attributed to one plant known to everyone, <u>Taraxacum</u> <u>officinale</u>, which means the "Official Remedy for Disorders." We call it the common dandelion. It is so well respected, in fact, that it appears in the U.S. National Formulatory, and in the Pharmacopeias of Hungary, Poland, Switzerland, and the Soviet Union. It is one of the top 6 herbs in the Chinese herbal medicine chest.

According to the USDA Bulletin #8, "Composition of Foods" (Haytowitz and Matthews 1984), dandelions rank in the top 4 green vegetables in overall nutritional value. Minnich, in "Gardening for Better Nutrition" ranks them, out of <u>all</u> vegetables, including grains, seeds and greens, as tied for 9th best. According to these data, dandelions are nature's richest green vegetable source of beta-carotene, from which Vitamin A is created, and the third richest source of Vitamin A of all foods, after cod-liver oil and beef liver! They also are particularly rich in fiber, potassium, iron, calcium, magnesium, phosphorus and the B vitamins, thiamine and riboflavin, and are a good source of protein.

These figures represent only those published by the USDA. Studies in Russia and Eastern Europe by Gerasimova, Racz, Vogel, and Marei (Hobbs 1985) indicate that dandelion is also rich in micronutrients such as copper, cobalt, zinc, boron, and molybdenum, as well as Vitamin D.

Much of what dandelions purportedly do in promoting good health could result from nutritional richness alone. Vogel considers the sodium in dandelions important in reducing inflammations of the liver. Gerasimova, the Russian chemist who analyzed the dandelion for, among other things, trace minerals, stated that "dandelion [is] an example of a harmonious combination of trace elements, vitamins and other biologically active substances in ratios optimal for a human organism" (Hobbs 1985).

Recent research, reported in the Natural Healing and Nutritional Annual, 1989 (Bricklin and Ferguson 1989) on the value of vitamins and minerals indicates that:

* Vitamin A is important in fighting cancers of epithelial tissue, including mouth and lung.

* Potassium rich foods, in adequate quantities, and particularly in balance with magnesium, helps keep blood pressure down and reduces risks of strokes;

* Fiber fights diabetes, lowers cholesterol, reduces cancer and heart disease risks, and assists in weight loss. High fiber vegetables take up lots of room, are low in calories, and slow down digestion so the food stays in the stomach longer and you feel full longer;

* Calcium in high concentrations can build strong bones and can lower blood pressure.

* B vitamins help reduce stress.

Throughout history, dandelions have had a reputation as being effective in promoting weight loss and laboratory research indicates that there is some support for this reputation. Controlled tests on laboratory mice and rats by the same Romanians indicated that a loss of up to 30% of body weight in 30 days was possible when the animals were fed dandelion extract with their food. Those on grass extract lost much less. The control group on plain water actually gained weight.

Beyond nutritional richness, however, are the active chemical constituents contained in dandelions which may have specific therapeutic effects on the body. These include, as reported by Hobbs (1985):

* Inulin, which converts to fructose in the presence of cold or hydrochloric acid in the stomach. Fructose forms glycogen in the liver without requiring insulin, resulting in a slower blood sugar rise, which makes it good for diabetics and hypoglycemics.

* Tof-CFr, a glucose polymer similar to lentinan, which Japanese researchers have found to act against cancer cells in laboratory mice; Lentinan is a yeast glucan (glucose polymer) that increases resistance against protozoal and viral infections.

* Pectin, which is anti-diarrheal and also forms ionic complexes with metal ions, which probably contributes to dandelion's reputation as a blood and gastrointestinal detoxifying herb. Pectin is prescribed regularly in Russia to remove heavy metals and radioactive elements from body tissues. Pectin can also lower cholesterol and, combined with Vitamin C, can lower it even more. Dandelion is a good source of both Pectin and Vitamin C.

* Coumestrol, an estrogen mimic, which possibly is responsible, at least in part, for stimulating milk flow and altering hormones.

* Apigenin and Luteolin, two flavonoid glycosides which have been demonstrated to have diuretic, anti-spasmodic, anti-oxidant and liver protecting actions and properties, and also to strengthen the heart and blood vessels. They also have anti-bacterial and anti-hypoglycemic properties, and, as estrogen mimics, may also stimulate milk production and alter hormones.

* Gallic Acid, which is anti-diarrheal and anti-bacterial;

* Linoleic and Linolenic Acid, which are essential fatty acids required by the body to produce prostaglandin, which regulate blood pressure, and such body processes as immune responses, which suppress inflammation. These fatty acids can lower chronic inflammation, such as proliferate arthritis, regulate blood pressure and the menstrual cycle, and prevent platelet aggregation.

* Choline, which has been shown to help improve memory;

*Several Sesquiterpene compounds, which are what make dandelions bitter. These may partly account for dandelions tonic effects on digestion, liver, spleen and gall bladder, and are highly anti-fungal.

* Several Triterpenes, which may contribute to bile or liver stimulation;

* Taraxasterol, which may contribute to liver and gall bladder health or to hormone altering.
These chemicals, individually, are not unique to dandelions, but the combination of them all in one plant, along with high levels of vitamins, minerals, carbohydrates, proteins and fiber account for the many claims made regarding the plant.

These claims include the following results of clinical and laboratory research, again as reported in Hobbs (1985):

* A doubling of bile output with leaf extracts, and a quadrupling of bile output with root extract. Bile assists with the emulsification, digestion and absorption of fats, in alkalinizing the intestines and in the prevention of putrefaction. This could explain the effectiveness of dandelion in reducing the effects of fatty foods (heartburn and acid indigestion).

* Italian researchers have demonstrated a reduction in serum cholesterol and urine bilirubin levels by as much as half, in humans with severe liver imbalances.

* Romanian scientists found diuretic effects with a strength approaching that of the potent diuretics Furosemide and Lasix, used for congestive heart failure and cirrhosis of the liver, with none of the serious side effects. They found that water extract of dandelion leaves, administered orally, because of its high potassium content, replaced serum potassium electrolytes lost in the urine, eliminating such side effects common with the synthetics as severe potassium depletion, hepatic coma in liver patients, circulatory collapse, and transmission through mothers' milk;

* In 1979 a Japanese patent was filed for a freeze-dried warm water extract of dandelion root for anti-tumor use. It was found that administration of the extract markedly inhibited growth of particular carcinoma cells within one week after treatment.

* Dental researchers at Indiana University in 1982 used dandelion extracts in antiplaque

preparations.

* In studies from 1941 to 1952, the French scientist Henri Leclerc demonstrated the effectiveness of dandelion on chronic liver problems related to bile stones. He found that roots gathered in late summer to fall, when they are rich in bitter, white milky latex, should be used for all liver treatments.

* In 1956, Chauvin demonstrated the antibacterial effects of dandelion pollen, which may validate the centuries old use of dandelion flowers in Korean folk medicine to prevent furuncles (boils, skin infections), tuberculosis, and edema and promote blood circulation. Also, Witt (1983) recommends dandelion tea to alleviate the water buildup in PMS (pre-menstrual syndrome).

There are many testimonials from those who have benefited from the use of dandelions in the treatment of what ailed them.

Robert Stickle, an internationally famous architect, was diagnosed as having a malignant melanoma 21 years ago, and was given, after radical surgery had not halted its spread, less than 2 years to live. He said, in a letter to Jeff Zullo, president of the Society for the Promotion of Dandelions, (June 23, 1986):

" I went on a search for the answer to my mortal problem, and [discovered] that perhaps it was a nutritional dilemma.... To me, cancer is primarily a liver failure manifestation. {Italians are very concerned about problems of the 'fegato']. [I discovered that] the cancer rate in native Italians is very low among the farming population (paesanos). When they get affluent and move to the city, it's the same as the rest of civilized man. Paesanos eat dandelions, make brew from the roots, and are healthy, often living to over 100 years."

He states that he began eating dandelion salad every day, and his improvement confounded the doctors. When he wrote the letter in 1986, 18 years had passed and there had been no recurrence of the melanoma.

A benefit, which comes from writing articles for national media is that you hear from people who have interesting stories to tell. I recently received a call from Peter Gruchawka, a 70-year-old gentleman from Manorville, NY, who reported that he had been diagnosed with diabetes melitis 3 months before and was put on 5 grams of Micronase. At the time, he had a 5+-sugar spillover in his urine. He took Micronesia for about a month before he learned, from his wife who is a nurse, that Micronase can do damage to the liver. He had read in "Herbal Medicine" by Diane Buchanan and "Back to Eden" by Jethro Kloss about the effectiveness of dandelions in controlling diabetes. Without saying anything to his doctors, he stopped taking Micronase and began drinking dandelion coffee each day. During the first week, his urinary sugar, measured night and morning, was erratic and unstable, but after a week, his sugar stabilized and when he called, he had been getting negative urine sugar readings for over a month. The doctors are amazed and can't explain it. An interesting side benefit to replacing Micronase with dandelion coffee is that, while Micronase damages the liver as a side effect, dandelions are particularly known for strengthening the liver.

According to Mr. Gruchawka, he changed nothing but the medication. He had cut out pastries and other sugars when he was diagnosed and started on Micronase, and has continued to do without those things while taking dandelion coffee.

And there is the importance of faith in the healing process, whether it is faith in God or faith in the curative properties of the herb being taken.

While dandelions, given all these variables, may never be proved to cure any specific ill, they are an extremely healthy green, which cannot in any way hurt you. Research on how much you would have to eat to cause harm indicates that eating grass is more dangerous than eating dandelions (Hobbs 1985). Therefore, with everything going for dandelions, it is highly probable that everyone can derive at least some nutritional benefit from them by eating or drinking them regularly.

The medical and pharmacological establishment is generally critical of claims regarding the use of herbs on disease, and their concerns need to be put in perspective.

Herbal medicines have been used very effectively far longer than synthetics, and many current pharmaceutical products have been derived from research on plants used as medicine by many cultures. The problem with plants, however, is that they are available to anyone. It is impossible to patent a plant, and thereby gain proprietary rights to it. As a consequence, pharmaceutical companies attempt to isolate the active properties from medicinal plants and synthesize them so that they can patent them. Many of the synthetics have serious side effects, which were not present in the natural plant product, often because other chemicals in the plant offset them (i.e. the large quantities of potassium in dandelions which allows for potassium replenishment when dandelion is used as a diuretic).

USDA botanist Dr. James Duke (1989) suggests that a proper and appropriate "herbal soup", filled with "vitamins, minerals, fibers and a whole host of bioactive compounds," from which the body can selectively strain the compounds it needs to restore itself to health, will be more effective than synthetic medicines containing a "very select and specialized compound or two plus filler, usually non-nutritive." This is especially true if the "herbal soup", in the form of a potent potherb like dandelion, is a regular part of the diet so that the appropriate bioactive substances are present in the right amounts when the body needs them'.

DOSAGES

Fluid extract, B.P., 1/2 to 2 drachms. Solid extract, B.P. 5 to 15 grains. Juice, B.P., 1 to 2 drachms. Leontodin, 2 to 4 grains.

---Dandelion Tea---

Infuse 1 oz. of Dandelion in a pint of boiling water for 10 minutes; decant, sweeten with honey, and drink several glasses in the course of the day. The use of this tea is efficacious in bilious affections, and is also much approved of in the treatment of dropsy.

Or take 2 oz. of freshly sliced Dandelion root, and boil in 2 pints of water until it comes to 1 pint; then add 1 oz. of compound tincture of Horseradish. Dose, from 2 to 4 oz. Use in a sluggish state of the liver.

Or 1 oz. Dandelion root, 1 oz. Black Horehound herb, 1/2 oz. Sweet Flag root, 1/4 oz. Mountain Flax. Simmer the whole in 3 pints of water down to 1 1/2 pint, strain and take a wineglassful after meals for biliousness and dizziness.

---For Gall Stones---

1 oz. Dandelion root, 1 oz. Parsley root, 1 oz. Balm herb, 1/2 oz. Ginger root, 1/2 oz. Liquorice root. Place in 2 quarts of water and gently simmer down to 1 quart, strain and take a wineglassful every two hours.

For a young child suffering from jaundice: 1 oz. Dandelion root, 1/2 oz. Ginger root, 1/2 oz. Caraway seed, 1/2 oz. Cinnamon bark, 1/4 oz. Senna leaves. Gently boil in 3 pints of water down to 1 1/2 pint, strain, dissolve 1/2 lb. sugar in hot liquid, bring to a boil again, skim all impurities that come to the surface when clear, put on one side to cool, and give frequently in teaspoonful doses.

---A Liver and Kidney Mixture---

1 oz. Broom tops, 1/2 oz. Juniper berries, 1/2 oz. Dandelion root, 1 1/2 pint water. Boil ingredients for 10 minutes, then strain and add a small quantity of cayenne. Dose, 1 tablespoonful, three times a day.

---A Medicine for Piles---

1 oz. Long-leaved Plantain, 1 oz. Dandelion root, 1/2 oz. Polypody root, 1 oz. Shepherd's Purse. Add 3 pints of water, boil down to half the quantity, strain, and add 1 oz. of tincture of Rhubarb. Dose, a wineglassful three times a day. Celandine ointment is to be applied at same time. In Derbyshire, the juice of the stalk is applied to remove warts.

ECHINACEA

LATIN NAME Echinacea purpurea

Kingdom: Plantae
Clade: Tracheophytes
Clade: Angiosperms
Clade: Eudicots
Clade: Asterids
Order: Asterales
Family: Asteraceae
Subfamily: Asteroideae
Supertribe: Helianthodae
Tribe: Heliantheae
Genus: *Echinacea*

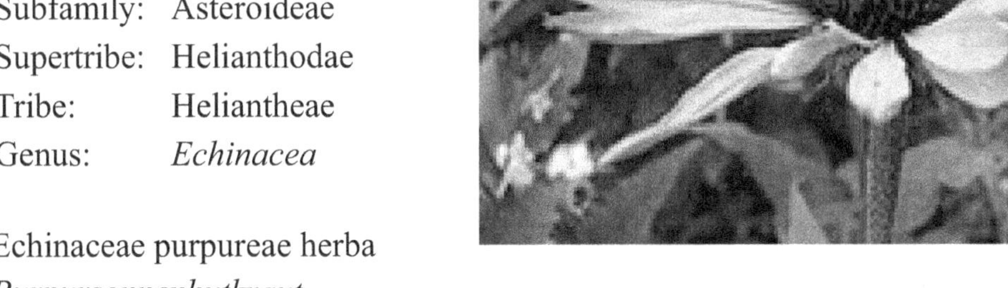

Echinaceae purpureae herba
Purpursonnenhutkraut

Name of Drug

Echinaceae purpureae herba, purple coneflower herb.

Composition of Drug

Purple coneflower herb consists of fresh, above-ground parts, harvested at flowering time, of *Echinacea purpurea* (L.) Moench [Fam.Asteraceae], as well as its preparations in effective dosage.

Use
Internal:

- Supportive therapy for colds and chronic infections of the respiratory tract and lower urinary tract.

External use:

- Poorly healing wounds and chronic ulcerations.

Contraindications
External:

- None known.

Internal:

- Progressive systemic diseases, such as tuberculosis, leucosis, collagenosis, multiple sclerosis.

No parenteral administration in case of tendencies to allergies, especially allergies to members of the composite family (Asteraceae), as well as in pregnancy.

Warning : The metabolic condition in diabetics can decline upon parenteral application.

Side Effects
Internal and external application:

- None known.

Parenteral application:

- Depending upon dosage, short-term fever reactions, nausea and vomiting can occur.

In individual cases, allergic reactions of the immediate type are possible.

Interactions with Other Drugs

None known.

Dosage

Unless otherwise prescribed:

Internal:
Daily dosage:

- 6 - 9 ml expressed juice;
- equivalent preparations.

Parenteral:

- Depends on individual kind and seriousness of condition as well as specific nature of the preparation.Parenteral application requires a gradation of dosage, especially for children; the manufacturer is required to show this information for the particular preparation.

External:

- Semi-solid preparations containing at least 15 percent pressed juice.

Mode of Administration

Pressed juice and galenical preparations for internal and external use.

Duration of Administration

Preparations for parenteral use:

- Not longer than 3 weeks.

Preparations for internal and external use:

- Not longer than 8 weeks.

Actions

In human and/or animal experiments, Echinacea preparations given internally or parenterally have produced immune effects. Among others, the number of white blood cells and spleen cells is increased, the capacity for phagocytosis by human granulocytes is activated, and the body temperature is elevated.

EYEBRIGHT

LATIN NAME Euphrasia officinalis

Kingdom: Plantae
Clade: Tracheophytes
Clade: Angiosperms
Clade: Eudicots
Clade: Asterids
Order: Lamiales
Family: Orobanchaceae
Tribe: Rhinantheae
Genus: *Euphrasia* L.

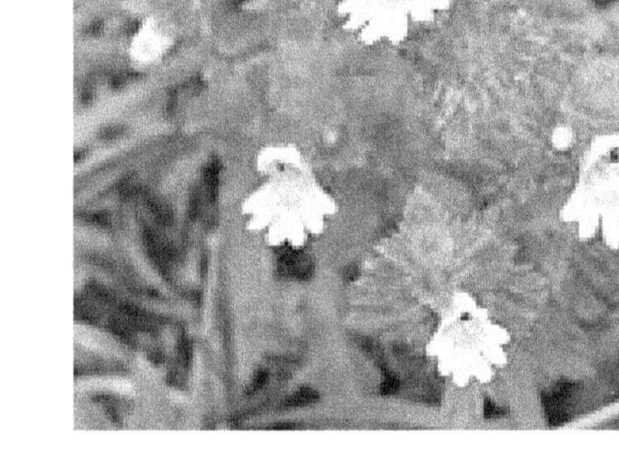

Name of Drug

Euphrasia officinalis, eyebright.
Euphrasiae herba, eyebright herb.

Composition of Drug

Eyebright consists of the whole plant of *Euphrasia officinalis* L.p.p.
[Fam. Scrophulariaceae] gathered during flowering season, as well as preparations thereof.

Eyebright herb consists of the fresh or dried, above-ground parts of *E.officinalis* L.p.p., as well as preparations thereof.

**Pharmacological Properties,
Pharmacokinetics, Toxicology**
Not known.

Clinical Data

Uses

Eyebright preparations are used externally as lotions, poultices, and eye-baths, for eye complaints associated with disorders and inflammation of the blood vessels, inflammation of the eyelids and conjunctiva, as a preventive measure against mucus and catarrh of the eyes, "glued" and inflamed eyes, for coughs, colds, catarrh, and as a stomachic and against skin conditions.

Activity for the indications listed has not been substantiated.

The effectiveness of the herb for its claimed uses is not documented.

Risks

None known.

HISTORY

The herb commonly known as eyebright has the Latin name *Euphrasis officinalis.* The French name is Casse-lunette and the German name is Augentrost which means consolation of the eyes. The name Euphrasis is derived from the Greek word Euphrosyne which means gladness. In Greek mythology, one of the three graces who was known for her joy and mirth was also named Euphrosyne. The herb may have been named after the grace Euphrosyne because the herb also brings joy and gladness to the person who is suffering from eye problems as this herb has many medicinal properties that are beneficial to the eye.

Another old tradition says that the Greek word Euphrosyne was given to the small finch known as a linnet. The story goes that the linnet was the first to use the leaf of the herb to help clear the sight of her young. The linnet then passed this knowledge on to mankind who named the herb in honor of the bird.

Although the eyebright herb has a name of Greek origin, the ancient herbalists such as Dioscorides and Pliny make no mention of this herb. It is not until the fourteenth century that we see it mentioned in Gordon's "Liticium Medicina," 1305, where it is considered medicine for the eye 'outwardly in a compound distilled water and inwardly as a syrup.' Matthaeus Sylvaticus, a physician of Mantua, recommended this herb for disorders of the eyes. A treatise on the virtues of eyebright, entitled "Vini Euphrasiati tantopere celebrati," was written by Arnoldus Villanovanus who said 'it hath restored sight to them that have been blind a long time.' Hildamus also believed that it would restore the sight of many people who were seventy or eighty years old.

In the sixteenth century the herbalists such as Tragus, Fuchsius, and Dodoens regarded eyebright as a specific in diseases of the eyes. In 1616, in the book "Countrie Farm," Markham says: 'Drinke everie morning a small drought of Eyebright wine' this was claimed to help the dimness of sight and restored old men's sight to read small letters without their spectacles when they could hardly read large letters with their spectacles before. In 1671, Salmon said that eyebright strengthens the head, eyes and memory and clears the sight. The famous seventeenth century herbalist Nicholas Culpepper said, 'if the herb was but as much used as it is neglected, it would half spoil the spectacle maker's trade and a man would think that reason should teach people to prefer the preservation of their natural before artificial spectacles, which that they may be instructed how to do… Being used in any of the ways, it strengthens the weak brain or memory.' He also said eyebright helped, 'all infirmities of the eyes that cause dimness of sight.'   In the eighteenth century eyebright tea was used, and there was a kind of ale called 'Eyebright Ale' used in Queen Elizabeth's time.

Poet's such as John Milton used Euphrasis in their poems and described the benefits of eyebright on the eye. In his poem "Paradise Lost", an angel gives Adam rue and eyebright to purge his sight. The Doctrine of Signatures was also credited as having prompted the use of eyebright for eye problems. One writer pointed out, 'the purple and yellow spots and stripes which are upon the flowers of the Eyebright doth very much resemble the diseases of the eye, as bloodshot, etc., by which signature it hath been found out that this herb is effectual for the curing of the same.'

Eyebright is not used in the orthodox medical profession today and they take pride in poking fun at the Doctrine of Signatures which eyebright is a ready example of. There has been a lack of research and scientific studies which also leads to their derision of eyebright. Even the Commission E of Germany that is open minded and recommends many herbs for use, does not recommend eyebright because of the lack of research and the problems of keeping the formulas sterile enough to use in the eyes. However, most modern herbalists highly recommend eyebright and they have many formulas that contain eyebright. Naturopaths and Homeopaths recommend and use eyebright formulas as well. Because eyebright seems to work for those who try it and because so many herbal companies are formulating formulas with eyebright, we are starting to see some research and small studies being done on the effects of eyebright by these herbal companies.

CHEMICAL CONSTITUENTS

The eyebright herb contains tannins, resins, volatile oil, and mannite. It also has iridoid glycosides, the favonoids rutin and quercetin, saponins, essential fatty acids, sterols, iron, silicon, traces of iodine, copper, and zinc, and the vitamins A, C, D, E and the B complex. The phytochemicals it contains are; aucubin, beta-carotene, caffeic-acid, catalpol, choline, ferulic-acid, gallotannins, geniposide, luproside, niacin, riboflavin, selenium, and thiamin.

MEDICINAL QUALITIES

Eyebright is slightly tonic and the actions are anti-catarrhal, anti-inflammatory, anti-septic, and astringent. The anti-catarrhal property of eyebright works first on the upper portion of the respiratory tract and then on the mucous structures of the throat and bronchial tubes. It is very beneficial if the discharge is thin and watery. The common cold, hay fever, and even measles are helped by eyebright. The bronchial and pulmonary irritation caused by measles is relieved by the use of this herb. When there is an earache, headache, or distress across the eyes, as in acute catarrhal affections, eyebright has a direct influence upon the lachrymal apparatus.   It has been recommended for use in epidemic influenza and when there is intestinal catarrhal as well.

The aucubin found in eyebright has an anti-inflammatory action which is useful when there is a cough, hoarseness, or sore throat. This also accounts for eyebrights well known reputation for soothing tired and inflamed eyes as well as improving weak eyesight with its cooling and detoxifying effect The other key nutrients responsible for this are niacin, riboflavin, cobalt, and silica.

The tannins act as astringents to help dry up secretions and relieve inflammation of the mucous membranes. This is helpful when treating conjunctivitis an inflammation of the protective membrane of the eyes, blepharitis an inflammation of the eyelids, and the catarrhal
conditions of the sinuses and nasal passages such as sinusitis and hay fever. The tannins and quercetin, a flavonoid found in eyebright are thought to reduce allergic responsiveness by inhibiting the release of histamines. 'It's a very good herb for relieving runny eyes, especially
when they're caused by allergies,' confirms Claire Gibson, N.D., a naturopathic physician based in Oakland, California.

The caffeic acid acts as an antiseptic in eyebright similar to goldenseal. This antiseptic property helps in fighting styes which is an inflammation of one or more of the sebaceous glands in the eyelid which is caused by the build up of toxic poisons and it will help other eye infections as well. The aucubin content also helps fight bacterial infections and liver toxicity. For this reason some herbalists use eyebright to treat jaundice and liver problems. Some studies say that eyebright has even been used to improve appetite, improve memory, help with vertigo, and cure epilepsy.

The vitamins B, C, E, beta carotene, copper, and selenium found in eyebright have been shown to improve clarity of eyesight by one or more lines on the eye chart over a 6 month period. The Vitamins B, E, and selenium were also shown to reduce cataracts over 5 months. In macular degeneration and diabetic retinopathy the disease was slowed by 70% by using the Vitamins A, C, E and selenium all of which are found in eyebright.

The antioxidant vitamins A, C, E, and beta carotene all lower the risk of cataract formation and are all found in eyebright. Even a slight deficiency of vitamin A can cause tired eyes, sensitivity to light, dry eyelids and susceptibility to infection. The vitamin A found in eyebright may be why it is said to decrease sensitivity to light. Vitamin A is also crucial to the formation of visual purple for darkness adaptation so eyebright would help with night time vision as well. A severe deficiency in vitamin A can cause ulceration and distortion of the cornea and result in blindness.

The antioxidant vitamin C protects the lens proteins and proteases from damage by sunlight as well as helps in the production and maintenance of collagen which is important in glaucoma. Vitamin C works best with the flavonoid quercetin both of which are found in eyebright. The antioxidant vitamin E which is found in eyebright has been used to improve visual acuity in nearsightedness, crossed eyes, macular degeneration and reduce cataract risk by 50%.

When the body is deficient in the vitamin B complex, eye muscles may become paralyzed, light sensitivity may develop as well as itching, burning, bloodshot, and watery eyes. Nearsightedness can result from stress and the B vitamins help protect the nerves from damage that is due to stress. Vitamin B-5 or pantothenic acid is an anti-stress vitamin. Vitamin B-1 or thiamin is important for intracellular eye metabolism and vitamin B-2 or riboflavin deficiency has been linked to cataracts. All of these B vitamins are found in eyebright and contribute to its remarkable effects on the eyes.

Zinc, copper, and selenium help protect against cataracts because they act as antioxidants. The selenium also is used in the production of the enzyme glutathione peroxidase that protects red blood cells and cell membranes from free-radical damage. Zinc also helps stop macular degeneration because it is vital for the normal lens function, night vision, and maintaining the retina of the eye since there is a higher concentration of zinc in the retina then in any other organ. All of these minerals are found in eyebright.

Eyebright has some unusual characteristics that other herbs don't possess. The volatile oil properties in the flowers are activated by sunlight and saturate the conjunctiva, cornea, sclerotic, chorloid, ciliary muscle and process, iris, suspensory ligament, both the posterior and anterior fluid chambers, lens, retina, optic nerve, and other miscellaneous tissue membranes.

The herb will then strengthen all of these and provide an elasticity or more resiliency to the optic nerve and devices responsible for sight. If any of these tissues have a laxity then it will help to tighten them up to normal again or if any are too tight it will help relax them. Eyebrights chemical constituents regulate the tensile strength of all the fibrous mass in the eyes by either tightening up or relaxing them as the case merits. Sunlight is the key to the eyebright herbs remarkable chemical conditioning performance. In the dark this chemical conditioning doesn't function.

DOSAGES

Historically a simple infusion was used externally to bathe the eyes with. It was made by infusing 1oz of the eyebright herb in a pint of boiling water and three to four times a day washing the eyes with it. If there was pain in the eyes this infusion was used warm and more frequently throughout the day. For ordinary use a cold application of the infusion worked just fine. However in Iceland it was the expressed juice that was used for the eye and in Scotland they made the infusion with milk and applied it to the eye with a feather dipped in the infusion.

For bronchial problems eyebright was combined with tobacco and smoked by the British and the American Indians. Homeopaths used a tincture of eyebright in wine and then combined 30 drops of the tincture with a wineglassful of rosewater which was used several times a day for inflamed eyes or for bronchial catarrh, hay fever, and colds.

A convenient way to take eyebright today is in capsule or tablet form. The formulas listed above range from taking two to eight capsules daily. You can also take eyebright internally as a tea and several cups of tea a day can be taken. When taking eyebright internally you can also use a tincture of eyebright in an alcohol or glycerin base and put 15-30 drops directly in the mouth or put them in a cup of water and drink it. By taking eyebright internally you are usually trying to get the benefit of the nutrients available in eyebright or use it for getting rid of congestion or allergies.

For external use of eyebright to help reduce inflammation, as an antiseptic, or as an astringent to tonify mucus membranes, you can make an infusion with the eyebright steeping it in hot water for at least 10 minutes. After straining the infusion you can use it to make an eye compress by soaking cloth in the infusion and placing it over the eyes for 20 minutes. You can also use the infusion to bathe the eyes with by pouring the cooled infusion into sterile eyecups and tipping the head back blink the eyes for several minutes and then repeat with another sterile cup for the other eye. Another way to bathe the eyes is to put 3-5 drops of an alcohol based eyebright tincture in boiling distilled water poured into the sterile eyecups and letting this cool before using it as an eyewash

FENNEL

LATIN NAME Foeniculum vulgare

Kingdom: Plantae
Clade: Tracheophytes
Clade: Angiosperms
Clade: Eudicots
Clade: Asterids
Order: Apiales
Family: Apiaceae
Genus: *Foeniculum*
Species: **F.vulgare**

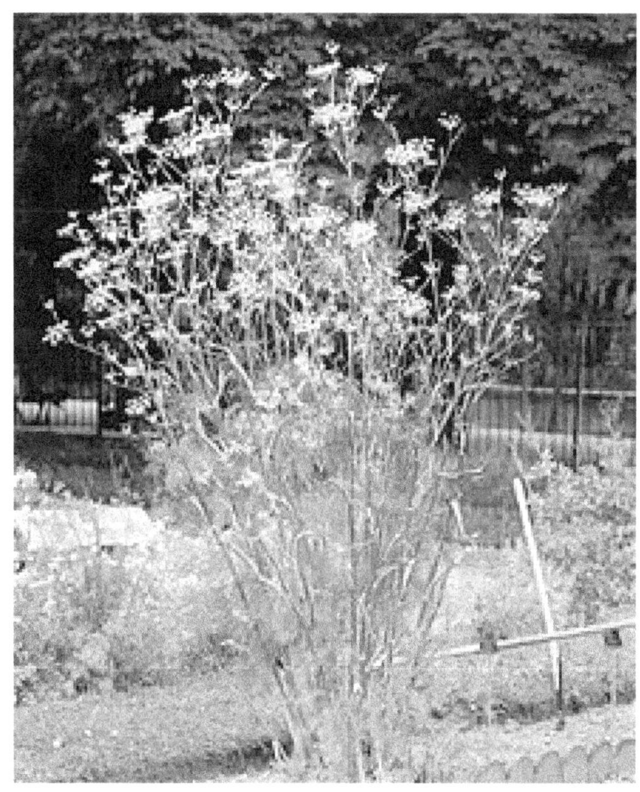

Fennel seed

Foeniculi fructus
Fenchel

Name of Drug

Foeniculi fructus , fennel seed.

Composition of Drug

Fennel seed consists of the dried, ripe fruits of *Foeniculum vulgare* Miller var. *vulgare* (Miller) Thellung [Fam.Apiaceae], as well as their preparations in effective dosage.

The seeds contain at least 4 percent essential oil with not more than 5 percent estragon.

Uses

Dyspepsias such as mild, spastic gastrointestinal afflictions, fullness, flatulence.

Catarrh of the upper respiratory tract.

Fennel syrup, fennel honey: catarrh of the upper respiratory tract in children.

Contraindications

Herb for infusions and preparations containing an equivalent amount of the essential oil:

- None known.

Other preparations:

- Pregnancy.

Side Effects

In individual cases allergic reactions of skin and respiratory tract.

Interactions with Other Drugs

None known.

Dosage

Unless otherwise prescribed:

Daily dosage:

- 5 - 7 g herb;
- 10 - 20 g fennel syrup or honey (*Erg. B.6*);
- 5 - 7.5 g compound fennel tincture;
- equivalent preparations.

Mode of Administration

Crushed or ground seeds for teas, tea-like products, as well as other galenical preparations for internal use.

Duration of Administration

Fennel preparations should not be used on a prolonged basis (several weeks) without consulting a physician or pharmacist.

Note: Fennel syrup, fennel honey: Diabetics must consider sugar content of bread exchange units according to manufacturer's information.

Actions

Promotes gastrointestinal motility, in higher concentrations acts as an antispasmodic.Experimentally, anethole and fenchone have been shown to have a secretolytic action in the respiratory tract; in the frog, aqueous fennel extracts raise the mucociliary activity of the ciliary epithelium.

GARLIC

LATIN NAME Allium sativum

Kingdom: Plantae
Clade: Tracheophytes
Clade: Angiosperms
Clade: Monocots
Order: Asparagales
Family: Amaryllidaceae
Subfamily: Allioideae
Genus: *Allium*
Species: **A. sativum**

Allii sativi bulbus
Knoblauchzwiebel

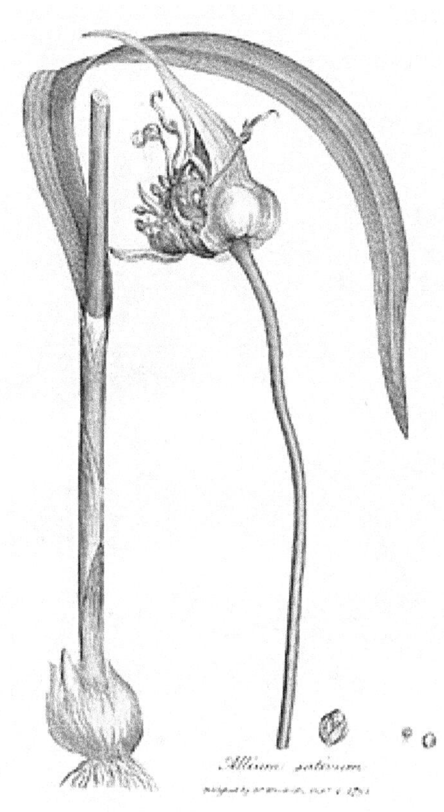

Name of Drug

Allii sativi bulbus, garlic clove.

Composition of Drug

Garlic bulbs, consisting of fresh or carefully
dried bulbs that consist of the main bulb with several secondary bulbs (cloves) of *Allium sativum* L. Fam. Alliaceae], as well as its preparations in effective dosage.

Garlic contains alliin and its degradation products and sulfur-containing essential oil.

Uses
Supportive to dietary measures at elevated levels of lipids in blood.

Preventative measures for age-dependent vascular changes.

Contraindications
None known.

Side Effects
In rare instances there may be gastrointestinal symptoms, changes to the flora of the intestine, or allergic reactions.

Note: The odor of garlic may pervade the breath and skin.

Interactions with Other Drugs

None known.

Dosage

Unless otherwise prescribed:

Average daily dosage:

- 4 g fresh garlic;
- equivalent preparations.

Mode of Administration

The minced bulb and preparations thereof for internal use.

Actions

Antibacterial
Antimycotic
Lipid-lowering
Inhibition of platelet aggregation
Prolongation of bleeding and clotting time
Enhancement of fibrinolytic activity

Garlic: Man's Best Friend in a Toxic World

Garlic has been known for centuries to function as a natural antibiotic. It destroys the unnecessary and harmful bacteria throughout the human system. It emulsifies cholesterol and loosens it from arterial walls. It is effective in arresting intestinal putrefaction; it is used against contagious diseases, high blood pressure, fevers, parasites, worms, nicotine poisoning, colic, and yeast infections. (Concern, April 1977, p. 7)

The brilliant Dr. Edward Shook, herbalist, pharmacist and one of our illustrious teachers, began his lectures on garlic with the phrase of the Gentle Shepherd, "Consider the Lilies. . . " Garlic is a member of the Liliaceae family which also includes the onion. This is Dr. Shook's botanical description of garlic:

Allium Sativum. Natural order. Liliaceae.

Common Names Garlic, poor man's treacle.

Part used. Bulb.

Description. The leaves are long, narrow, and much like grass.

The bulb (the only part used) is compound, consisting of numerous bulblets, commonly called "cloves," grouped together between the membrane scales, and enclosed within a whitish skin which holds them as in a sac. The whitish flowers are located at the end of stalks growing directly out of the bulb. They are grouped together in globular umbels with spathes surrounding them.

It will pay us handsomely to consider this lily because it is one of nature's great masterpieces as a safe and certain remedy for many of man's serious and devastating diseases.

This wonderful herb has been used from very ancient times both as food and medicine.

Theophrastus, the Greek philosopher (born 372 BC) relates that garlic was placed by the ancient Greeks on piles of stone at the crossroads as a feast for Hecate (literally a feast for the gods.)

Virgil, the Roman poet (70 BC) in his eclogues states that garlic was part of the entertainment served by Nestor to his guest Machaon. He also tells us that it was owing to the virtues of garlic that Ulysses owed his escape from being changed by Circe into a pig like each of his companions.

Galen speaks very highly of it, eulogizing it as the "theriac" or "heal all."
Chaucer calls it "theriac" as do several old English botanists and herbalists.

Pliny gives an exceedingly long list of complaints in which it was considered beneficial.

The name garlic is of very ancient Anglo-Saxon origin being derived from gar (a spear) and lac (a plant) in reference to the shape of its leaves. It is one of the oldest medicinal remedies known to man, which has been cultivated and used from time immemorial in the treatment of many diseases. Both its romantic history and its very remarkable curative virtues are vastly interesting and educational to all earnest and honest physicians, and it is notable that it stands out today as one of our greatest and most important therapeutic agents.

It is alterative, diaphoretic, diuretic, expectorant, antispasmodic, antiasthmatic, stimulant, antiseptic, disinfectant, tonic, nervine, antiphthisic, germicide, and vermicide. Chemical Constituents: Volatile oil (25 percent), mucilage (35 percent), albumen, sugar, starch, fibrin, and 50 percent water. The oil is a rather complex substance, of a strong, intensely penetrating odor and consists of allyl compounds of sulfur. It will be seen that this remarkable herb is heavily laden with organic sulfur, but no oxygen is found in the oil. Yet, it is the action of oxygen when the skin is taken off the cloves that releases the sulfur by combining with an allyl group to form allyloxide, which is also a pungent liquid having a sulfur odor.

Many marvelous effects and healing powers have been claimed for garlic. It is probable that none of them were exaggerated. I, myself, have seen it cure tuberculosis, asthma, bronchitis, several skin diseases, stomach ulcers, leg ulcers, athletes foot, furunculosis, abscesses, epilepsy, and special affinity for the respiratory tract, lungs, bronchi, and so forth, though it diffuses itself through the whole system and wherever there is pus, it is a certain and safe remedy. The use of garlic in the World War as an antiseptic was most sensational. In 1916, the British government asked for tons of the bulbs offering one shilling a pound for as much as could be produced. A great quantity of it was used for the control of suppuration in wounds. The raw juice was expressed, diluted with water, and put on swabs of sterilized sphagnum moss which was applied to the wounds. Where this treatment was given, it has been proved that there has never been one single case of sepsis of septic results. Consequently, the lives of tens of thousands have been saved by this one miraculous herb. That was nearly many years ago, and still we do not find garlic as an official remedy in the United States Pharmacopeia. This is one of the most disgraceful facts connected with the so-called regular practice of medicine, and proves beyond all doubt that their practice is neither ethical, moral, or even humane; otherwise, such a miracle of healing power would never have been discarded as it was.

In olden days, garlic was employed as a specific for leprosy, psoriasis and several forms of exanthematous skin diseases. It was also believed to have most beneficial results in smallpox applied to the soles of the feet in a linen cloth renewed daily.

Those unacquainted with garlic might think this was merely superstition; but, as a matter of fact, it is quite true. If chopped or minced fresh garlic is placed on the soles of the feet and allowed to remain there for some time, it will not be long before the odor of garlic can be detected on the breath; and cases of purulent disease in different parts of the body have been reported completely cured by simply keeping an application of garlic to the soles of the feet, and renewing it once or twice a day.

We positively know that organic sulfur is a universal antiseptic, whether taken internally or applied outwardly to any part of the body. It has been authoritatively reported that tuberculosis has been successfully treated by inhalation of the freshly expressed juice of garlic, diluted with equal quantities of water.

Garlic was the principal ingredient in the famous Four Thieves Vinegar which was adapted so successfully at Marseilles for protection against the plague when it prevailed there in 1772. This originated, it is said, with four thieves who confessed that, while protected by the liberal use of aromatic garlic vinegar during the plague, they plundered the dead bodies of the victims with complete safety. It is stated that during an outbreak of infectious fever in certain poor quarters of London early in the last century, the French priests who constantly used garlic in all their dishes visited the very worst cases with impunity, while the English clergy caught the infection, and in many instances, fell victims to the disease. Another instance of the remarkable penetrating power of garlic is the fact that the expressed juice of fresh garlic mixed with olive oil and rubbed on the chest, throat, and between the shoulder blades gives great relief in whooping cough, asthma, bronchitis and dyspnea, according to an English physician who has used it with success for many years. It also has a reputation for safely reducing high blood pressure, and in this relation we have an exceedingly valuable formula.

Boiling garlic reduces its active virtues considerably. Vinegar and water both extract its curative principles, though vinegar alone seems to be more effective for that purpose. Expressed fresh juice of garlic contains all of its many virtues. The following priceless formulas will cover its therapeutic applications completely for asthma, bronchitis, catarrhal conditions of the mucous membranes, phthisis, tuberculosis, coughs, dyspnea, heart weakness, internal ulcerations, and so forth.

Garlic Syrup

Peel 1 pound of fresh garlic, then chop or mince. Put into a wide mouthed jar and add equal parts of vinegar and distilled water to just cover the garlic. Close tightly, shake well, then let stand in a cool place for four days, thoroughly shaking once or twice a day. Now, add one pint of glycerine, shake well, and let stand another day. Strain with pressure, then filter liquid through a muslin or linen cloth. Add three pounds of pure honey, and stir till thoroughly blended. Put into jars, seal tightly, and store in a cool place.

In order to cover the pungent odor of the garlic, in case it is objectionable, do the following:

In place of macerating the garlic in equal parts of vinegar and distilled water, as directed above, use 1 quart of vinegar in which 3 ounces of powdered caraway seed and 3 ounces of sweet fennel seed have been slowly boiled for 15 minutes, while closely covered. Strain and when cold, add 1 pint of glycerine. Use this in the above formula instead of the vinegar and distilled water mixture.

This is much more acceptable to those who have an antipathy to the smell and taste of garlic. Of course, the 3 pounds of honey are also added after the filtering process. The deviation in no way affects the curative properties of the garlic, while it helps materially to disperse gas and flatus. We use aromatic vinegar in our own preparation of this formula, which is one of the most meritorious and useful remedies to have on hand. It is harmless, and very effective in the above mentioned cases, and will please and astonish both you and the patient.

Dose: For asthma and coughs: 1 teaspoonful with or without water every 15 minutes until spasm is controlled; then 1 teaspoonful every 2 or 3 hours for the rest of the day. After that, 1 teaspoonful 3 or 4 times a day is usually sufficient.

For tuberculosis, cardiac asthma and dyspnea: 1 dessertspoonful to a tablespoonful 3 or 4 times a day between meals.

Children: (8 to 15 years) one half of the above dose; (5 to 8 years) one quarter dose; (1 to 4 years) one eighth in a little water or honey

Garlic has also been used successfully in dropsy. The above formula may be used with benefit, but the following will be found to be much more prompt and effective, especially where the heart is much involved.

Dropsy with Heart Involvement.

Boil 8 ounces lily of the valley root (cut) (Convallaria majalis) in 3 pints of distilled water for 20 minutes. Strain then boil slowly till reduced to 1 pint. Set aside to cool, and while still warm, add 8 ounces of expressed garlic juice, 8 ounces of brown cane sugar, and 1 pint of glycerine. When cold, bottle and keep in a coot place.
This is one of the most potent remedies for dropsy and heart disease ever devised.

Dose: 1 teaspoonful to a dessertspoonful in water, as required. The dose should be regulated and given every 3 hours to bring about diuresis. Also, a slowing of the heart action, and an increase in the tone of its contraction. After this effect has been produced, administer 1 teaspoonful in water 3 or 4 times a day.

Garlic for outward application: For eczema, pityriasis, psoriasis, ulcers, cancers, swollen glands, tubercular joints, necrosis and all purulent conditions that are accessible, we recommend the following formula:

These garlic formulas we have given you are priceless. It will pay you to study them, and utilize them with confidence whenever occasion arises."
--(Shook, 1978; reprint. pp. 69-73)

Dioscorides, a second century physician and herbalist who traveled with the army of Alexander the Great, has the following to say on the subject of garlic. Dioscorides was translated into middle English by a scholar of the middle ages:

SKORODON Allium Sativum
LEUKOSKORODON Allium Ampeloprasum
OPHIOSKORODON Allium Scorodoprasum
ELAPHOSKORODON Allium subhirsutum

Garlic

Garluk (some call it Geboscome againe Elaphoboscum, the Latins Allium) some of it is Satiue & growes in gardens & this in Egypt, being only but of one head as the teeke, sweet, inclining to a purple colour. But elsewhere, it is compacted of many white cloues, the cloues that therein (the Greeks) call Aglithai. But there is another wilde kinde, called Ophioscorodon. (that is Serpent's Garlick). It hath a sharp, warning biting quanitie, expelling of flatulencies, and disturbing of the belly, and drying of the stomach causing of thirst & puffing vp, breeding of boyies in ye outsyde of the body, dulling the sight of the eyes. And the same thinges don also, (as we should say, Hart's garlick). Being eaten, it driues out the broade wormes, and drawes away the vrine. It is good, as none other thing, for such as are bitten of vipers, or of the Haemorrhous, who being taken presently after, or else that being beaten small in wine & soe dranek. It is applyed also by ye way of Cataplasme both for the same purposes profitably, as also layd on upon such as are bitten of mad dogge. Being eaten, it is good against the chaunge of waters (fauces expediende, easdeings asperas leniendo.) It doth cleare the arteries & being eaten either raw or sod, it doth assuage old coughes. Being dranck with decoction of Origanum, it cloth kill lice and nitts. But being burnt, and tempered with bony it cloth cure the sugillationes oculorum, and Alopeciae being anointed on, but for the Alopeciae (it must be applyed) with vnguentum Nardinum. And with salt & oyle it cloth heale ye eruptiones papularum. It doth take away also the Vitiligines, & the Lichenes, & the Lentigenes, and the running ulcers of the head, and the Furfures & ye Lepras, with hony. Being sod with Taeda and Franckincense, & kept in the mouth it doth assuage the paine of ye teeth. And with figge leaues & Cummin it is a Cataplasme for such as are bitten of the Mygale. But the leafes decoction is an insession that brings downe the Menstrua & the Secondas. It is also taken by way of suffumigation for ye same purpose. But the stamping that is made of it and ye black olive together, called Myrton, cloth moue the vrine & open ye mouths of ye veins & it is good also for the Hydropicall."

(Dioscorides, Book 11, pp. 188-91, under the heading of "Sharp Herbs.")

Let's go into some interesting historical facts on garlic, a most revered patriarchal herb:

"Garlic, a cousin of the lily originated in Central Asia or India, where the early peoples enjoyed eating raw garlic as an enhancement to their meals. They also enjoyed longevity, and the lowest incidence of cancer on the planet." (Messegue, 1979, p. 132)

The builders of the pyramids of Egypt were paid in the coin of the realm; onions and garlic, a valuable commodity.

These builders of the pyramids of Cheops, a Fourth Dynasty Pharaoh, consumed great quantities of garlic. It was during these times that garlic was elevated to the rank of a deity.

The Ebers Papyrus, 1500 BC, one of the earliest herbal pharmacological documents we know, mentions garlic used in external applications for wounds.

Here is a quotation from the Bible:

"We remember the fish which we did eat in Egypt for Nought, the cucumbers, and the melons, and the leeks, and the onions, and the garlic." (Numbers 11:5)

According to Helen Noyes Webster, who interpreted the above quotation in her book, Herbs, How to Grow Them and How to Use Them, the Israelites traveling with Moses obviously missed the garlic when they went toward the Promised Land. If Moses had carried garlic, the Israelites may have been able to avoid intestinal putrefaction from eating the desert's available lizards and snakes.

Homer mentions garlic in his famous Odyssey. The deity Mercury, or Hermes, gave garlic to Odysseus as a protection against the goddess Circe's evil sorcery in which she turned men to swine. The athletes of the original Olympic games in ancient Greece traditionally chewed a clove of garlic before participating in the games. Galen, an early Greek doctor, spoke of garlic as the panacea of the common man. Hippocrates prescribed the eating of garlic for uterine tumors. The Vikings and the Phoenicians always carried garlic on their ocean voyages.
The crusaders brought garlic back to France. (In those days, it was a common law that two men's lives could be sacrificed in order to save a 100 lb. sack of peppercorns.)

A French herbalist, Messegue, born in Gascony, France, states that all the children born in that province are baptized with a clove of garlic on the lips. The emperor Charlemagne recommended that his subjects cultivate garlic. King Henry IV of France was baptized with a clove of garlic on his lips, and although he was said to have chewed a clove of raw garlic every morning upon arising, he was still very popular with the ladies.

The National Cancer Institute central files show that the incidence of cancer is extremely low in France where garlic consumption is the greatest and that garlic eaters in Bulgaria do not have cancer. It is reported in a textbook on pharmacognosy that a physician in British Columbia has successfully treated malignant situations by prescribing the eating of garlic.

The prophet Mohammed recommend that garlic be applied externally on the sting of the scorpion or the bite of the viper in the 7th century.

"The herb becomes the teacher. Men stray after false goals while the herb he treads (or in these days, stomps upon) knows much much more."

The above quote was written by Henry Vaughn, the early 17th century poet and mystic, as well as Hermetic philosopher during the days when the Doctrine of Signatures was popular. The Doctrine of Signatures was the method by which the ancients recognized the usage of a plant. According to Nicholas Culpeper, the 17th century English Physician and Herbalist, "and by the icon or image of every herb, man first found out their virtues. Modern writers laugh at them for it, but I wonder in my heart how the virtues of herbs first came to be known, if not by their signatures. The moderns have then from the writings of the ancients--the ancients had no writings to have them from."

The 17th century "moderns" felt that garlic, with its hollow stalk, helps afflictions of the windpipe. We know this to be a truth; that garlic is an antihistamine, and has been successfully used in bronchial and pulmonary disorders. As we examine some of the virtues of garlic, we find that the claims of the old Doctrine of Signatures will be far surpassed.

The National Dispensatory of 1887 gives us a fine description of the constituents of garlic at a period in our medical history when Syrupus Alli was an official U.S. preparation.

Constituents.--Besides the cellular tissue, garlic contains between 50 and 60 percent of water, 35 percent of mucilage some albumen, sugar, starch, and about 1 percent of volatile oil, to which its odor and taste are due. In its crude state, oil of garlic is of a dark brown-yellow color, heavier than water, of a very interesting taste, and consists of oxide and sulphides of allyl. The rectified oil consists mainly of the sulphide, $(C_3H_5)_2S$, is colorless, lighter than water and may be obtained artificially by treating an alcoholic solution of potassium sulphide with allyl iodide. It dissolves easily in alcohol and ether, and sparingly in water ... Garlic, macerated in water or vinegar, yields its virtues to these liquids.--(p. 154)

They also describe its physiological action and medicinal uses:

Physiological action and Medical Uses--Garlic as well as leek and onion, is a stimulant to the part to which it is directly applied and to be the whole system. Its odorous element may be perceived on the breath and its taste in the mouth when the bruised bulb has been applied to the skin. When eaten raw, its odor "hales from many parts of the body, and, given to nursing women, it taints their milk, so that their infants refuse the breast. It reddens the skin, and may even vesicate it. Internally, it stimulates the digestive organs, and is everywhere used, but principally in southern countries, as a condiment for various kinds of food. The odor or garlic is popularly employed to revive persons from a swoon or from hysterical insensibility. It is a vermifuge not to be neglected in the treatment of lumbricoid worms when given by the mouth, and for destroying ascarides when administered by the rectum. Many cases of dropsy, particularly of anasarea produced by cold, have been cured by a diet of bread and raw onions. This regimen will sometimes produce copious diuresis. Onions boiled in milk have been used successfully for a like purpose. Bruised cloves of garlic and poultices of boiled onion are admirable remedies for chronic bronchitis in children. They should be applied over the whole front of the chest. Internally, garlic is a very useful agent in the same affection. It is also a domestic remedy for whooping cough. Onion poultices are particularly applicable to abscesses; the core of a roasted onion relieves earache when introduced into the auditory canal. Onion and garlic cataplasms applied to the perineum relieve strangury. The dose of bruised or chopped garlic or of the expressed juice is about 30 grains (Gm 2). (p.154-155)

Frances Ward published this summary of garlic in her post-World War II book, British Herbs:

"GARLIC Allium Sativum, Amaryllidaceae

Anyone who travels in Italian buses might be forgiven for deciding never to grow this unpleasant smelling plant, and one can quite appreciate the decision of the old Greeks that people who ate Garlic should not be allowed in the temples of Cybele.
But from early times it has been considered a very useful medicine, and in the Middle Ages in Britain it was believed to be, either by itself by itself, as a 'simple', or mixed with other herbs, one of the cures for leprosy. Lepers were often called 'pilgarlics', as they were made to peel their own garlic, certainly a mark of identity and a means of segregation!

Throughout the ages it was held to have antiseptic properties, and during the 1914-18 War, sterilized Sphagnum Moss soaked in Garlic juice was used for suppurating wounds, a reminder of the old method of treating leprous sores. From time to time, even in modern days, Garlic has been claimed to have marvelous properties; now, in addition to its stimulating powers, it is held to be beneficial in digestive complaints and for coughs, colds and asthma.

Cultivation of Garlic is a fairly easy matter, though it needs a finely sifted soil similar to that of an onion-bed. The cloves should be set about 2 in. in the ground about February or March, and lightly covered with soil. The bulbs may usually be lifted during August. There is generally a demand for Garlic from druggists, and good prices have been paid for it." (Ward, 1949, p. 159).

It in the medical literature we find several references to garlic as a therapeutic agent.

Phytocides of garlic suppress the proteinases (cathepsin) in malignant tumors of humans (postoperative material) and of experimental animals. These phytocides also inhibit cathepsin in the liver of cancerous animals, the activity of which increases during malignant growth. This action was detected by adding garlic extract to inoculated Ehrlich carcinoma. The results may be useful in further studies on garlic in the diet of cancer patients." (p. 140)

Joseph A. Di Paolo and Christopher Carruthers of the Roswell Park Memorial Institute of Buffalo, New York, wrote an article in Cancer Research, 1960. The title is, "The effect of Allicin From Garlic on Tumor Growth." By the way, Allicin is responsible for the odor in garlic, so the new odorless garlic isn't quite as effective as regular garlic. For those fortunate souls who can ingest raw garlic; the garlic breath can be obliterated by chewing on a raw clove (not a garlic clove, but the spice clove), or putting a drop of peppermint of spearmint oil on the tongue.

Chester J. Cavallito and John Hays Bailey writing in the Journal of the Chemical Society, Volume 66, November, 1944, discuss the antibacterial principle of garlic, allicin. They isolated allicin, a colorless oil, from garlic cloves and found it to be effective against the following bacteria strains both gram positive and gram negative:

Organism
STAPHYLOCOCCUS AUREUS
STREPTOCOCCUS HEMOLYTICUS
STREPTOCOCCUS VIRIDANS
B. SUBTILIS
B. TYPHOSUS
B. PARATHYPHOSUS A
B. PARATHYPHOSUS B
B. PARATYPHOSUS KUNZENDORF
B. MORGANI
B. ENTERIDITIS
B. TYPHI-MURIUM
B. DYSENTERIAE SHIGA
B. DYSENTERIAE FLEXNER
B. DYSENTERIAE SONNE
V. CHOLERAE
(P. 1951)

H. Dold and A. Knapp, German Researchers writing in Chemotherapy section of Biological Abstracts in the 1950's discovered that garlic was effective against Streptococci, Escherichia coli, Bacillius prdigiosis, B. proteus, B. Subtilis, Shigelia paradysenteriae Flexner, Eberthelia typhosa, Salmonella enteritidis and Vibrio cholerae. It was more effective when crushed than sliced. It in addition, garlic exhibited some bacterial action even through the air. Bacteria could not be made resistant to the garlic either. The antibacterial action of garlic juice became somewhat weaker after having been stored in the ice box for 8 days and after boiling for 10 minutes. Remember, too, that when garlic is cooked above 130 degrees F., the enzymes in it are destroyed, and the organic sulphur in the garlic now becomes a harmful form of inorganic sulphur.

A most unique article appeared in the Chinese Medical Journal in May of 1977;

"GARLIC SLICE IT IN REPAIRING EARDRUM PERFORATION"

by Hsu Wei-cheng

Teaching Research Group of Ear, Nose and Throat Department, Inner Mongolia Medical College, Huhehot

"Clinical use of fresh garlic was satisfactory in repairing eardrum perforations in 18 cases (1 having perforation in both ears) except 1 with irreversible chronic otitis media. The time required for healing by this method was 16 days in 12 cases with perforations smaller than half of the eardrum pars tensa and 28 days in 6 cases with perforations larger than half of it. 10-19 db hearing was gained after treatment.
Of the 18 cases, 6 had increased exudate in the middle ear during the latter part of the garlic treatment. Exudation stopped quickly after treatment was discontinued and anti-inflammatory measures were taken. It in 4 of these, healing took place soon after exudation was checked and in 2 it was necessary to repeat garlic application before the wound healed completely...

This method is indicated in adult's traumatic eardrum perforations within 3 weeks of injury provided there is no infection, perforation is not larger than half of the pars tensa and there is sufficient eardrum left around the perforation edges. It in cases where the duration of perforation is over one month and its edges have already become cicatrized, repairing with fresh garlic slice can only be started after 50% trichloro-acetic-acid has been used to cauterize the edge (repeat the cauterization every few days, if necessary), until the formation of whitish ring (0.1-0.2 mm width) and reddish granulation.

Prepare a fresh clove of garlic carefully, peel it but leave the transparent epithelium-layer tightly attached. The external auditory canal is sterilized routinely. Slice off a very thin piece of the garlic clove (about 0.2 mm thick) shaping it just large enough to cover the perforation. Keep the epithelium-layer attached to the garlic slice and insert it into the ear canal and carefully push it against the eardrum so that its cut surface hugs the peroration while the epithelial layer covered surface faces the external auditory meatus. Pack the external auditory meatus with an alcohol moistened cotton ball. Forceful blowing of the nose is prohibited and water should not be allowed into the ear canal in order to prevent infection. Usually the garlic slice should be replaced once or twice a week until healing is complete. Stop treatment when the middle ear becomes inflamed with excessive exudate and start anti-inflammatory treatment.

Garlic is a strong stimulant which hastens growth of new granulation, contains allin (C6H11O3NS) which rapidly breaks down to yield the antibiotic allicin (C6H10OS2) in the presence of enzyme allinase and water." (Chinese Med. Journal, 3 (3); pp. 204-205).

"With garlic, the patient himself is doctor, pharmacologist, nurse, and pharmaceutical manufacturer all in one."
--Yoshio Kato

Yoshio Kato of the Oyama Garlic Laboratory in Japan has written a very comprehensive booklet entitled, Garlic, The Unknown Miracle Worker. It in it he describes a unique process of garlic juice therapy known as FLOW-LEBEN. in his own words:

"FLOW-LEBEN is a total therapy system of medical application, particularly the external application of garlic. Application for the patents has been made in ten countries. Already the patents have been granted in four countries. (The Republic of China, Italy, France, Germany and the United Kingdom.)

It is very well known that garlic contains all the elements except Vitamin D. It is also known that garlic essence warms the body and promotes better circulation of the blood .... Aillin, an oily substance contained in garlic, diluted as much as 200 times can kill typhoid germs.

Another study reported that garlic juice diluted 30-40 times stops the growth of certain types of bacteria in a nutrient media--garlic has strong germicidal properties which are not found in other plants. When aneurinase bacteria grow in the body, the majority of the internally produced vitamin B1 is spoiled by this bacteria--garlic shows antipyretic effects when it, diluted with water, is applied externally to a person's body at times of high fever.

FLOW-LEBEN is the only system in the world by which we can obtain the maximum effects from garlic. The first unit was completed in 1970. It in this clinic, various concentrations of garlic-water solution are sprayed on the bodies of patients by means of atmospheric pressure compressed air (2 to 7 lbs.) shot through atomizing nozzles. Hydraulic pressure is employed in the newer models. This process stimulates the body's metabolism and removes cholesterol from the blood. Various functional disorders are eliminated and skin diseases are also cured by the germicidal effect of garlic."(Kato, 1973, pp. 173-175)

The unique and very deluxe treatment has been effective in treatment of ringworm, skin cancer, frostbite, and other skin disorders using a 100% solution of garlic juice.

Richard Lucas in Nature's Medicines, published in 1966, presents the history of the Four Thieves Vinegar:

"It in Marseilles, a garlic-vinegar preparation known as the Four Thieves was credited with protecting many of the people when a plague struck that city (1722). Some say that the preparation originated with four thieves who confessed that they used it with complete protection against the plague while they robbed the bodies of the dead. Others claim that a man named Richard Forthave developed and sold the preparation, and that the "medicine" was originally referred to as Forthave's. However, with the passing of time, his surname became corrupted to Four Thieves." (Lucas, 1966, p. 38)

We now have the modern version of the formula. It is known as the Super Garlic Immune formula. It consists of fresh garlic, apple cider vinegar, pure vegetable glycerine, U.S.P., honey, garlic juice, fresh comfrey root, wormwood, lobelia, marshmallow root, oak bark, black walnut bark, mullein, skullcap, and uva-ursi. We recommend that you have several gallons of the preparation on hand in storage and hope that you will not need it. But, at the time of writing this article, a radio broadcast informed us of a case of Bubonic Plague with ensuing death in Lake Tahoe, U.S.A. The medical authorities were trying to locate all of the persons with whom the late subject came in contact in hopes of isolating the infection so the general public would not become exposed to this disease. The plague, related to the Black Plague in Europe during the 1300's, left people dead in their tracks and hanging out of windows waving goodbye to their friends. According to Herman Hesse, a German Writer, Goldmund was a young man who left a 14th century monastery and became a vagabond. He enjoyed the merriment of the wanderer as he traveled through Europe tasting the pleasures of love and life. All this was to change as Hesse describes the character's feeling of powerlessness and horror as he wanders throughout plague-stricken towns, cities, and rural areas observing the Hand of Death had reached everywhere; striking people regardless of their social standing or age. He describes a grotesque scene in a farm cottage where an entire family lay frozen after the throes of death.

The best insurance in the world against the "predicted coming plagues" and "killing diseases" is to have the body in a good healthy condition. Disease germs are merely scavengers and can only live on toxins, mucus and residue from junk foods. They cannot and will not be damage healthy cell structure. Therein lies the key! Have a healthy, clean body and disease germs will by-pass you--wanting nothing to do with your body, because it would be "obnoxiously clean" (in their language) and no filth for them to live on.

If the plague, or some other epidemic hits before you are in a good healthy condition, it is good to have an aid for a fast cleaning.

While lecturing in Snowflake, Arizona one night, one of the group asked if we had an Super Garlic Immune formula, and I was prompted to give them a "certain combination" of herbs to use.

The people there were very impressed to go right to work and prepare this liquid, having it read for use. We had told them that plagues come at unexpected times and it could be tomorrow or maybe even years away, but expect the unexpected and be ready now. If the formula was still unused, from "no need" years later, we could all be happy but "TIS BETTER SAFE THAN SORRY".

These good people made it up in gallon lots and had it on hand. Months later while speaking in Tucson, Arizona, someone asked for the "Super Garlic Immune remedy." I was surprised and asked where they had heard of it, as we had only given it out once. We were informed that a plague-like condition or flu had hit the Snowflake area and when other aids failed, this combination of herbs in liquid form performed its job with amazing speed.

At our next series of lectures in Snowflake, some time later, we heard one testimony after another about the many different types of ailments that were given quick relief by using this formula. The formula has now spread in many areas from coast to coast and is being used with good results. A man picked us up at an airport on the west coast a short time ago, and on the floor of his car was a bottle with liquid in it. When asked what it was he said, "oh, that's your Super Garlic Immune remedy, we never travel without it as it works good on about any sickness that comes up while we are traveling. We are also never without a bottle of it at home."

Super Garlic Immune Formula is available in The Cold Sheet Treatment book.

Because of the wonders we have told you about in this article of the greatness of garlic, it is easy to see how it fits in this formula. Drop a culture of almost any known disease germ into "apple juice" or "apple cider vinegar" an it will die immediately. The ingredients found in "black walnut" are one of the few-known herbal-destroyers of fungus. Marshmallow is the enemy of gangrene and peritonitis. It is a "softening emollient" that will aid in removal of the inorganic deposits broken up by the "solvent" gravel root. Wormwood relieves pain and kills pin-worms and other unwanted parasites, etc. Oak bark tones and firms up the cells in the muscles, cartilage, and flesh. It is also an aid in rebuilding the circulatory system and feeding it. Scullcap is one of the finest nerve repairing and rebuilding aids. It works especially well on the spinal cord--the trunkline for health to the entire body. Comfrey is the cell-proliferant that causes the good cells to multiply rapidly and push out the waste and dead-cell structure, being supplied with the wonderful allantoin. Lobelia is the Lord's great catalyst to combine the herbal entities to a "smoothly-operating whole."

Garlic is a handy herb that will grow right in your own yard, taking very little space, but which should be in everybody's yard. Any time of the year it is needed, one can go out and dig up the bulb. This can be done in spring, summer, or fall, in an emergency, but the best harvest time is autumn, when the leaves have died down. After shaking off the dirt, the bulbs can be put into a mesh bag and hung in the shade where the cool air can circulate through the bulbs.

The single buttons or cloves, that make up the bulb, can be planted in the fall and by going through the winter will come up the following year in the form of a bulb, with a number of cloves or buttons. When planted in the spring, they will generally be just a larger button by fall and not become a bulb. Some people will put the garlic buttons into the refrigerator (not freezer) and keep cold for a few weeks, bring them out into room temperature for several weeks, and repeat this process several times. Thus, the garlic now believes it has gone through several winters and it mature enough to develop from a clove into a bulb. Rather sneaky we would say, but if it works, fine!

Garlic can be planted around rose bushes and other aphid infested plants and the aphids will disappear. Gardeners have reported to us that they plant garlic between the rows of cauliflower, tomatoes, etc., and the garlic will discourage plant-destroying bugs, cut worms, etc. Here "you can have your cake and eat it too" for you can get the value of garden-assistance from this herb during the growing season, and then thin them out in the fall to use as a food and a healing herb during the winter.

The reason for garlic's miraculous type of healing is in its creation, and this will be explained in more detail further along in this article. Briefly now, this is what happens: The garlic clove contains a very high amount of sulphur; sulphur is one of the best minerals to be used as an oxygen carrier. Oxygen is the breath of life and sulphur will carry the oxygen in the body directly to the infected area. Germs cannot live in a good supply of oxygen, therefore, the infection is cleared quickly. This is an organic wonder, so garlic may be termed 'a wonder herb'.

Medical science discovered that sulphur caused this rapid healing, so in World War II, flowers of sulphur (an inorganic mined-mineral) was substituted for the garlic. The army used sulfa for practically every ailment from "falling hair to fallen arches."

Wonderful results were reported to us and we were told to use it in ever increasing amounts.

The difference in the healings of the garlic and the inorganic, manmade remedies is that garlic does its job and the excess of the organic materials not being used in healing the infection is easily passed as harmless vegetable fiber from the body. No harm and certainly nothing but good could result from using this powerful, yet harmless, herb. But, with the man-made sulfa drug we used, (this 'wonder drug' healing or the infection), the inorganic flowers of sulphur remained in the body. This inorganic mineral eventually combined with the urine and formed a substance that cut up the urinary tract, causing bed wetters. Many soldiers and other servicemen were given medical discharges, because of "bed wetting". This habit was acquired while in the service after the use of sulfa drugs. It is a well-known fact that too much sulfa drug has also caused other problems. The sulphur in the garlic will assist in healing the urinary tract after its infection-clearing job, instead of damaging it.

Following are various other uses of garlic. Many people have been helped in ridding the body of worms by inserting a peeled button of garlic as high as possible into the rectum. Do this just before retiring at night and it will come out with the first bowel movement in the morning. (This is also a fine aid in adjusting high blood pressure and low blood pressure). Many mothers find it easier to insert the peeled button of garlic (into the child's rectum) after the child is asleep at night.

Here is a very successful routine for removal of these unwanted growths called moles, or warts. Take a button of garlic, slice or cut in two, and placed the cup area over a wart of mole. Tape it on, and as it dries out put a fresh piece. Many users have reported good results.

Massage painful joints and areas with Oil of Garlic, massage it thoroughly. Massage in thoroughly oil of garlic a number of times a day for rough hands.

To make oil of garlic place chopped or grated garlic in a bottle, glass servicing dish or baking dish, (an inch or more of the garlic), and cover with olive oil so that the oil is a half inch or so above the garlic. Keep in a warm place or in the sun two to three days. Strain with muslin or any good cotton material (no synthetics) and bottle the oil. Keep in a cool place.

I remember one time we were called out to a house in the wee hours of the morning. This call was to see a little boy, under the age of two years, that had double pneumonia. The physician on the case had informed the parents that nothing more could be done and he would come back in the morning to sign the child's death certificate. Seeing as it was well under forty degrees below zero and nearly fifty miles from ambulance service, the parents were told that the boy, if taken by car to a hospital, would surely die. These parents tried to get other doctors, but at that time of night, and in such a remote area, no one would offer help. A friend told them about us, then living in Evanston, Wyoming, and to try to call us. Having been told of the boy's condition we went expecting to give him the cold-sheet treatment. Upon arriving there we found that the plumbing was frozen and there was not running water in the house. We found enough in the toilet tank above the bowl to give the little chap an enema. We were not able to give the cold sheet treatment (no water) so only the garlic paste was made up and applied. This was done after a complete massage of the body and the feet. After oiling the feet up to the ankles, thoroughly, and massaging the olive oil in well, a half-inch thickness of the garlic paste was applied to the soles of his feet. (This is put on only the soles and not up onto the sides). Then gauze was placed over to cover the paste, bandages to hold it into place, and a loose white cotton sock was pulled over the bandages to hold them securely.

Garlic paste is made by taking freshly peeled buttons of garlic and garlic about half and half with Vaseline. This amount can vary, according to the toughness of the feet, more Vaseline for tender feet, less for thicker skin. Many of the health minded readers will be shocked by our using a low-vibration ointment like Vaseline instead of using anhydrous lanolin or some lighter more organic type. The reasoning for this is that the lighter type ointments will penetrate more quickly into the skin, but the Vaseline will hold the garlic on the ointment form. This will also keep the garlic from blistering as easily. (A garlic blister looks bad, but does not hurt and heals back quickly.) The little boy was running an extremely high fever and was delirious when he was covered and put back into bed. (This was well after 2:00 a.m.). We assured the parents the child would be all right and would get well. A few days later we were called again by these parents. They told us that the doctor came back to sign the death certificate that next morning, but the little boy was sitting in his high chair, drinking some juice and breathing normally as if nothing had happened the night before. The doctor became so angry and demanded to know the name of the other doctor who had taken over the case before it had been released by him. He wanted a hearing by "the board" to have the other doctor thrown out of practice for going "against procedure" by taking over a case without written release. The parents asked if his "release" was the death of their child? He probably changed his mind because we were not brought before a hearing.

I had forgotten this case until nearly twenty years had passed. One evening, after a lecture in another state, a fine-looking young fellow in his early twenties came up to the podium and shook my hand vigorously, saying he had always wanted to meet me. His mother had told him of our long trip in sub-zero weather at night to their house, of using the natural methods on, and saving his life. He stated that he enjoyed living so much he had been looking forward to meeting me.

That paid off for a cold night out on a house call by far more than the small fee that was charged.

GINGER

Ginger root

LATIN NAME Zingiber officinale

Kingdom: Plantae
Clade: Tracheophytes
Clade: Angiosperms
Clade: Monocots
Clade: Commelinids
Order: Zingiberales
Family: Zingiberaceae
Genus: *Zingiber*
Species: **Z. officinale**

Zingiberis rhizoma
Ingwerwurzelstock

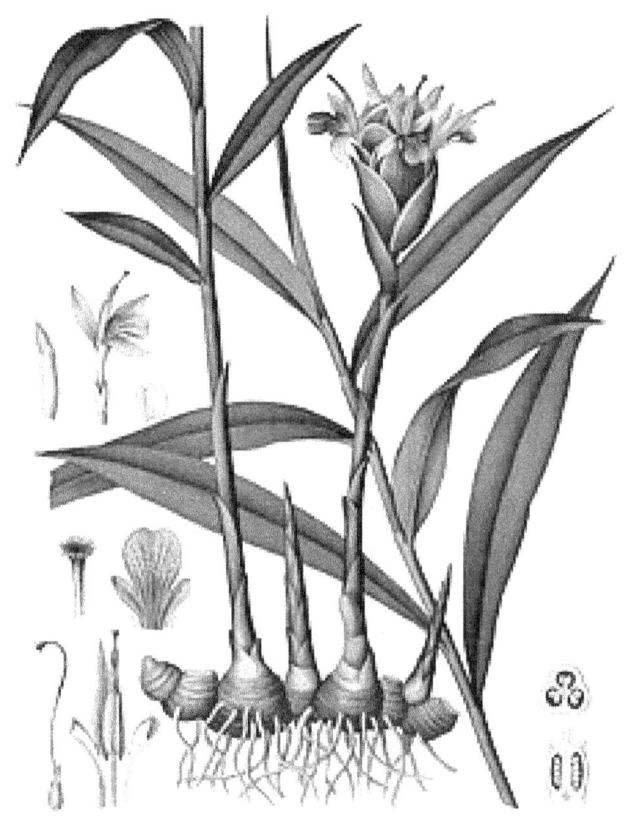

Name of Drug

Zingiberis rhizoma, ginger root.

Composition of Drug

Ginger root consists of the peeled, finger-long, fresh or dried rhizome of *Zingiber officinale* Roscoe [Fam.Zingiberaceae], as well as its preparations in effective dosage

The rhizome contains essential oil and pungent principles.

Uses
Dyspepsia, prevention of motion sickness.

Contraindications
With gallstones, only to be used after consultation with a physician.

Note: No administration for morning sickness during pregnancy.

[**Ed.note:**A review of clinical literature could not justify this caution. There is no evidence that ginger causes harm to the mother or fetus.

Side Effects
None known.

Interactions with Other Drugs

None known.

Dosage

Daily dosage:

- 2 - 4 g rhizome;
- equivalent preparations.

Mode of Administration

Chopped or comminuted rhizome and dry extracts for teas, other galenical preparations for internal use.

Actions

Antiemetic
Positively inotropic
Promoting secretion of saliva and gastric juices
Cholagogue

In animals:

- antispasmodic

In humans:

- increase in tonus and peristalsis in intestines.

HISTORY

What a humble herb, to be so grand, so mighty in strength, so hard working, all for such little recognition.   This is an herb to be discovered, experienced and enjoyed in abundance! There is far too little celebration, understanding and appreciation for the wonder of ginger, but this has not always been the case.

From its origin to the present, ginger is the world's most widely cultivated herb. Testimonials of both the medicinal and economic importance of ginger have been recorded as far back as five thousand-year-old Greek literature to 200 B.C. Ancient literature from the Middle East, Asia and Europe write of its impact. Chinese records chronicle the immense wealth associated with growing acres of ginger. Trade in spices like ginger could easily be associated with one's wealth and power. In the Middle Ages, as little as just one pound was worth 1 shilling and 7 pence, approximately equivalent to the price of a sheep. Having such a rich history, it's easy to see how explorers like Marco Polo and Vasco da Gama were careful to document the cultivation of ginger.

The historical reverence for and usage of ginger is simply staggering. Ginger had great historic, medicinal value as a spiritual beverage, aphrodisiac, digestive aid, etc. Traditional Chinese and Ayurvedic Indian systems viewed ginger as a healing gift from God. Chinese pharmacopeias claim long term use of fresh ginger as putting a person in contact with the spiritual advantages. Writings of the Koran describe ginger as a beverage of the holiest heavenly spirits. Its healing heritage is unmatched in the history of medicine.

Throughout history, ginger is reported for its value as an aphrodisiac. The list of references of ginger's sexual tonic properties is impressive, including endorsements by the Greek Dioscorides; a citation in Arabia's *A Thousand and One Nights,* John Gerard's prescriptive herbal; and Italy's famed University of Salerno medical school prescribed that a rule for happy life in old age was to "eat ginger, and you will love and be loved as in your youth."

Ginger's value as an aphrodisiac is undoubtedly connected to its widespread use as a systemic tonic, hormone balancer, energy enhancer, and agent for improving the appetite and circulation. It is no wonder that ginger is so widely used as a prerequisite for a healthy sexual appetite.

As a digestive aid, Confucius wrote as far back as 500 B.C. of never being without ginger when he ate. In the famous *De Materia Medica* 77 A.D. Dioscorides recorded that ginger "warms and softens the stomach".[1] Virtually every culture has recorded the virtues of ginger as a digestive aid. Bruce Cost, wrote of ginger's use as the "Alka-Seltzer of the Roman Empire".[2] Ginger was part of the Revolutionary War soldier's diet. In U.S. early twentieth century, ginger was named the herb of choice for digestive support.

Either alone or in combination with other herbs, ginger has been the herb of choice for thousands of years. As a testimony to its numerous usages, it remains a component of more than
50% of all traditional herbal remedies.[3]

The Japanese soothed spinal and joint pain with it. The Chinese found it helpful with tooth aches, symptoms of a cold, flu and hangover. Progressive early-twentieth century U.S. physicians prescribed ginger for painful menstruation.

Years before British surgeon Dr. James Lind discovered that lime could prevent scurvy; fifth-century Chinese sailors were using ginger's vitamin C nutritive value for the same purpose on long voyages.

The cultural outlook on aphrodisiacs in the seventeenth century was another factor in the reduction of its usage as a therapeutic agent. Over time, the widespread use of ginger to retard spoilage and disguise taste was superseded by modern refrigeration. As time passed, ginger came to be thought of as a relic of the past; a reminder of a more primitive time.

1.   Pursegtlove , J.W., Brown, E.G., Green, C. L., and Robbins, S.R.J. Spices. Vol. 2. London and New York: 1981 ,447-532.

2.   Cost, Ginger, East to West. 169.

3.   Lad and Frawley, Yoga of Herbs b. Sakai, Y.m et al. :"Effects of medicinal plant extracts from Chinese herbal medicines on the mutagenic activity of benzo(a)pyrene." *Mutation Research* 206 (1988): 327-34.

CHEMICAL CONSTITUENTS

Zingiber officinale is the botanical name of ginger. It is botanically correct to refer to ginger as a rhizome rather than a root. Ginger can therefore be propagated from budded sections. Ginger is one of the world's top ten favored spices. Yet surprisingly, its tremendous medicinal value is virtually unknown.

Ginger can be divided into four principle parts: taste or pungency, essential oil or fragrance, macro/micro-nutrients, and synergists. An oily-resinous substance dissected from the plant comprising 5 to 10 percent of the plant is called ginerol.[4]

This oleoresin was then broken down into close to thirty elements. Gingerols or zingiberene may be responsible for taste and scent respectively. In fact, within ginger there are hundreds of ingredients that are referred to as synergists. These interact to make the plant as a whole the powerful healer that it is.

There may be dozens of different complex chemical interactions allowing ginger to prevent or benefit conditions like heart attacks, arthritis and ulcers. There are more than four hundred taste, fragrance, nutrient and synergistic constituents interacting to create an endless number of medicinal benefits.

One gram of one of ginger's principle constituent, zingibain, can actually tenderize as much as twenty pounds of meat. The obvious impact or effect is improved digestion. This enzyme can enhance the effectiveness of other antibacterial elements by as much as 50%. The enzyme zingibain can aid immunity to the effect of digesting parasites and their eggs, and is associated with anti-inflammatory activity. This is due in part to the fact that ginger acts as an antioxidant with more than twelve constituents superior to vitamin E.[5] This action empowers ginger to help neutralize free radicals which are widely recognized as participation or being responsible for the inflammation process.

Each of ginger's 477 constituents could be listed. This impressive list includes the well known ascorbic acid, caffeic acid, capsaicin, beta-sitosterol, beta-carotene, curcumin, lecithin, limonene, selenium and tryptophan. It is nothing less than an exercise in complete and utter futility to try and isolate the "active" element from ginger.

4   Felter, H. W., and Lloyd, J. U. *King's American Dispensatory*. Portland, Ore.: Eclectic Medical, 1983, 2110.

5.   a. Govindarajan, V.S. "Ginger –Chemistry, technology, and quality evaluation: Part 2.: *Critical Reviews in Food Science and Nutrition* 17, no. 8 (1082): 189-258 (p. 230), citing Hirahara, F. "Antioxidative activity of various spices on oils and fatrs. Antioxidative activity towards oxidation on strorage and heating.,: *Japanese Journal of Nutrition* 32, no. 1 (1974): 1; Food Sci Technol Abstr. 7, nol. 3 (1975): T 126.   b-j listed in Notes and References chapter 3 #20 page 131 of GINGER Common Spice & Wonder Drug by Paul Sdchulick.

MEDICINAL QUALITIES

Ginger is probably best known as a digestive aid. It effectiveness in this area is so impressive that if this was ginger's only virtue, it would be worth its weight in gold on this point alone. However the list of both, medicinal and culinary benefits of this unassuming plant are incredible.

It is estimated that 80% of persons over the age of fifty suffer from osteoarthritis.[6] Amazingly more than 100 different diseases are grouped under the designation of arthritis.[7] Though these all have a different title, they all have one thing in common, inflammation. This is precisely where ginger shines. Ginger is a stimulant and anti inflammatory herb.

Numerous studies have been performed comparing ginger to aspirin for pain relief. Not only did ginger require a smaller dosage for the same pain relief accomplishment; unlike its counterpart, it did the job with no side effects.[8]

Many physicians also recommend a daily intake of aspirin to check clogged arteries and reduce the number of potentially fatal situations as a result of this problem. Clogged arteries are the cause of more than one-half of all deaths in the United States annually. When there is an excess of platelet-generated thromboxanes there is an increase in blood viscosity and aggregation leading to potentially lethal clotting. Is aspirin the best answer to this common life threatening phenomenon? Looking at the measure of total mortality rate will help us determine aspirin's true effectiveness. Some of the largest studies have shown that regular aspirin consumers suffer a higher mortality rate, experience more bleeding ulcers, joint discomfort and a potentially compromised immune system increase.[9]

An outpatient cardiology clinic in an Israeli hospital now encourages all of their patients to take one-half teaspoon of ginger daily. This is because ginger inhibits the same blood thickening enzyme as aspirin and does this naturally without the side effect of aspirin. This "wonder drug" herb has an additional benefit to the circulatory system and is remarkable, even transcending the potential of many modern cardiovascular drugs. With heart disease the #1 killer in America, is it any wonder that ginger is growing in popularity?

A group of Cornell Medical school researchers published an article in the *New England Journal of Medicine* in 1980 confirmed that ginger completely inhibited the potentially life-threatening process of platelet aggregation.[10] Because of ginger's many constituents, it offers synergistic cardiovascular features producing antioxidant effects which include strengthening the muscle and lowering serum cholesterol.[11] Ginger, in fact, actually decreases or interferes with cholesterol biosynthesis.[12]

Additionally, ginger may boast of having ulcer preventing properties. At least six anti-ulcer constituents from ginger have been isolated and identified.[13] It is nothing short of mind boggling how ginger can treat two opposites and balance the system. Ginger protects while stimulating, treats constipation and diarrhea while relieving nausea, inhibits toxic bacteria while promoting friendly species of bacteria. All of the above, once more, with no side effects!

Ginger has an ancient reputation as a carrier herb enhancing the absorption of other herbs. *You are what you eat* is an old adage, but are you what you eat or what you absorb?

Dr. Christopher said, "Ginger is generally combined with herbs going into the abdominal area, because it is a carrier. Ginger is an herb which accentuates so many herbs."

Environmental exposure is believed to be responsible for as many as 80% of all cancers.[14] Ginger contains at least two other properties that could positively influence the outcome of the patient's cancer; stimulation of immunity and inhibition of platelet aggregation. Studies in Montreal and Tokyo in1955 and 1979 concluded that ginger does indeed enhance immunity.[15]

Of particular note to diabetics is ginger's ability to regulate blood sugar[16] and increase circulation.[17] The increase in circulation is also a boon to the reproductive system. Researchers have concluded there is a significant increase in the sperm motility (swimming ability) and sperm content associated with ginger consumption.[18] As a result of this, ginger has long been prized for its ability to increase fertility.

Amazingly, among industrialized nations, we place close to the lowest in life expectancy (fifteenth) and highest in all cancer and heart disease rates. This should be a flashing red flag to us that our health care system is drastically wrong – not to mention a bad investment.

"We don't know what we're doing in medicine. Perhaps one-quarter to one-third of medical services may be of little or no benefit to patients."[19]

"The scientific basis of medicine is much weaker than most patients or even physicians realize; this leads to treatment based on uncertainty."[20]

6. Murray, M., and Pizzorno, J. *Encyclopedia of Natural Medicine*. Rocklin, Calif.: Pima Publishing, 1991,447.

7. Beasley, J. D., and Swift, J.J. The *Kellogg Report. The Impact of Nutition, Environment & Lifestyle on the Health of Americans.* Institute of Health Policy, Bard College, Annandale on Hudson, New York, 1989, 7G:353.

8. *GINGER Common Spice & Wonder Drug* 3rd edition, Chart page 64

9. The Aspirin Myocardial Infarction Study Research Group. *"The aspirin myocardial infarction study: Final results." Circulation* 62 (6, Pt 2.) (Dec. 1980): V79-84

10. Dorso, C., et al. "Chinese food and platelets." New *England Journal of Medicine* 303, no. 13 (1980): 756-57

11. Govindarajan, V.S. "Ginger-Chemistry, technology, and quality evaluation: Part 2." *Critical Reviews in Food Scienceoan Nutrition* 17, no. 3 (1982): 189-258 (p. 230), citing Gujral, S., et al. "Effect of Ginger *(Zingiber officinale*

roscoe) oleoresin on serum and hepatic cholesteros levels in cholesterol-fed rats." *Nutrition Reports International* 17, no. 2 (1978):

12. Sambaiah, K., and Srinivasan, K. *Die Nahrung* 1 (1991): 47-51

13. Shiba, M., et al. "Antiulcer furanogermenone extraction from ginger." *Chemical Abstracts* 196, no. 6 (1987) b. Yamahara, J., Hatakeyama, S., Taniguchi, K.m kawamura, M., and Yoshikawa, M. "Stomachic principles in ginger. II.."

Yakugaku Zasshi (Journal of the Pharmaceutical Society of Japan) 112, no. 9 (Sept. 1992): 645-55

14. Ames, B. *"Dietary carcinogens and anticarcinogens."* Science 23 (Sept. 19830: 1256-64

15. A. Duke, J. "The joy of ginger.*" American Health*, May 1988. b. Yamazaki, M.m and Nishimnura, T. "Induction of neutrophil accumulation by vegetable juice." *Bioscience Biotechnology Biochemistry* 1 (1992)" 150-151.

16. Mascolo, N., Jain, R., Jain, S. C., and Capasso, F. "Ethnopharmacologic investigation of ginger (Zingiber officinale)." Journal of Ethnopharmacology 27, nos. 1-2 (Nov. 1989): 129-140 b. Srivastava, K.C.mand Mustafa, T.

"Pharmacological effects of spices" Eicosanoid modulating activities and their significance in human health." Bio Medical Reviews (Bulgaria) 2 (1993): 15-29

17. Same as #16

18. Chart page 70 of GINGER Common Spice & Wonder Drug

19. Dr David Eddy, Director, Duke University Health Policy Research

20. C. Everett Koop, M.D., Former U.S. Surgeon General.

DOSAGES

<u>Compound of Turkey Rhubarb and Ginger</u>

Preparation: Mix the powders thoroughly together until uniform.
Dosage: Stir ¼-1/2 teaspoon of the compound powder into 2 fluid ounces of water; stir and drink, powder and all. Children: Do not give to infants under 5 because it is too powerfully a stimulant.

<u>Hepatic</u>

Preparation: Mix thoroughly.
Dosage: 1 teaspoonful 2-3 times daily.

<u>Menstrual problems (dysmenorrheal, amenorrhea)</u>

Preparation: When powders are used, stir 1 teaspoonful of the mix in 1 cupful of hot water, cover with a lid and steep 10 minutes. When herbs are used, steep 1 ounce of the mixture in 1 pint of boiling hot water, cover and let stand 10 to 15 minutes; keep warm.

Dosage: When powders are used, drink the cupful warm, leaving sediments; when the herbs are used, give 2 fluid ounces every 4 hours.

Gravel Kidney and Bladder problems

Preparation: Mix thoroughly. Infuse 2 ounces of powder in 1 quart of boiling hot water; cover and let stand until cool; strain.

Dosage: 3 Tablespoonfuls 4 to 5 times daily.

Bronchial Catarrh

Preparation: Infuse the herbs in 1 quart of boiling hot water, cover tightly and keep warm for 20 minutes; strain, sweeten to taste; allow to cool, bottle and keep in a cool place.

Dosage: 1-2 tablespoons 3 to 4 times daily.

GINKGO

Ginkgo Biloba Leaf

LATIN NAME Ginkgo biloba

Kingdom: Plantae
Clade: Tracheophytes
Division: Ginkgophyta
Class: Ginkgoopsida
Order: Ginkgoales
Family: Ginkgoaceae
Genus: *Ginkgo*
Species: **G. biloba**

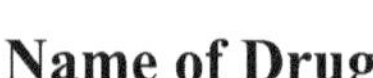

Ginkgo folium
Ginkgo biloba bltter

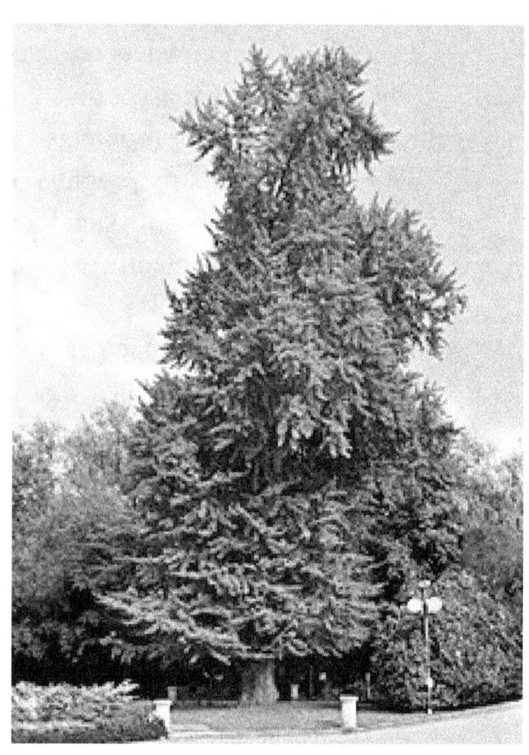

Name of Drug

Dry extract (35 - 67:1) from *Ginkgo biloba* L.leaf [Fam.Ginkgoaceae], extracted with acetone/water. Active Ingredient Classification ASK No.05939.

Composition of Drug

A dry extract from the dried leaf of *Ginkgo biloba* L manufactured using acetone/water and subsequent purification steps without addition of concentrates or isolated ingredients.

The drug/extract ratio is 35 - 67:1, on average 50:1.

The extract is characterized by:

22 - 27 percent flavonone glycosides, determined as quercetin and kaempferol, including isorhamnetin (via HPLC) and calculated as flavones with a molar mass of $MMr = 756.7$ (quercetin glycosides) and $Mr = 740.7$ (kaempferol glycosides); 5 - 7 percent terpene lactones, of which approximately 2.8 - 3.4 percent consists of ginkgolides A, B, and C, as well as approximately 2.6 - 3.2 percent bilobalide; below 5 ppm ginkgolic acids.

The given ranges include manufacturing and analytical variances.

Pharmacological Properties, Pharmacokinetics, Toxicology

The following pharmacological effects have been established experimentally:

- Improvement of hypoxic tolerance, particularly in the cerebral tissue.
- Inhibition of the development of traumatically or toxically induced cerebral edema, and acceleration of its regression.
- Reduction of retinal edema and of cellular lesions in the retina.
- Inhibition in age-related reduction of muscarinergic cholinoceptors and 2-adrenoceptors as well as stimulation of choline uptake in the hippocampus.
- Increased memory performance and learning capacity.
- Improvement in the compensation of disturbed equilibrium.
- Improvement of blood flow, particularly in the region of microcirculation.
- Improvement of the rheological properties of the blood.
- Inactivation of toxic oxygen radicals (flavonoids).
- Antagonism of the platelet-activating factor/PAF (ginkgolides).
- Neuroprotective effect (ginkgolides A and B, bilobalide).

The pharmacokinetics have been investigated both in animal experiments and in trials involving humans. An absorption rate of 60 percent was found in rats for a radioactively labeled extract (as specified under Composition of Drug). In humans after application of an extract specified as above, absolute bioavailability was 98 - 100 percent for ginkgolide A, 79 - 93 percent for ginkgolide B and at least 70 percent for bilobalide.

Both the acute and the chronic toxicity of an extract as specified under Composition of Drug is very low; accordingly, the LD_{50} in the mouse was 7725 mg/kg body weight after oral application and 1100 mg/kg body weight after intravenous application.

Investigations with this extract as specified above showed no effects which were either mutagenic, carcinogenic, or toxic to reproduction.

No evaluation was performed on the transferability of the experimental results to extracts other than those investigated.

[**Ed.note:**This statement refers to the fact that only a few proprietary ginkgo extracts were used in the studies upon which this monograph is based. Whether these results can be extrapolated to other ginkgo extracts is uncertain. SeeIntroduction]

Clinical Data

Uses
(a) For symptomatic treatment of disturbed performance in organic brain syndrome within the regimen of a therapeutic concept in cases of demential syndromes with the following principal symptoms:

Memory deficits, disturbances in concentration, depressive emotional condition, dizziness, tinnitus, and headache.

The primary target groups are dementia syndromes, including primary degenerative dementia, vascular dementia, and mixed forms of both.

Note: Prior to starting treatment with ginkgo extract, clarification should be obtained as to whether the pathological symptoms encountered are not based on an underlying disease requiring a specific treatment.

(b) Improvement of pain-free walking distance in peripheral arterial occlusive disease in Stage II of Fontaine (intermittent claudication) in a regimen of physical therapeutic measures, in particular walking exercise.

(c) Vertigo and tinnitus (ringing in the ear) of vascular and involutional origin.

Contraindications
Hypersensitivity to *Ginkgo biloba* preparations.

Side Effects
Very seldom stomach or intestinal upsets, headaches, or allergic skin reaction.

Special Cautions in Use

None known.

Use During Pregnancy and Lactation

No restrictions known.

Interactions with Other Drugs

None known.

Dosage and Administration

Unless otherwise prescribed:

Daily dosages:

Indication (a):

- 120 - 240 mg native dry extract in 2 or 3 doses.

Indications (b) and (c):

- 120 - 160 mg native dry extract in 2 or 3 doses.

Mode of Administration

In liquid or solid pharmaceutical forms, for oral intake.

Duration of Administration

Indication (a):

- Length of administration should be judged according to the severity of symptoms and should extend at least 8 weeks in the case of chronic illness.

Administration for more than 3 months should be reviewed as to justification for continued administration.

Indication (b):

- Improvement of ambulatory range requires administration for not less than 6 weeks.

Indication (c):

- Administration for more than 6 - 8 weeks has no therapeutic benefit.

Overdosage

None known.

Special Warnings

None.

Effects on Operators of Vehicles and Machinery

None known.

HISTORY

Ginkgo biloba is a "living fossil" as was stated by Charles Darwin (1959). It is the oldest living tree species in the world. The Ginkgo species dates all the way back to the Permian Period some 286 to 248 million years ago. Ginkgos began increasing in number a great deal in the middle of the Jurassic Period through the Cretaceous Period approximately 213million to 66.4 million years ago. During this era of the first flowering plants and the height of the Dinosaurs, fossils revealed several different Ginkgo species. These species were common and outspread in Asia, Europe, and America. This era along with its incredible kingdom of plants and animals ended with complete extinction. Scientists had thought that Ginkgo, along with the rest of the prehistoric plants and animals, had too ceased to exist. It was not until 1691 that Englebert Kaempfer (1651-1692), a German Physician and Botanist, made a most amazing discovery in China. Ginkgo had somehow survived the devastating Ice Age, although it was not quite the same as its ancient ancestors. Due to environmental changes, the ancient Ginkgo had evolved. Today, *Ginkgo biloba* is the only surviving member of the Ginkgo family. This survival is said to be owed to its remarkable adaptability, resistance to disease, and to Buddhist monks who cultivated and preserved the trees on sacred grounds. In fact one particular story tells of a rather large, ancient Ginkgo tree in Hiroshima. It sat 1.1 km away from the where an atomic bomb landed on August 6th 1945 during the end of World War II destroying a religious temple. The tree continued to bud after the blast with no major deformations. After the war they considered cutting down the tree to rebuild the temple. Instead, the temple was rebuilt and adjusted around the giant Ginkgo tree with the front stairs splitting on either side of it. Engraved on the tree is "No more Hiroshima" and peoples prayers for peace.[1] Interestingly, four atomic bombed Ginkgo trees are still alive today.

In 1778 Ginkgo was brought into North America by William Hamilton for his own personal garden. Credit for its popularity is given to Frank Lloyd Wright, a well known architect of the 20th century. It was a favorite of his and soon made its way into city landscapes across the United States.[2] Modern day streets of New York City are still lined with the beautiful trees and it has become popular in landscapes worldwide.

Landscape is not the only use mankind has found for this primeval plant. The recorded medicinal uses of Ginkgo in China can be tracked back nearly 5000 years, chiefly as a treatment for asthma.[3] The use of Ginkgo nuts has been recorded in Japanese text books since 1492. They were used at weddings and tea ceremonies as sweets and deserts. Medicinal uses of the seeds were not recorded until around 1578 in the 'Great Herbal' or *Pen tsao kang mu* by Li Shin-chen. The leaves were later used for medicinal purposes in Asia but became more of a western medicine practice in the 1950's. The first extract from the leaves was produced in 1965 by Dr. Willmar Schwabe. Since that time, the eminence of Ginkgo biloba has spread and its medicinal properties are desired through out populations all over the world. Ginkgo is today the most widely used herbal treatment for mind enhancement as well as treatment for other various diseases.

CHEMICAL CONSTITUENTS

Ginkgo contains many different substances. Most of them fall into two categories Flavnoids and Terpenoids or Terpene lactoids.

Flavnoids are naturally occurring substances that function as anti-oxidants (scavenge free radicals-damaging compounds in the body that alter cell membranes, tamper with DNA, and even cause cell death) also found in fruits and vegetables. They enhance the immune system in the body and interfere with tumor formation. The type of flavonoid in Ginkgo is called Ginkgolide. Ginkgolides are very unique compounds exclusive to Ginkgo and are broken down into separate ginkgolides A, B, C, J, and M. Each Ginkgolide has a different degree of potency. Ginkgolide B is considered the most active. Other flavnoids present are quercitin (which is one of the most studied flavnoids and is a stronger antioxidant than vitamin E), and kaempferol.

Terpene lactones are the active constituents that give ginkgo a bitter strong flavor and helps increase blood circulation.

Other components present are Amino Acid-6hydrozykynurenic acid, Dimeric flavones (bilobetin, ginkgetin, isoginkgetin, scieadopitysin), Proanthocyanidins, ginkgolic acid, ascorbic acid, carotenoids, and Bilobalide.

MEDICINAL QUALITIES

Ginkgo biloba is the most frequently prescribed herbal medicine worldwide. Over 1.5 million prescriptions of ginkgo leaf extract per month are being dispensed by doctors in Europe (especially Germany and France) for various complaints including vertigo, tinnitus, short term memory loss, etc.[1] In the United States, Ginkgo is not prescribed by medical physicians but is still considered a nutritional food supplement. In my personal opinion this is good because it is still available to be used freely and is not regulated by health officials. However, it is sad that because it is not prescribed its strength and abilities to make immense improvements on ones health is underutilized.

Ginkgo has been used and is still used for a numerous amount of health complaints and diseases. Its primary properties are considered to be antibacterial, antifungal, antioxidant, antitussive, astringent, circulatory stimulant, expectorant, kidney tonic, rejuvenative, and sedative.   Ginkgo's most powerful effect is on the circulatory system. Ginkgo flavnoids directly dilate the smallest segment of the circulating system, the micro capillaries, which increase blood circulation and oxygen levels in the body. This is one of the main reasons it is so effective in certain ailments. Ginkgo also contains constituents that inhibit platelet activity factor (PAF), which is a common allergen in the body. Physical stress, and poor diet can over stimulate PAF production; in other words blood clotting. Platelets become excessively sticky causing them to cling to the blood vessel wall or to each other. The clot may stay attached to the vessel or break loose and float around the bloodstream until it encounters a vessel that it can not pass through. Blood clotting can be responsible for a large variety of devastating diseases. Ginkgo acts similar to Aspirin in the way that it thins the blood and reduces stickiness.

Below are several instances in which Ginkgo biloba has been effective in certain health and disease concerns. In order to understand why Ginkgo is effective in treating these particular diseases, we must first understand what causes the disease. Therefore, each disease will be followed by a brief description of the cause and then an explanation of how and why Ginkgo is effective.

Ginkgo biloba is highly sought after due to its medicinal properties and ability towards mind enhancement. Both Age related degenerative diseases such as Alzheimer's as well as improving simple mind tasks such as Short term memory.

Alzheimer's disease

Alzheimer's disease is a degenerative brain disorder that manifests itself by progressive mental deterioration, loss of memory and cognitive functions, and the inability to carryout activities of daily life. This state of mind is often medically referred to as **Dementia.** In the United States, five percent of the population over the age of sixty-five suffers from severe dementia, while another ten percent of the population suffers from mild to moderate dementia.

Although there are many contributors to the cause of Alzheimer's, there are mainly two that are treatable with Ginkgo; free radical damage and oxidative damage. Because of its antioxidant properties Ginkgo improves blood circulation and increases oxygen levels in brain tissues. These antioxidants also scavenge and fight free radicals (highly reactive chemicals that attack molecules crucial for cell function causing damage in the brain and other tissues). As a result cell longevity and membrane stability is increased. It also increases metabolism and regulates neurotransmitters that are directly related to brain function. Other effects were demonstrated in a double blind study using EEG (test used to detect and record the electrical activity generated by the brain). This study showed that Ginkgo increases alpha rythem (which is the bio feedback frequency associated with mental alertness) and decreases the theta rhythm (which is related to the lack of attention) in elderly who were showing signs of mental deterioration.

Other studies have shown that Ginkgo extract is not only able to increase the functional capacity of the brain; it also has been known to normalize the acetylcholine receptors in the hippocampus (the area of the brain most affected by Alzheimer's disease) of aged animals, to increase cholinergic transmission (neurotransmitters), and to address many of the other major elements of Alzheimer's disease.

Many clinical studies have been done proving the positive effects that Ginkgo has on Alzheimer's patients. It has been proven that Ginkgo is most affective in early signs of Alzheimer's and in the case of Alzheimer's prevention.

Cognitive and Memory Improvement

Since Ginkgo increases oxygen flow to the brain, enhances glucose uptake and utilization of glucose (boosting brain metabolism and energy), it is also being researched for its role in senility, forgetfulness, headaches, improving alertness, and memory and mental performance.

Hindmarch (1988) reported on the effects of oral administration of the standardized Ginkgo biloba extract (GBE) on the short term memory of healthy young volunteers ages 25-40 years. In a double-blind cross-over trial, Hindmarch found that, one hour following a single oral 600 mg dose of GBE, short –term memory parameters were significantly improved compared with controls. According to Hindmarch, the battery tests indicate a specific activity on central cognitive processes and he proposes the use of GBE in cases and conditions where memory problems are a feature.

Ginkgo is often added to nutrition bars, fruit smoothies, and other healthy snacks in order to achieve such results as improving cognitive and memory ability. Since I have begun to study herbs, I have had the largest number of individuals inquire about Ginkgo biloba than any other herb. I would assume that its popularity can be credited to its paramount ability of improving ones mind and capacity to retain information and think more clearly is an element to be desired by all. I always encourage individuals to put it to the test themselves and get back with me. Positive feedback has been returned by a majority of these individuals. Besides an increase in mind enhancement, other agreeable results have been achieved as well.

Vascular Disease or Intermittent Claudication

Vascular diseases refer to diseases of blood vessels outside the heart and brain. It is often a narrowing of vessels that carry blood to the legs, arms stomach or kidneys. Because of narrowed vessels to the legs blood flow is decreased and the disease impairs ones ability to walk causing a great deal of pain in the legs. Other complications become factors of health due to vascular diseases.

Intermittent Claudication is similar to vascular disease in that it too is caused by inadequate blood oxygen flow to the leg muscles. It commonly occurs during exercise or walking. Symptoms are pain in the legs, muscle cramping, and lameness. The simple task of walking becomes unbearable to some.

Due to the same antioxidant properties that assist with brain function, ginkgo seems to offer the same protection to vascular disorders. It increases blood flow, assists oxygen in being more thoroughly distributed to blood vessels and muscle tissue. It helps maintain integrity and permeability of cell walls by inhibiting lipid peroxidation (lipids breaking down to form free radicals). It also helps tone and nourishes vascular organs.

Other circulation disorders can also be treated with Ginkgo such as hemorrhoids, varicose veins, insufficient circulation as a result of a stroke or skull injury, etc.

Depression and Anxiety

I recently chose Ginkgo to add to a formula I created to naturally assist the body in overcoming Depression and Anxiety. I carefully chose Ginkgo in my formula for its brain and oxygen enhancers. A clear mind is very important in controlling mood and depression. Besides a clear mind, Ginkgo also helps stabilize mood and balance serotonin it the system. Serotonin is a chemical neurotransmitter in the brain and systems that controls emotions, behavior and thought. Such abilities combined with several other select herbs provide a powerful combination that has in my experience, proved to be affective.

Tinnitus

In the United States, an estimated 17 million people have or have had tinnitus to one degree or another. Tinnitus is not a disease. It is a symptom of nerve damage and certain blood vessel disorders. It creates the perception of ringing, hissing, or other sound in the ears or head when no external sound is present. In 1986, Christopher Hobbs proved the effectiveness of Ginkgo as a tinnitus treatment. Ringing disappeared in thirty-five percent of the patients tested, with a distinct improvement in seventy days. When 350 other patients with hearing loss and tinnitus due advance in age were treated with ginkgo extract, the success rate for improved hearing and tinnitus was eighty-two percent.[9] Many patients taking Ginkgo for tinnitus, claim that it is inexpensive compared to other available treatments and that there are few side effects.

Eyesight, Glaucoma, Cataracts, and Macular Degeneration

Simply taking Ginkgo on a regular basis helps improve eyesight and can protect your eyes from a serious eye condition.

Glaucoma is a term used to describe a group of eye conditions usually involving increased pressure within the eyeball but does not have to. It can be related to damage to the optic nerve and retina. This is known as normal-tension Glaucoma. It is this form of Glaucoma that Ginkgo is most effective. Glaucoma is usually a condition that comes with age and can cause blindness in the worst case.

Cataracts are defined by a clouding or darkening of the lens in the eye causing blurry, hazy or distorted vision. It is a naturally occurring condition in the elderly but can also be caused by over exposure to ultraviolet rays.

Macular degeneration is an abnormality of blood supply to the light sensitive portion of the eye, or the macula. As a result, deterioration in the macula takes place causing a loss of focusing ability and central vision.

The flavnoids in Ginkgo helps to thin blood. Red blood cells become more flexible making it easier for them to move through the fine capillaries and increases blood supply to the retinal capillaries.   This can slow retinal deterioiation, and results in an increase of visual acuity and preservation. Antioxidants present in ginkgo also protect the eyes.

Counter Impotence

This is another malfunction of the body due to inadequate blood oxygen flow and atherosclerosis (hardening and clogging of arteries) of the penis.

There have been several studies over the last fifteen years to see what effects Ginkgo may have on this disorder. For example, in 1991 a study published in the *Journal of Sex Education and Therapy* evaluated the effect of Ginkgo leaf extract in the treatment of erectile dysfunction in fifty patients. The men diagnosed with arterial erectile impotence received 240 mg of ginkgo leaf extract daily for a period of nine months. The patients were divided into two groups based on their response to conventional therapies. Twenty of the patients had previously experienced some success with conventional drug therapies. The second group had not experienced erection following conventional therapies. Following treatment with the ginkgo leaf extract, all patients in the first group (twenty men) regained full, sufficient, and spontaneous erections following six months of treatment. Improvement continued through the nine-month treatment period. Nineteen of the thirty patients in the second group responded positively to the treatment, while eleven remained impotent. No side effects were reported in the study. This was only the second study published on the use of ginkgo leaf extracts in the treatment of impotence. [10] In another study, ultrasound examinations of sixty impotent men who took Ginkgo biloba showed improved penile blood circulation after just six weeks. After six months, fifty percent of the patients had regained potency. Studies continue to investigate Ginkgo in the treatment of impotence and the findings are quite satisfactory.

Relief from Asthma Attacks

Asthma is a lung disease in which tightening of the air passages can provoke wheezing and difficulty breathing. It is usually of allergic origin.

Ginkgo has been used for Asthma in China for a very long time. Ginkgo inhibits the activity of eosinophils (a type of white blood cells active in fighting parasites and allergies); an action attributed to Ginkgolide B. It seems to relieve the airway spasms and wheezing associated with this lung disease. In a trial conducted in Belgium, six out to ten children with sever asthma were found to improve "dramatically" within the first three to four days of taking Ginkgo. Three others in this same group made huge improvements but still required some other therapy.

Ginkgo is recommended for asthma treatment but not in the case of an acute attack.

Reduce the risk of Heart Attack or Stroke

Heart attack is the death of heart muscle due to loss of blood supply. The loss of blood supply is usually caused by complete blockage of a coronary artery, on the arteries that supplies blood to the heart. Heart attack is often fatal.

By inhibiting the inappropriate formation of blood clots by platelets and increasing overall blood flow and oxygenation, Ginkgo is and ideal herb for preventing and treating heart attack. (Ginkgo is not recommended to stop an acute heart attack. In this case Emergency Medical Attention is immediately required.)

A Stroke occurs when an artery in the brain becomes blocked or when a blood vessel breaks, interrupting the flow to an area in the brain. When a stroke occurs, it kills brain cells in the surrounding area. These brain cells control different functions such as moving a limb or speech. When those nerve cells are lost, so is the function.

By inhibiting the inappropriate formation of blood clots by platelets and increasing overall blood flow and oxygenation, Ginkgo is an ideal herb for preventing and treating heart attack and stroke. (Ginkgo is not recommended to stop an occurring heart attack or stroke. In case of Emergency, Medical care should be sought out immediately)

Other and New Breakthroughs

New studies and applications are being discovered for the use and positive effects of Ginkgo biloba.   Some other diseases that are currently being tested and treated with Ginkgo are Vitilgo-a common auto immune skin disease, Protection from cell phone induced brain damage, anti-aging, toxic shock, improvement of social behaviors, and preventing the rejection of transplanted organs.

DOSAGES

Ginkgo leaves were originally applied as a topical skin treatment. The medicinal properties of the leaf extract when taken orally are what have made ginkgo one of the best selling herbal dietary supplements.[1]

Although it grows in your backyard, the leaf extracts are recommended to be pharmacologically standardized to deliver the most benefits. Tea made from the leaves does not contain enough of the active ingredients (Ginkgo flavone glycocydes and terpene lactone) to be as effective. Ginkgo is one botanical that is difficult to produce as a home remedy because the active photochemical need to be extracted. It takes an estimated 50 fresh leaves to yield one standard dose of the extract.[2] Herbalists may have a different opinion on the preparation of Ginkgo biloba.

Recommended doses may vary according to what is stated by your personal health care professional as well as the particularly disease being treated and its severity.   A "standard" daily dose is anywhere from 40-120 mg of Ginkgo Extract (GBE) per day. Standard GBE contains at least 24% flavone glycides (to maximize the herb's antioxidant and anti-clotting potential) and 6% terpene lactones (for improved blood flow and nerve protection).

Nutritional supplement: 40 mg GBE 3 times per day

    Alzheimer's disease: 80 – 240 mg GBE 2-3 times per day
    Asthma: 40 mg GBE 3 times per day when asthma is acute
    Allergies: 40 mg GBE 3 times per day or 60 mg GBE 2 times per day.
    Eyes: 40-60 mg of GBE 2-3 times per day
    Depression: 60 mg GBE 2 times per day
    Impotence: 60 mg 3 times per day
    Stroke: 80 mg GBE 3 times per day
    Tinnitus: 80 mg GBE 3 times per day

The dosage amounts of other forms of Ginkgo besides GBE are not as well established. The doses would vary as did the doses of GBE. As was stated before, studies show that other forms are not as effective in treatments but can be used. A daily dose would be similar to GBE as it would be consistent with taking doses 2-3 times daily as a tonic.

There are few known reports of the use of Ginkgo in Pediatric use of ginkgo. Therefore it is not currently recommended for children. On the contrary, side effects are rare. Because of the general overall safety of the herb, it may be used for children (with smaller doses) in certain and necessary cases.

It commonly takes four to six weeks, and in some cases up till twelve weeks, to notice the herbs effects.

---

[1] Blumenthal, Mark. *The ABC clinical guide to Herbs*. (Austin TX: American Botanical Council, 2003)
[2] Ginkgo biloba

GINSENG

LATIN NAME Panax quinquefolius

Kingdom: Plantae
Clade: Tracheophytes
Clade: Angiosperms
Clade: Eudicots
Clade: Asterids
Order: Apiales
Family: Araliaceae
Subfamily: Aralioideae
Genus: *Panax*

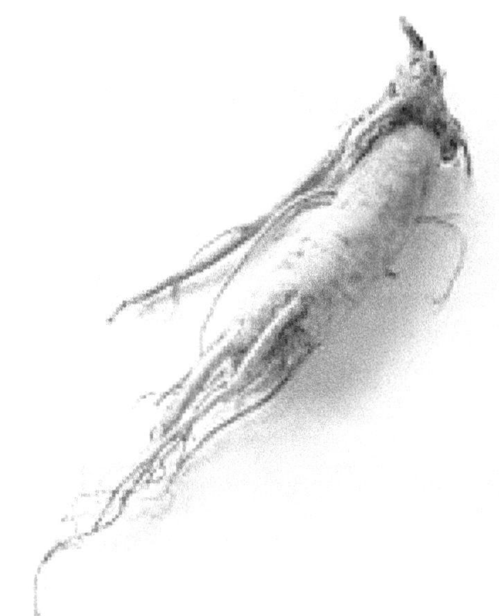

Name of Drug

Ginseng radix, ginseng root.

Composition of Drug

Ginseng root consists of the dried main and lateral root and root hairs of *Panax ginseng* C.A.Meyer [Fam. Araliaceae], as well as their preparations in effective dosage.

The root contains at least 1.5 percent ginsenosides, calculated as ginsenoside Rg1.

Uses
As tonic for invigoration and fortification in times of fatigue and debility, for declining capacity for work and concentration, also during convalescence.

Contraindications
None known.

Side Effects
None known.

Interactions with Other Drugs

None known.

Dosage

Unless otherwise prescribed:

Daily dosage:

- 1 - 2 g of root;
- equivalent preparations.

Mode of Administration

Cut root for teas, powder and galenical preparations for internal use.

Duration of Administration

Generally up to 3 months.

A repeated course is feasible.

Action

In various stress models, e.g., an immobilization test and the coldness test, the resistance of laboratory test animals (rodents) was increased.

HISTORY

World renowned medicinal plant expert, Stephen Fulder PhD. in his excellent book, *"The Ginseng Book, Nature's Ancient Healer"* mentions how ginseng is spoken of in the Vedas, which are ancient books of scripture from India, approximately 5,000 years old. He tells us that the Vedas have many 'health hymns" and they speak about Ginseng in this way.

"The root which is dug from the earth and strengthens the nerves. The strength of the horse, the mule, the goat, the ram, moreover the strength of the bull it bestows on him. This herb will make thee so full of lusty strength that thou shalt, when excited, exhale heat as a thing of fire." [1] Ginseng is spoken of as a brother of Soma, another highly revered life giving plant, both were believed to have magical powers.

In Korea gatherers would purify themselves for a week, remaining clean and chaste before they went to search for the revered plant. The leaves of Ginseng were said to give off a glow in the moonlight. The gatherers would shoot an arrow into the place where they saw the glow and retrieve the arrow next day along with the plant. The va-pang suis, were the shang diggers, the ginseng hunters. Some were employed by the Emperor, and others risked their lives for the honor and wealth it brought to them. This was a very hazardous profession. Bandits called "The White Swans' would wait to attack the prospectors and steal their treasures, or torture them to find out where the ginseng was. The bandits had a strange code of ethics whereby they would give the victim a red flag to carry so that they would not be attacked again. It seemed they felt it only fair not to be stolen from twice in one day.   The va-pang suis, were also in danger from panthers and tigers who hunted the root.   The ginseng hunters would go into the forest armed only with a stick and the belief that no evil could come to them if they were pure of heart. These hunters would pray to the spirit of the panther and tiger and most of all to the spirit of the mountain. The fact that they found the root was testimony to them that they were indeed of pure heart and they would set up an altar, say prayers and give thanks for the root. This purity also protected them from the legendary spirit inside the root, which could appear and disappear at will, leading those who were evil further into the forest to be lost forever.

Ginseng has grown wild for generations in certain parts of the world. It was originally the name of several medicinal plants but is now often associated with the genus Panax. Panax is native to the Asian continent and it is believed to have been originally used as a source of food when it was first discovered over 5,000 years ago in the mountains of Manchuria, China.

Soon it became revered for its health and life giving properties.   *Its human shape became a powerful symbol of divine harmony on earth.*" [2]   In 221 B.C. 3,000 foot soldiers were sent by the emperor Shongtjie to find wild ginseng. Any who returned empty handed were beheaded. Ginseng grew wild for generations in some areas of the world. After the scouring of the mountains and forests, the plant is nearly extinct and wild ginseng is extremely expensive.

"Panax is derived from the Greek word Panakos meaning 'All Healing' also known as "Wonder of the World" and the "Root of Heaven" [3] It was the name given to the herb by the botanist and explorer, Carl Anton Mayer. The word ginseng is derived from 'jen shen' and according to Stephen Fulder PhD, it means a "*Crystallization of the essence of the earth (shen) in the form of a man (jen)"* [4] or more simply 'man root'. The Chinese term of *rénshen* also means the same. This refers to the root's characteristic forked shape, which resemble a body with the legs of a man.   Other names are magical herb, divine root, blood like, five fingers, red berry and root of life. It is referred to as the kingly herb.   Panax ginseng is native to Asia and Panax Quinquefolius is the American ginseng. Quinquefolius refers to the leaves which have five lobes and are said to resemble a hand.

The earliest mention of it comes from a book of the Chien Han Era (33-48 B.C.). *"Later about 500 A.D. a book called the "Sheng Nung Pen Ts'ao Ching" (the book of herbs by Sheng Nung) makes mention of it.* "[5] Li Yenwen, the father of Li Shizhen (author of Bencao Gangmu published in 1596 A.D.) includes this passage in his ginseng treatise.

Used fresh, ginseng displays a cool nature. When it is used after preparation [steamed, red ginseng], its nature is warm. The slight sweet taste strengthens the yang; the somewhat bitter taste strengthens the yin. Nature [xing] controls the genesis of things: their origin is in heaven; tastes control the completion of things; their origin is in the earth. Nature and taste, genesis and completion are realizations of yin and yang. The cool nature of fresh ginseng expresses the yang influence of spring, namely, of genesis and development. This is the yang of heaven. It has the nature of rising. Sweet is a taste that has been formed through transformation of moisture and earth. These are the yang influences of earth. They have the nature of floating. The somewhat bitter taste has been formed through reciprocal interaction of fire and earth. These are the yin influences of earth. They have the nature of descending in the body. [

The first European reference was in 1643 in the writings, "Relations della Grande Monarchia Cina" which was published in Rome. In 1709 the root was again written of in "The Memoir of the Royal Academy in Paris", by a Jesuit named Father Jartoux who had returned to Europe from an assignment in China. In 1711 the memoir was translated into English in "The Philosophical Transactions of the Royal Society of London." Five years later, another Jesuit, Father Joseph Francois Lafitau, who had been sent to a mission in Canada, read Jartous writings. Realizing that Canada was on the same latitude as the area in China where ginseng grew he began to wonder if the plant grew in his own vicinity. After considerable seeking for the plant Father Lafitau came across wild ginseng near Montreal, growing by a house he was building. He had earlier employed a Native American woman to look for the plant without success. He took his findings to her and she verified it as the plant of this species which the Indians used.

With the discovery of ginseng , a thriving ginseng trade had begun, which was second only to Canada's fur trade. John Jacob Astor, was a business man in the fur trade. He sold a boatload of ginseng to China.   Daniel Boone was also reported to have dug for the plant and sold many tons. It was speculated that Davy Crockett did the same.   The China Empress was the first American ship to deliver ginseng to China, in 1784. By 1800, the United States was doing more trade with Canton that with the whole of China in 1925. "Ton upon ton of wild ginseng was dug and exported." [7]

Soon after the discovery of ginseng in Canada, French-Canadian traders and native North Americans collected roots to export to China. In the 1700's Chinese merchants refused to do business after receiving poorly harvested shipment of dried roots. This put an end for a while to the thriving export of ginseng. Trade switched to the British colonies. American ginseng was also discovered in central New York and Vermont and Massachusetts and in western New England in the mid 1700's.   In Amsterdam and London, middlemen waited to make large profits as they dealt in the ginseng which arrived by boat.   As the trade of ginseng expanded, with huge monetary rewards, the destruction of the forests led to over harvesting and scarcity of the plant, with a resulting price increase. This is when cultivation in shaded areas began. *Now the plant is threatened and is controlled by the International CITES Treaty".* [8] The plant is only harvested wild in a few states, and then it is at a certain season which is mandated, requiring a license. The ginseng berries are immediately planted to re-grow more ginseng.

NATIVE AMERICAN USE

North Americans Indians used ginseng in many of their herbal formulas. They considered it to be one of their most sacred herbs. They were using American ginseng for medicinal purposes well before its commercial development in the 18th century. It was used as a headache cure, to cure croup, soothe eyes, and as a poultice for wounds as well as many other medicinal uses. On being showing a drawing of the ginseng plant by the Jesuit priest, Lafitau, the native Indians took him to a similar plant which they called "Garantequen"

The Creek Indians called ginseng "White medicine" they used it for fevers, boiling it with ginger and then mixing it with alcohol before administering it to the patient. This would cause the patient to sweat. They also used it in many other preparations, including stoppage of bleeding from wounds.   It was also used in magic to ward off evil. It was believed that evil spirits caused illness. When a Creek Indian passed through a graveyard he would chew ginseng and spit it out in four directions to protect himself from evil. Ginseng was also used to keep a person alive when they had been shot. Ginseng was especially used by the Cherokees for headaches. Ginseng and wild tobacco was considered to save someone's life if they had apoplexy.

The Cherokees believed that the number four was a number of special magical significance and so they would pass by the first three plants before digging up the fourth.   Before they did this they would build an altar and give thanks and they would leave an offering in return, similar to the ritual which the va-pang suis would perform in the Orient.

In the Chippewa culture It was believed that ginseng had the power to revive the dying, along with a ceremony where the person's soul was asked to stay. A traditional song would be sung to those who were deathly ill. It was called "the White Swan". They would then blow through a reed into a decoction of ginseng. The dying person would drink this decoction.

Ginseng was highly favored by the Mide medicine men being used on occasion to 'bring people back to life'. It was also considered excellent for stomach ailments. The Pawnee Indians used it with other herbs as a love potion. *"The Seminole Indians also used it as a Love Medicine, rubbing it on their body and clothes to bring back a divorced wife"*.

The Sioux benefited from its trade rather than its medicinal uses. They never used the herb itself much but they gathered and prepared it, and Sioux ginseng fetched unusually large prices.

MODERN SCIENCE

Modern science with randomized and double blind tests finds it difficult to prove hard scientific evidence for the important uses of ginseng. It is prized as an adaptogen but this property is also extremely difficult to prove scientifically. Comparative, randomized, double blind government studies simply indicate it to be 'a promising dietary supplement'.

I cannot help but think that we are so eager to prove scientific facts and to make new drugs and more money that the standard which the medical profession is supposed to live by "First do no harm." is becoming lost in a craving for new and better drugs. We lose sight of God's pharmacy and the effective yet safer means of healing, which, when coupled with a healthy lifestyle can have a powerful healing effect upon us. The Hippocratic Oath states: *"I will follow that system of regimen which, according to my ability and judgment, I consider for the benefit of my patients, and abstain from whatever is deleterious and mischievous.   I will give no deadly medicine to anyone... Into whatever house I enter, I will go into them for the benefit of the sick, and will abstain from every voluntary act of mischief and corruption..."* [10] Yet what have these new drugs truly accomplished? The reward often comes in the form of fame, money and prestige for large corporations. There can be respite from illness, drugs are without a doubt very powerful, but the respite is often temporary and none of them are without the price of side effects, which are often serious, and at times life threatening.

The week of April 17th 2006, C.N.N. reported details of a healthy man who took part in a pharmaceutical study to test a drug for leukemia. As a result of these tests, he is now critically ill waiting to see which parts of his fingers and toes he will lose. He suffered multiple organ failure and he was unconscious for three weeks. Tests on animals were supposed to have shown very few side effects, the company later admitted this was untrue. If only this was an isolated incident with otherwise great success in the medical profession. But this is only one of thousands of iatrogenic diseases, illness and heartache brought about by the misuse of the medical profession and their often blatant disregard for the Hippocratic oath.   I saw a large highway advertisement this week which read, "All Doctors Are Healers. Not All Healers Are Doctors."

The Journal of the American Medical Association July 26th 2000, itself carries the real truth of these statements. It states that medical mistakes, infections, and pharmaceutical drugs are the third leading cause of death. In one year, two hundred and eighty four thousand died under the supervision of the medical profession - from iatrogenic diseases - doctor induced diseases, not the illness they came in from. One hundred and six thousand of that number died taking the properly prescribed therapeutic dose of pharmacy medication. That did not include interactions, overdoses, or mis-prescribed drugs. We lost approximately 4,000 people at the World Trade Center, on September 11th 2001, but we lose over a 1,000 a day by following today's medical system. Despite the lack of modern medicine's approval ginseng continues to be widely used and valued.

CHEMICAL CONSTITUENTS

The main active ingredients in the Panax species are a group of dammarane-type triterpenoid glycosides. They are referred to as saponins. And termed ginsenosides. In Russia they are termed Panaxosides. These are in the ginseng root. There are more than thirty ginsenosides. One of them is an oleanolic acid derivative.

It is the type and composition of the ginsenosides which give their different qualities. There are eight main ginsenosides and the composition in American and Asian is quite different. There are many more ginsenosides in American ginseng than there are in Asian ginseng. *The most abundant ginsenoside in both species is ginsenoside Rb1. This ginsenoside is reported to have a sedative effect. Ginsenoside Rg1 is said to have a stimulant effect. The levels of Rg1 in Asian ginseng are much higher than in American ginseng. Asian ginseng also contains ginsenosides Rf and Rg2, whereas American ginseng is virtually devoid of these ginsenosides. Pseudoginsenoside F11 is noted in American ginseng, but it is almost absent from Asian ginseng.*

"The root of ginseng contains a resin, sugar, starch, mucilage, a saponin, a volatile oil and several steroid compounds."

Ginsenosides , as noted in the medicinal properties, are powerful adaptogens. Also containing strong antioxidant components they help the body to recover from stress, fatigue and illness.   Saponins are anti inflammatory, analgesic, anticonvulsant and they also help to regulate cholesterol and blood sugar levels.

Panaxtriol is one of several steroid compounds found in ginseng. These compounds are remarkably similar to anabolic steroids which are found in the human body. This suggests a safe alternative for athletes to use, instead of synthetic steroids.

Another component found in ginseng root is germanium. Germanium has a powerful hydrogenating effect on the body and especially on organs such as the liver. It is said that a trained herbalist should be able to tell the quality of ginseng by the smell and appearance and taste. It is difficult to judge if it has been made into a capsule. Freeze drying is said to preserve the ginsenosides better than any other method followed second by air drying.

MEDICINAL QUALITIES

GINSENG LATEST MEDICINAL PROPERTIES

As we have seen, through generations of time, ginseng has been considered a remarkable herb, endowed with magical powers and held as sacred by certain cultures.
Credited mainly with tonic properties of longevity, endurance strength memory improvement and aphrodisiac qualities,

Below are some of the other benefits ascribed to ginseng.

Longevity

Memory improvement
Stress reduction
Normalization of blood pressure.
Immune system enhancement
Normalization of blood sugar.
Libido enhancement.
Lowering of cholesterol

Other recognized uses are for gastric disturbances, lack of appetite, lowering of blood sugar and cholesterol levels, increasing resistance to disease, stimulating and increasing endocrine activity, supporting liver function, shock, chronic illness, nausea and vomiting, impotence and sterility, rheumatism and mental health, diabetes, as well as helping with the effects of alcohol or drugs. Christopher Hobbs notes its promise in helping with those who suffer from chronic fatigue syndrome. *"Through a number of psychometric tests designed to evaluate psychological and physical status, it was determined that the patients were improved in many of the areas studied, especially levels of attention and concentration. The change was statistically significant."*

He also mentions ginsengs ability to relieve hangover symptoms because of increased alcohol clearance from the body.

Known as a universal remedy Ginseng herb has wide usage, especially in the Orient. Alternative medicine is widely used by many people looking for an effective and safe way not only to heal from illness, but also to prevent illness. When a plant resembles a part of the human anatomy, it is said to be beneficial for that particular part of the body. As ginseng resembles a man it is believed to be beneficial for the whole system. As man is made up of many elements so ginseng is believed to synergistically restore health and harmony to the body. This harmony is expressed as Yin and Yang in the Chinese culture and is held to be essential to a healthy body and a peaceful spirit.

The philosophies of Yin and Yang, say that Yin, which is feminine, cool, and soothing, and Yang, which is masculine, hot, and aggressive, must be balanced within a healthy human body. The energy flow of Chi is said to balance these two elements. Chinese medicine uses a preventative approach to keep the body balanced and healthy while the Western approach is to control and cure diseases. Asian ginseng is believed to be Yang-rich and is used to replenish Chi in the body. It is taken to prevent conditions such as poor blood circulation, slow metabolism, poor digestion and lack of vitality. American ginseng is considered to have more Yin than Asian ginseng. It is prescribed for quite different conditions such as high blood pressure and the hot feelings associated with menopause. Ginseng is often taken regularly to help the body cope with stress, increase physical stamina, reduce fatigue and improve mental capacity. It is also used for alcohol detoxification, and has been shown to reduce the effects of anemia by stimulating erythropoiesis (the formation or production of red blood cells). Other applications include radio-protection, protection against cancer and boosting the immune system. Taking ginseng is thought to reduce the effects of diabetes and hypertension (arteriosclerosis), protect liver function, enhance sexual function and slow the process of ageing.

Soviet researchers pioneered the study of ginseng, which is considered to be the primary resistogen, and some other plants of the "ginseng group". A sizable volume of literature was published as a result of their studies. Soviet scholars were the first to establish the fact that many araliaceous plants are resistogens (adaptogens).

Lazarev, a Russian pharmacologist, in 1947. defined "adaptogens" as agents which help to counteract adverse effects of a physical, chemical or biological stressor by generating nonspecific resistance.
Vaxa Homeopathic medicinals state, " *Adaptogens are specific plant extracts that control excess Cortisol levels during times of stress. Cortisol in excess amounts is highly toxic, attacks muscle mass and organs, lengthens recovery time, and diminishes strength as well as the immune system.   To be considered an adaptogen, plant extracts had to meet three key criteria. First, they had to be totally non-toxic to human cells. Second, they had to support cells at a healthy state. And lastly, they had to help the body adapt to stress*.
Besides being an adaptogen ginseng is also a cardiotonic, sedative, sialogogue, tonic, stomachic, and panacea.

CANCER STUDY.

Beth Israel Deaconess Medical Center and Harvard Medical School, Boston, Mass were involved in a study which showed that American ginseng had a synergistic effect on the suppression of cell growth in a cancer study.

CANCER CELL PROLIFERATION

At the University of Southern Illinois University School of Medicine in Carbondale, mice are injected subcutaneously (beneath the skin) with human breast cancer cells. When fed American Ginseng extract, they produced smaller tumors which spread more slowly than in the control mice. Dr. Laura Murphy who is working on these tests also found that ginsenoside Rc had a strong anti-proliferation effect on human breast cancer cells growing in petri dishes. Another study by Dr. Murphy showed that prostate cancer in mice is inhibited when they are fed an extract of American ginseng. It appeared that prostate cells were more sensitive to the use of ginseng than breast cancer cells.

STUDIES FOR ALZHEIMER'S DISEASE

Dr. Lawrence Wang, Ph.D. FRSC Professor & Presidential Advisor, International Affairs, University of Alberta studied ginseng usage for the treatment of Alzheimer's disease. The success of these studies have led to patented products.

REDUCTION OF BLOOD SUGAR

A study from St. Michael's hospital and the University of Toronto showed that ginseng reduced blood sugar levels.

DOSAGE

Ginseng comes in root and powder form, in tincture and in tablets, or encapsulated.

Most research studies suggest a standardized extract of Panax ginseng in a dosage of 200mg per day. The dry root can be chewed and a dosage of 0.5 to 2 g is suggested on a short term basis. Ginseng can also be taken in tea form, at this amount, but it is said to be very low in ginsenosides. Capsules are usually given in divided doses at 100 to 600 mg per day. If taking casules make sure they are standardized to ginsenoside content. You want at least five percent. Ginseng is usually taken for long periods. Some sources suggest a two week rest from ginseng every two to three weeks. This may depend on the health and temperament of the person taking it, as Chinese medicine looks at each individual.

If taking a tincture, take half a teaspoon in a little warm water three times a day for at least a month or two then stop for a week or two and try again if wished. [20]

As a general rule, acute ailments are treated for 1-30 days, although something such as influenza if it is caught early enough may only require a one or two day approach. For those illnesses which have persisted for a long time (chronic diseases) the treatment needs to be combined with healthy strategies, such as changes in diet, exercise and lowering stress. Most chronic ailments, such as an autoimmune or degenerative disease, can be brought under control when a high dosage is followed with a treatment of approximately three months. If the client cannot tolerate the herb and a lower dose needs to be used then this increases the time of recovery. Sometimes, herbs need to be taken for an indefinite period, especially if there is irreversible damage which cannot be entirely reversed, or where ailments have been left a very long time without being effectively treated. Some remedies from China are labeled with only the herbal ingredients and yet they have western drugs within them. The ingredients may be in Chinese and so it is important to be aware of this if dealing with imported products.

GOLDEN SEAL

LATIN NAME Hydrastis canadensis

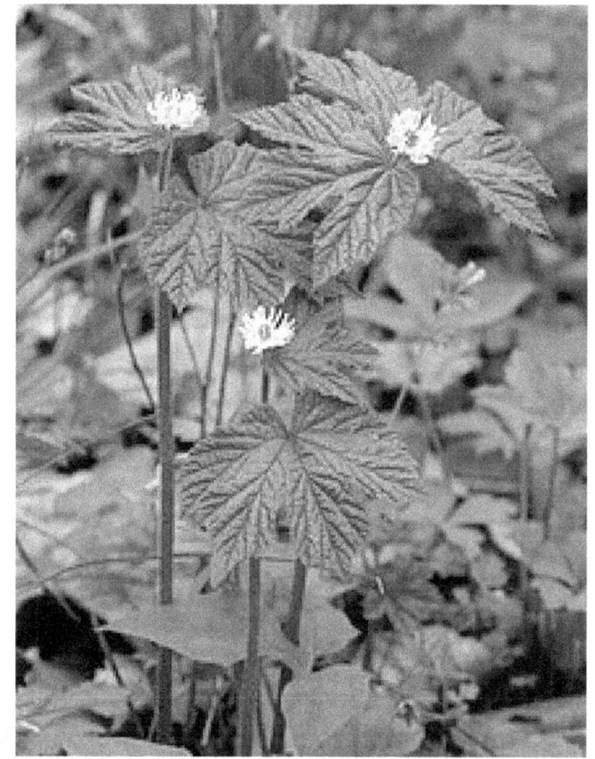

Kingdom:	Plantae
Clade:	Tracheophytes
Clade:	Angiosperms
Clade:	Eudicots
Order:	Ranunculales
Family:	Ranunculaceae
Subfamily:	Hydrastidoideae
Genus:	*Hydrastis* L.
Species:	***H. canadensis***

Goldenseal (***Hydrastis canadensis***), also called **orangeroot** or **yellow puccoon**, is a perennial herb in the buttercup family Ranunculaceae, native to southeastern Canada and the eastern United States. It may be distinguished by its thick, yellow knotted rootstock. The stem is purplish and hairy above ground and yellow below ground where it connects to the yellow rhizome. Goldenseal reproduces both clonally through the rhizome and sexually, with clonal division more frequent than asexual reproduction. It takes between 4 and 5 years for a plant to reach sexual maturity, i.e. the point at which it produces flowers. Plants in the first stage, when the seed erupts and cotyledons emerge, can remain in this state one or more years. The second vegetative stage occurs during years two and three (and sometimes longer) and is characterized by the development of a single leaf and absence of a well developed stem. Finally, the third stage is reproductive, at which point flowering and fruiting occurs. This last stage takes between 4 and 5 years to develop.

A second species from Japan, previously listed as *Hydrastis palmatum*, is now usually classified in another genus, as *Glaucidium palmatum*.

Traditional use

At the time of the European colonization of the Americas, goldenseal was in extensive use among certain Native American tribes of North America, both as a medicine and as a coloring material. Benjamin Smith Barton, in his first edition of *Collections for an Essay Toward a Materia Medica of the United States* (1798), refers to the Cherokee use of goldenseal as a cancer treatment. Later, he calls attention to its properties as a bitter tonic, and as a local wash for ophthalmia. It became a favorite of the Eclectics from the time of Constantine Raffinesque in the 1830s. Tribes also used goldenseal for digestive issues, as an eyewash, as a diuretic and as a bitter.

In the early 20th century, it was used as a yellow dye, astringent, and insect repellent.

Constituents and modern pharmacology

Goldenseal contains the isoquinoline alkaloids hydrastine, berberine, berberastine, hydrastinine, tetrahydroberberastine, canadine and canalidine. A related compound, 8-oxotetrahydrothalifendine, was identified in one study. The *United States Pharmacopoeia* requires goldenseal sold as a supplement to have hydrastine concentrations of at least 2% and berberine concentrations of at least 2.5%. The requirements in Europe are that hydrastine concentrations be at least 2.5% and that berberine concentrations at least 3%. The hydrastine concentrations of goldenseal plants range between 1.5% and 5%, while the berberine concentrations are usually between 0.5% and 4.5%. Goldenseal is harvested for its rhizomes because the concentrations of hydrastine and berberine in the shoots do not meet these requirements. Berberine and hydrastine act as quaternary bases and are poorly soluble in water but freely soluble in alcohol. The herb seems to have synergistic antibacterial activity over berberine *in vitro*, possibly as a result of efflux pump inhibitory activity.

Endangered status

Goldenseal became popular in the mid-nineteenth century. By 1905, the herb was much less plentiful because of overharvesting and habitat destruction. Wild goldenseal is listed in Appendix II of the Convention on International Trade in Endangered Species of Wild Fauna and Flora (CITES), which by definition means harvest from public land is prohibited and may require a permit to export, although trade of the plants is not deemed to be detrimental to the wildlife population and is otherwise unregulated. The U.S. Fish and Wildlife Service recommends that diggers and harvesters track sales and harvests and prove legality of all harvests.

Canada, as well as 17 of the 27 U.S. states where goldenseal grows natively, have declared it as threatened, vulnerable or uncommon. More than 60 million goldenseal plants are picked each year without being replaced. Although goldenseal's geographical range is wide, it is found in small quantities in these habitats.The core of the herb's range is in the Ohio River Valley, but its population there has decreased by almost half. The process of mountain top removal mining has recently put the wild goldenseal population at major risk from loss of habitat.

Many herbalists urge caution in choosing products containing goldenseal, as they may have been harvested in an unsustainable manner rather than having been organically cultivated.[*citation needed*]

There are several berberine-containing plants that can serve as useful alternatives, including Chinese coptis, yellowroot or Oregon grape root.

5 Health Benefits of Goldenseal

Goldenseal is an impressive herbal remedy with many health benefits:

1. Improves Digestive Issues

Goldenseal is an excellent digestive aid since it is very bitter, which stimulates the appetite, aids digestion and encourages bile secretion. It contains berberine, which has been used in Traditional Chinese Medicine (TCM) and **Ayurvedic medicine** for thousands of years to treat dysentery and infectious diarrhea. This is not surprising since berberine has shown antimicrobial activity against certain pathogens that cause bacterial diarrhea, including *E. coli* and *V. cholera* as shown by a randomized controlled clinical trial back in 1987 involving 165 adults with acute diarrhea due to those two bacterial offenders.

Goldenseal can also be helpful to people experiencing small intestine bacterial overgrowth **(SIBO) symptoms**. Current conventional treatment of SIBO is limited to oral antibiotics with inconsistent success. The objective of a study published by *Global Advances in Health and Medicine* was to determine the remission rate of SIBO using an antibiotic versus an herbal remedy. Researchers found that the herbal treatment, which included berberine, worked just as well as antibiotic treatment and was equally safe.

Some people also use it for stomach swelling (gastritis), peptic ulcers, **ulcerative colitis**, diarrhea, **constipation**, hemorrhoids and intestinal gas. Another impressive study found that among several herbs tested in vitro, goldenseal extract was the most active in inhibiting the growth of *H. pylori*, a type of bacteria which can lead to gastritis, ulcers and even stomach cancer.

As you can see, goldenseal may be able to help a wide range of problems when it comes to the gastrointestinal system.

2. Natural Antibiotic & Immune System Booster

Goldenseal is often found in herbal remedies for allergies, colds, and the flu because of its natural antibiotic and immune-boosting capabilities. Scientific research suggests that medicinal plants like goldenseal and **echinacea** may enhance immune function by increasing antigen-specific antibody production. A product containing goldenseal and echinacea is an awesome **natural bronchitis remedy.**

Additionally, research at the University of Texas-Houston Medical School has shown goldenseal's medicinal effectiveness as an immune stimulant may be due to its ability to reduce the pro-inflammatory response, which indirectly leads to the limiting of clinical symptoms during infection.

There haven't been any clinical (human) studies to date, but goldenseal is also sometimes recommended to treat **urinary tract infections (UTIs),** which are caused by bacterial overgrowth in the bladder's interior walls. The berberine may actually prevent infection-causing bacteria from binding to urinary tract walls.

3. Fights Cancer

According to Memorial Sloan Kettering Cancer Center, the berberine in goldenseal has been found to induce cell cycle arrest and apoptosis (programmed cell death) in cancer cells in multiple studies. For example, one in vitro study published in the journal *Phytomedicine* found that berberine inhibited the growth of breast cancer cells to a greater extent than doxorubicin (a chemotherapy drug).

Berberine alkaloids have also been shown during in vivo studies to have potent cancer cell killing activity against tumor cells. In vivo research has also been performed on a series of human malignant brain tumor cells and rat brain tumor cells in which berberine was used alone at a dose of 150 mcg/ml and had an average cancer cell kill rate of 91 percent. In contrast, the chemotherapy drug carmustine had a cell kill rate of only 43 percent. The rats treated with berberine at 10 mg/kg had an 81 percent kill rate.

Research will continue, but so far goldenseal showing some noteworthy anticancer abilities.

4. Aids Eye & Mouth Problems

Goldenseal is also commonly used as a mouthwash for sore throats, gum complaints, and canker sores (small ulcers in the mouth). For any of these concerns, a goldenseal mouth rinse can help by reducing inflammation and getting rid of any nasty bacteria.

You can purchase a mouthwash that already contains goldenseal or you can easily make some mouthwash at home. Simply make a cup of goldenseal tea and let it cool down before using it to rinse your mouth. Or you can add five drops of liquid goldenseal extract to eight ounces of warm water with a teaspoon of salt and mix well.

Goldenseal has been utilized as an eyewash for eye inflammation and eye infections like **conjunctivitis** or "pink eye." Since the use of it in the eyes is somewhat controversial, consult a health care practitioner before using it in this way.

5. Boosts Heart Health

The cardiovascular effects of the berberine found in goldenseal suggest its possible clinical usefulness in the treatment of arrhythmias and/or heart failure. For this reason, goldenseal is believed to possibly be helpful for chronic congestive heart failure (CHF) and heart function in general.

An animal model study published in the *Journal of Lipid Research* also demonstrates that the root extract is highly effective in regulation of the liver's LDL ("bad" cholesterol) receptors and in reducing plasma cholesterol. Overall, the findings identified goldenseal as a natural LDL-lowering agent.

In combination with a healthy diet and lifestyle, goldenseal may help to **lower cholesterol naturally** and boost heart health.

Recommended Use of Goldenseal

Goldenseal can easily be found in tea or supplement form at your local health store or online. Depending on which product you purchase, make sure to read the label for each brand's recommended dosage.

For the powdered root and rhizome, four to six grams per day in tablet or capsule form is sometimes recommended. For liquid herbal extracts, a typical recommended dosage is two milliliters (40 drops) in two ounces of water or juice three to five times per day.

HAWTHORNE BERRY

Hawthorn Leaf and berry

LATIN NAME Crataegus monogyna

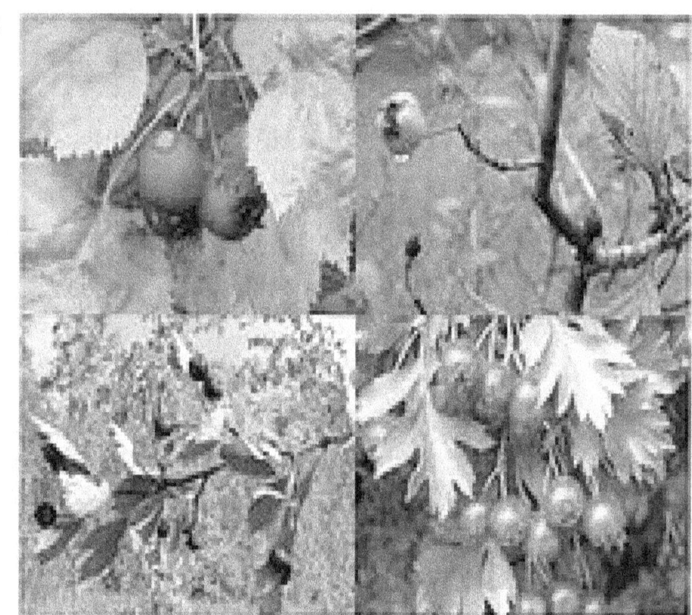

Kingdom: Plantae
Clade: Tracheophytes
Clade: Angiosperms
Clade: Eudicots
Clade: Rosids
Order: Rosales
Family: Rosaceae
Subfamily: Amygdaloideae
Tribe: Maleae
Subtribe: Malinae
Genus: *Crataegus* Tourn. *ex* L.

Crataegi folium cum flore
Weidornbltter mit Blten

Name of Drug

Crataegi folium cum flore, hawthorn leaf with flowers.

Composition of Drug

Hawthorn leaf with flower, consisting of dried flowering twig tips of *Crataegus monogyna* Jaquin emend. Lindman or *C.aevigata* (Poiret) de Candolle [Fam. Rosaceae], or other members of the *Crataegus* genus cited in a valid pharmacopeia as well as preparations from them in an effective dosage.

The drug contains flavonoids (flavones, flavonols) including hyperoside, vitexinrhamnose, rutin, and vitexin and oligomeric procyanidins (n=2 to n=8 catechins and/or epicatechins).

Pharmacological Properties, Pharmacokinetics, Toxicology

The following pharmacodynamic effects have been established in isolated organs or in animal experimentation with preparations from hawthorn leaf with flower (hydroalcoholic extract with defined content of oligomeric procyanidins and/or flavonoids: macerates, fresh plant extract) and with individual fractions (oligomeric procyanidins, biogenic amines): Positive inotropic effect, positive dromotropic effect, negative bathmotropic effect, increased coronary and myocardial circulatory perfusion, reduction in peripheral vascular resistance.

In cases of cardiac insufficiency according to Stage II New York Heart Association (NYHA), an improvement of subjective findings as well as an increase in cardiac work tolerance, a decrease in pressure/heart rate product, an increase in the ejection fraction and a rise in the anaerobic threshold have been established in human pharmacological studies following the administration of 160 to 900 mg aqueous-alcoholic extract per day (adjusted to oligomeric procyanidins and/or flavonoids) over periods lasting up to 56 days.

The pharmacokinetics of the drug have been investigated only in animal studies, and no scientific results are available in the context of human pharmacokinetics.

Investigations of acute toxicity using a hydroalcoholic dry extract (drug/extract ratio 5:1, standardized for oligomeric procyanidins) are available, according to which no fatal events occurred after oral or peritoneal administration in mice or rats in doses of up to 3 g per kg of body weight.

Symptoms of intoxication with an intraperitoneal administration of 3 g/kg body weight include sedation, piloerection, dyspnea, and tremor.

The oral administration of powdered herb at individual doses of 3 g per kg body weight in rats and 5 g per kg body weight in mice produce no fatal reactions.

No toxic effects were observed after oral administration of 30, 90, and 300 mg aqueous/ethanolic dry extract per kg body weight in rats and dogs over a period of 26 weeks. For this extract, the "no effect" dose was 300 mg per kg body weight in rats and dogs for 26 weeks. No fatal events and no toxic effects were observed after the oral administration of 300 and 600 mg drug powder per kg body weight over a period of four weeks.

No experimental data are available concerning embryonic and fetal toxicity, fertility, and post-natal development.

Although they have indeed produced different results, more recent studies are now available as regards testing the mutagenicity of *Crataegus* preparations. It is assumed that the mutagenic activity demonstrated on Salmonella is based on the quercetin content, and the induction of SCE particularly on the presence of flavone-C-glycosides as well as of flavone aglycones. By comparison with the quantity of quercetin ingested with the food, however, the content of quercetin in the drug is so low that a risk for humans may be practically excluded.

No experimental data are available regarding carcinogenicity. The findings regarding gene toxicity and mutagenicity give no indication of carcinogenic risk of the drug in human use.

Clinical Data

Uses
Decreasing cardiac output as described in functional Stage II of NYHA.*

Contraindications
None known.

Side Effects
None known.

Special Caution for Use

A physician must be consulted in cases where symptoms continue unchanged for longer than six weeks or in case of swelling of the legs. Medical diagnosis is absolutely necessary when pains occur in the region of the heart, spreading out to the arms, upper abdomen or the area around the neck, or in cases of respiratory distress (dyspnea).

Use During Pregnancy and Lactation

None known.

Interactions with Other Drugs

None known.

Dosage and Administration

Unless otherwise prescribed:

- 160 - 900 mg native, water-ethanol extract (ethanol 45 percent v/v or methanol 70 percent v/v, drug-extract ratio = 4 - 7:1, with defined flavonoid or procyanidin content), corresponding to 30 - 168.7 mg procyanidins, calculated as epicatechin, or 3.5 - 19.8 mg flavonoids, calculated as hyperoside in accordance with *DAB* 10, in two or three individual doses.

Hawthorn fluidextract *DAB* 10:

- Equivalent individual or daily dosage must be confirmed by clinical-pharmacological experiment or clinical study.

Mode of Administration

Liquid or dry pharmaceutical forms, for oral intake.

Duration of Administration

6 weeks minimum.

Overdosage

Not known.

Special Warnings

None.

Effects on Operators of Vehicles and Machinery

None.

Note: The drug as well as aqueous, aqueous-ethanolic, and wine-based extracts and fresh juice from the plant are traditionally taken orally as a tonic and strengthener of the cardiac/circulatory functions. This information is based exclusively on tradition and long-term experience.

*[**Ed.note:** Stages I and II of NYHA refer to stages of heart disease in the New York Heart Association's 1994 *Revisions to Classification of Functional Capacity and Objective Assessment of Patients with Diseases of the Heart:* "Patients with cardiac disease but without resulting limitations of physical activity. They are comfortable at rest. Ordinary physical activity results in fatigue, palpitation, dyspnea, or anginal pain." Monopreparations of hawthorn flower, fruit, and leaf are discussed in the Unapproved Herbs section.

JUNIPER BERRY

LATIN NAME Juniperus *communis*

Kingdom: Plantae
Clade: Tracheophytes
Division: Pinophyta
Class: Pinopsida
Order: Pinales
Family: Cupressaceae
Genus: *Juniperus*
Section: *Juniperus* sect. *Juniperus*
Subsection: *Juniperus* subsect. *Juniperus*
Species: ***J. communis***

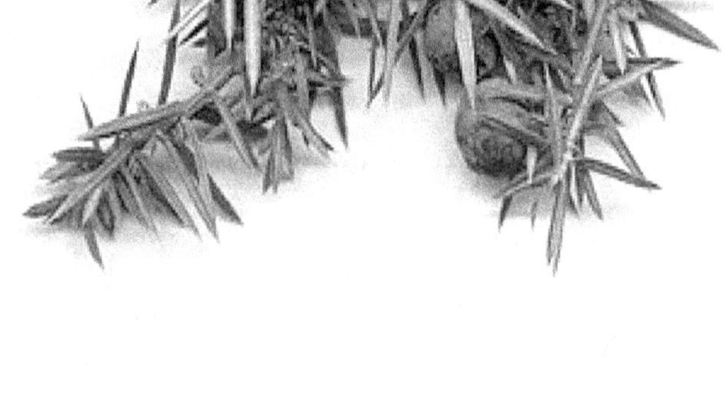

Juniperi fructus
Wacholderbeeren

Name of Drug

Juniperi fructus, juniper berry.

Composition of Drug

Juniper berry is the ripe, fresh or dried spherical ovulate cone ("berry") of *Juniper communis* L.[Fam.Cupressaceae], as well as its preparations in effective dosage. Juniper berry contains at least 1 percent (v/w) volatile oil in reference to the dried drug.

Main ingredients of the volatile oil are terpene hydrocarbons such as a-pinene, -pinene, myrcene, sabinene, thujone, and limonene. Also contained are sesquiterpene hydrocarbons such as caryophyllene, cadinene, and elemene and terpene alcohols such as 4-terpineol.

Furthermore, juniper berries contain flavonoid glycosides, tannins, sugar and resin- and wax-containing compounds.

Uses
Dyspepsia.

Contraindications
Pregnancy and inflammation of the kidneys.

Side Effects

Prolonged usage or overdosing may cause kidney damage.

Interactions with Other Drugs

None known.

Dosage

Unless otherwise prescribed:

Daily dose:

- 2 to a maximum of 10 g of the dried juniper fruit, corresponding to 20 - 100 mg of the essential oil.

Mode of Administration

Whole, crushed, or powdered drug for infusions and decoctions, alcohol extracts, and in wine. Essential oil. Liquid and solid medicinal forms only for oral application.

Warning: Combinations with other plant drugs in teas and similar preparations for treating bladder and kidney diseases may be helpful.

Action

Animal experiments have shown an increase in urine excretion as well as a direct effect on smooth muscle contraction.

KAVA KAVA

LATIN NAME Piper methysticum

Kingdom: Plantae
Clade: Tracheophytes
Clade: Angiosperms
Clade: Magnoliids
Order: Piperales
Family: Piperaceae
Genus: *Piper*
Species: ***P. methysticum***

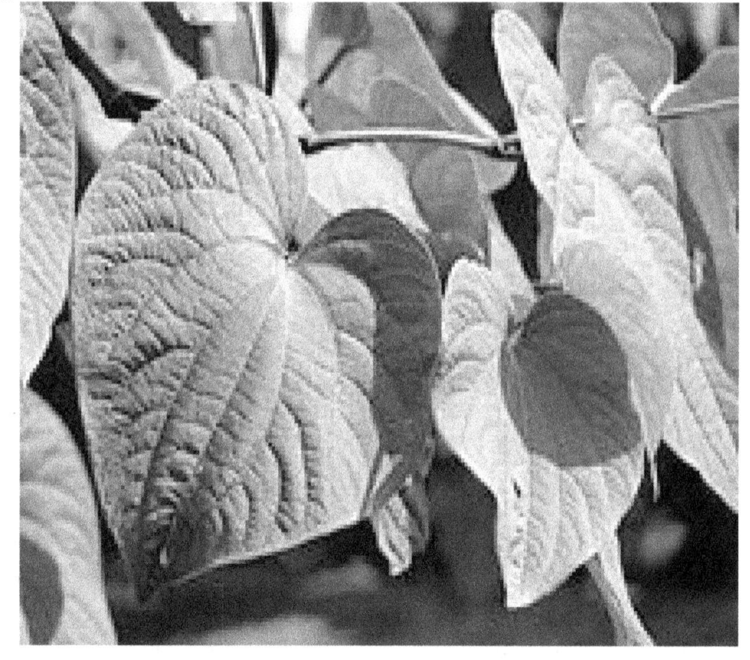

Piperis methystici rhizoma
Kava-kava-Wurzelstock

Name of Drug

Piperis methystici rhizoma, kava
kava rhizome (root).

Composition of Drug

Kava kava rhizome consists of the dried rhizomes of *Piper methysticum* G. Forster
[Fam. Piperaceae], as well as their preparations in effective dosage.

The drug contains kava-pyrones (kawain).

Uses
Conditions of nervous anxiety, stress, and restlessness.

Contraindications
Pregnancy, nursing, endogenous depression.

Side Effects
None known.

Note: Extended continuous intake can cause a temporary yellow discoloration of skin,
hair and nails. In this case, further application of this drug must be discontinued. In rare
cases, allergic skin reactions can occur. Also, accommodative disturbances, such as
enlargement of the pupils and disturbances of the oculomotor equilibrium, have been
described.

Interactions with Other Drugs

Potentiation of effectiveness is possible for substances acting on the central nervous system, such as alcohol, barbiturates and psychopharmacological agents.

Dosage

Unless otherwise prescribed:

Daily dosage:

- Herb and preparations equivalent to 60 - 120 mg kava pyrones.

Mode of Administration

Comminuted rhizome and other galenical preparations for oral use.

Duration of Administration

Not more than 3 months without medical advice.

Note: Even when administered within its prescribed dosages, this herb may adversely affect motor reflexes and judgment for driving and/or operating heavy machinery.

Actions

Anti-anxiety

In animal experiments a potentiation of narcosis (sedation), anticonvulsive, antispasmodic, and central muscular relaxant effects were described.

HISTORY

It is thought that the frequent consumption of Kava Kava is partially why the people of the South Pacific Islands are known as the happiest and friendliest people in the world. Traditionally on the islands it is used before important religious rites and other ceremonies. Kava Kava was always served at full formal ceremonies, meetings of village elders and chiefs, and at the less formal kava circle common at social occasions. The full Kava Kava ceremony was reserved for very honored guests. The guests are led to a platform. A group of young men arrive dressed in ceremonial attire, carrying a bowl of prepared Kava Kava and any necessary utensils. The bowl is placed between the guests and the preparers. The Kava Kava is placed in a cup by a specially selected individual, the cup bearer, who then turns and faces the visitor and delivers the beverage to the chief guest. The guest is instructed to hold the cup with both hands and drink from it. If the whole cup is drained without stopping, everyone says "a maca" (which means *it is empty*) and claps three times with cupped hands. The cup bearer then refills the cup and proceeds to serve the next person in rank or importance. These ceremonies still take place today. In 1992 Hillary Clinton participated in a Kava Kava ceremony conducted by the Samoan community on Oahu, Hawaii. Pope John Paul II also participated in a Kava Kava ceremony when he visited the Pacific.

A description of the classic process of Kava Kava preparation was given in 1777 by George Forster, a young naturalist on Captain James Cook's second Pacific voyage:

[Kava] is made in the most disgustful manner that can be imagined, from the juice contained in the roots of a species of pepper-tree. This root is cut small, and the pieces chewed by several people, who spit the macerated mass into a bowl, where some water (milk) of coconuts is poured upon it. They then strain it through a quantity of fibers of coconuts, squeezing the chips, till all their juices mix with the coconut-milk; and the whole liquor is decanted into another bowl. They swallow this nauseous stuff as fast as possible; and some old topers value themselves on being able to empty a great number of bowls.

Upon discovery of Kava Kava, James Cook gave it the name "intoxicating pepper."

Some cultures preferred the Kava Kava mixture to be prepared by young children or young women. According to Lebot, Merlin and Lindstrom, who have done a lot of research on Kava, a preferred traditional way of preparing the beverage is the ceremony as conducted in Samoa: 'which required the girl who chewed and infused the kava to sit cross-legged and bare-breasted on a mat behind the kava bowl, with flowers carefully arranged in her hair and her hips swathed in a grass skirt. This presented an image of beauty that added to the aesthetic dimension of kava preparation.' (Rudgley)

The Samoan's say that Kava Kava originated when a Samoan girl went to Fiji, where she married a great chief. After some time, she returned to Samoa, but before she left Fiji she noticed two plants growing side by side on a hill. A rat was chewing on one of the plants, and had fallen asleep. She decided that the plant must be a comforting food, and took it back to Samoa with her. This plant was Sugar cane. Then she noticed that the rat awoke, and began to chew the root of another plant-Kava Kava. The rat became bold, strong and more energetic. She decided to take this plant back to Samoa as well. The plants grew very well in Samoa, and soon a chief from a neighboring island exchanged two laying hens for the roots of the two plants. This is how Samoa explains the spread of sugar cane and Kava Kava.

In Tonga, there is a more grisly explanation for the origin of Kava Kava. The legend is told of a great chief named Loau, who lived on the island of Eua Iki and was visited by his servant, Feva Anga. Feva wanted to serve a great feast for the chief, but it was a time of great famine. In desperation, he and his wife killed and cooked their only daughter. The chief recognized the human flesh in the food when it was served, and would not eat it. He told Feva to bury his daughter and to bring him the plant that would spring forth. On receiving the mature plant, Loau instructed that a drink be prepared from it and consumed with due ceremony. That plant was Kava Kava.

Colonial governments and missionaries were so disgusted with the traditional preparation of Kava Kava, that they made this process illegal, and forced the natives to prepare the beverage by grinding or grating the root stock. There seems to have been no difference in the medicinal action of the grated root versus the chewed root. Fortunately, today we can get Kava Kava in a more sanitary condition, through commercially available extracts and capsules; extracted with machinery rather than human mastication.

Interestingly enough, the Island Communities of the Pacific were one of the few areas of the world that did not have alcoholic beverages before European contact in the eighteenth century. The use of Kava Kava began to decline when alcohol showed up.

Kava Kava was also of great religious significance and was seen to connect the user with the ancestors and the gods. It was not merely an offering or sacrifice to the spirits but a way of gaining access to the spirit world. It was used in healing ceremonies and to obtain hidden or esoteric knowledge. In Hawaii native priests would read the bubbles on the surface of a kava brew to predict the sex of an unborn child or the cause of illnesses, much like fortune tellers reading tea leaves. Hawaiians also use Kava Kava at ceremonies where children are named, and also when young girls are initiated into traditional hula and chanting. Being presented with a Kava Kava root means that you have been welcomed and that a gesture of peace has been made. By 1948, Hawaiians were no longer drinking Kava Kava on a regular basis. More than a dozen varieties of Kava Kava are known on Hawaii.

Kava Kava has become an important cash crop to the Pacific Islands. It is particularly suitable for the traditional practices of subsistence farmers. These farmers than sell their Kava Kava crops to dealers who export the plants to supplement manufacturers.

CHEMICAL QUALITIES

Kavalactones have been deemed the primary active compounds in Kava Kava based on detailed scientific investigations over the past 110 years. Kavalactones have been shown to be quite effective in treating anxiety and depression. A recent double-blind study had fifty-eight patients who were suffering from anxiety that received either 100mg of Kava Kava extract or a placebo three times daily for four weeks. The group that took the Kava Kava extract showed significant improvements in several psychological assessments. Symptoms of anxiety, such as nervousness, heart palpitations, chest pains, headache, dizziness, and feelings of gastric elimination were either completely eliminated or greatly reduced. The most amazing part of this study is that this was achieved without side effects.

Kavalactones appear to act primarily on the limbic system-an ancient part of the brain that affects all other brain activities and is the principal seat of the emotions. It is thought that the kavalactones promote sleep by altering the way in which the limbic system modulates emotional processes. It appears that many of the laboratory models used to identify how a substance provides a calming effect are simply not sophisticated enough to evaluate the kavalactones fully.

Kavalactones also may protect the brain against damage due to ischemia, a condition in which there is not enough oxygen-rich blood supplied to the brain. The effectiveness of the kavalactones is said to be due to their ability to limit the area affected by necrosis as a result of the reduction of the blood supply.

Another chemical constituent of Kava Kava is Kawain. According to James Duke's web-site, Kawain has quite a long list of medicinal actions, including: anesthetic, anti-convulsant, anti-dote, anti-imflammatory, anti-septic, anti-spasmodic, fungicide, myorelaxant, sedative, and tranquilizer. Piper methysticum is listed as the plant species with the highest amount of Kawain in it.
Piper methysticum is also listed as being the plant species with the highest amount of methysticin in it. This is also an anesthetic, anti-convulsant, anti-dote, anti-imflammatory, anti-spasmodic, myorelaxant. In addition, it is also neuroprotective. Yangonin, which is also highest in piper methysticum, is also anesthetic, anti-imflammatory, anti-spasmodic and myorelxant. In addition, yangonin is also anti-bacterial. There seems to be a lot more going on inside of Kava Kava than just relaxant activities.

A couple of important constituents in Kava Kava are dihydrokavain and dihydromethysticin. These constituents have analgesic effectiveness comparable to that of aspirin. Although Kava Kava has been described as a narcotic, it is non-addictive. In addition, unlike aspirin, Kava Kava does not cause ulcers.

MEDICINAL QUALITIES

Kava Kava induces a pleasant sense of tranquility and sociability after it is consumed. With moderate use of Kava Kava, the consumer remains in control of his moral conscious and reason. He attains a state of well-being and contentment, free of physical or psychological excitement. He never becomes angry, unpleasant, quarrelsome or noisy, as happens with alcohol. When consumption becomes excessive, the limbs become tired, the muscles no longer seem to respond, walking becomes slow and unsteady, and the consumer appears partially inebriated, and often falls asleep. Unlike alcohol, drinkers of Kava Kava do not experience hangovers. The Kava Kava drinker will awaken having recovered normal physical and mental capabilities. When consumed in large amounts, Kava Kava imparts a euphoric state. This could be why some people regard Kava Kava as an aphrodisiac.

Kava is anti-septic, anesthetic, narcotic, and a diuretic. It has been used for both acute and chronic gonorrhea, vaginitis, syphilis, leucorrhoea, nocturnal incontinence, urinary infections, irritable bladder, gout, rheumatism, bronchial ailments, and other ailments resulting from heart trouble. Dr. John R. Christopher recommended Kava Kava as a cardiac stimulant. Kava Kava has been recommended for insomnia, depression and anxiety. Kava Kava works on the central nervous system, and promotes relaxation to those suffering from anxiety or depression. Because of the relaxant properties of Kava Kava, it is beneficial in treating menstrual cramps as the Kava Kava will relax the uterus.

Kava Kava is an excellent anti-anxiety herb. Many people who have anxiety report that the anxious feelings leave or diminish when they begin taking Kava Kava. Studies have been done to show that Kava Kava is far superior to a placebo when treating anxiety, but are sadly lacking to show that Kava Kava is superior to anti-anxiety medication, such as Valium. Unlike many popular prescription drugs, Kava reduces anxiety but does not impair mental function or cause sedation. In a double-blind crossover study conducted in Switzerland, the effects of Kava on short-term memory were compared with those of the anti-anxiety and muscle relaxant drug Oxazepam. While the drug was found to impair short-term memory, Kava actually improved it slightly. And, when you look at the possible side effects of Kava Kava versus anti-anxiety drugs, it is easy to see that Kava Kava is a safer choice for almost everyone.

Kava Kava has long been used by Pacific Islanders as a pain reliever. Kava Kava will help relax tired, sore muscles. It also helps to provide a restful sleep to those suffering from insomnia or restlessness. James Duke mentions that when you chew the leaves of Kava Kava your mouth goes numb. As a result, this plant might be used to relieve the painful symptoms of sore throat, sore gums, canker sores, or even toothache. In Hawaii, children were given buds of Kava Kava to chew on when they were teething. Quite possibly, Kava Kava could be used as a local anesthetic. Kava Kava can be used in place of aspirin, acetaminophen, and ibuprofen. Due to its anti-inflammatory properties, Kava Kava could be useful in treating gout and cystitis. Dr. John R. Christopher recommended that Kava Kava be used to prevent, relieve or even cure rheumatism. He also recommended it in any other cases where you would need an anti-inflammatory herb.

Kava Kava can be used externally for ringworm and athlete's foot. Traditionally, Kava Kava was given to feverish or restless children to help them go to sleep.

Kava Kava has been traditionally used by Hawaiian healers to help sufferers of asthma. More studies need to be done to prove Kava Kava's efficacy as a treatment for asthma. Dr. Christopher mentions in his writings that Kava Kava can be used for broncho-pulmonary ailments.

Dr. Christopher recommended using Kava Kava to treat kidney infections, or other urinary disorders. He also mentioned its properties as a blood-cleansing herb, and also as a diaphoretic. Kava Kava has also been used to calm down enraged animals, although the exact properties of the herb that influence this action are not known.

High doses of Kava Kava are unnecessary, and should be discouraged, as a small amount will give the desired medicinal effect. A few people have reported blood in the urine, shortness of breath, increased red blood cell volume, and decreased platelet counts after consuming large doses of Kava Kava. However, these reports are suspect because the subjects also reported heavy alcohol and cigarette usage in addition to the Kava Kava. A few cases have been reported of people with Parkinsons's disease being adversely affected by Kava Kava.

The continued use of Kava Kava in large doses will result in inflammation of the body and eyes, and can cause leprous ulcers; the skin becoming parched and peeling off in scales. This condition is known as Kani, named by the Pacific Islanders. At one time, it was thought that Kani was caused by an interference of Niacin. However, in one double-blind, placebo-controlled study no therapeutic effect with Niacinide (100 milligrams daily) could be demonstrated. The only known was to deal with Kani is to reduce or cease consumption of Kava Kava.

DOSAGE

There are several different ways to take Kava Kava. The traditional way is to drink it as the Pacific Islanders do, preferably no more than three cups a day. For those of us who tend to get our herbs from herb stores instead of chewed up and spit into a bowl by old men, there are extracts and capsules to choose from. The standard dosage is one dropper of tincture three times a day, or two capsules three times a day. However, you can increase your dosage if you find it necessary. A full bottle of extract a day would be too much, but two to three full droppers three times a day should not lead to an increase in liver toxicity. Sixty capsules of Kava Kava would be too much, but five capsules three times a day should not have any affect on the liver either. Some people find that they only need to take Kava Kava right before bed, while others find it necessary to take it as a preventative measure to keep their anxiety at bay. Dr. Christopher said the best way to use Kava Kava was by grinding the root and making an infusion.

For toothache or other mouth problems, you would chew a couple of leaves until your mouth achieved a numbing effect.   To use it as a local anesthetic or pain reliever you could apply a liniment of Kava Kava externally.

Or, you could make your own traditional preparation of Kava Kava by chewing a small amount of the root. When you have a sufficient amount chewed up, put the pieces of Kava Kava into a bowl and mash them with a cup of fresh water. Strain the liquid through a cloth to remove the woody material. Sugar cane juice or honey can be added to sweeten the drink.

One of the debates about Kava Kava dosage is standardized extracts versus non-standardized extracts. The School of Natural Healing favors non-standardized extracts, as you will receive the benefit from the whole plant, not just the chemicals that man has decided are the most beneficial. When standardized Kava Kava is mentioned, it means that the kavalactone levels have been standardized, occasionally up to seventy percent! A double-blind study was done with a seventy percent standardized extract of Kava Kava. Twenty-nine patients were given 100 milligrams of Kava Kava extract three times a day, and twenty-nine patients were given a placebo three times a day. Therapeutic effectiveness was measured using standard psychological assessments. Over a four-week period, it was shown that the individuals taking the Kava Kava extract had a statistically significant reduction in symptoms of anxiety, including feelings of nervousness, somatic complaints such as heart palpitations, chest pains, headache, dizziness, and feelings of gastric irritation. No side effects were reported.

LICORICE ROOT

LATIN NAME Glycyrrhiza *glabra*

Kingdom: Plantae
(unranked): Angiosperms
(unranked): Eudicots
(unranked): Rosids
Order: Fabales
Family: Fabaceae
Subfamily: Faboideae
Genus: *Glycyrrhiza*
Species: **G. glabra**

Liquiritiae radix
Sholzwurzel

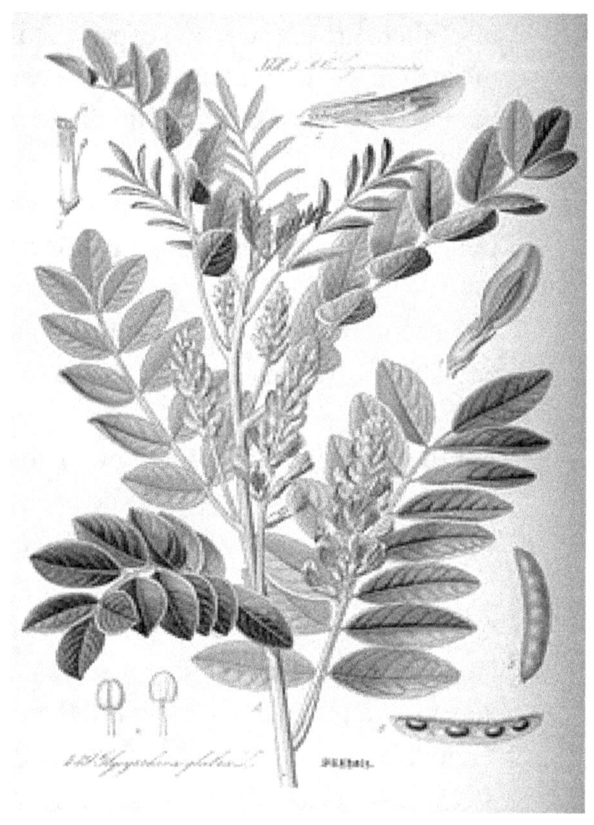

Name of Drug

Liquiritiae radix, licorice root.

Composition of Drug

Licorice root consists of unpeeled, dried roots and stolons of *Glycyrrhiza glabra* L. [Fam.Fabaceae], as well as their preparations in effective dosage.The unpeeled roots contain at least 4 percent glycyrrhizic acid and 25 percent water-soluble matter.Licorice root also consists of peeled, dried roots and stolons of *G.glabra* L.[Fam.Fabaceae], as well as their preparations in effective dosage. The peeled roots contain at least 20 percent water-soluble matter.

The root contains several flavonoids of flavanone and isoflavanone derivatives in addition to the potassium and calcium salts of the glycyrrhizic acid. It also contains phytosterols and coumarins.

Uses
For catarrhs of the upper respiratory tract and gastric/duodenal ulcers.

Contraindications
Cholestatic liver disorders, liver cirrhosis, hypertonia, hypokalemia, severe kidney insufficiency, pregnancy.

Side Effects

On prolonged use and with higher doses, mineralocorticoid effects may occur in the form of sodium and water retention and potassium loss, accompanied by hypertension, edema, and hypokalemia, and, in rare cases, myoglobinuria.

Interactions with Other Drugs

Potassium loss due to other drugs, e.g., thiazide diuretics, can be increased. With potassium loss, sensitivity to digitalis glycosides increases.

Dosage

Unless otherwise prescribed:

Average daily dosage:

- About 5 - 15 g of root, equivalent to 200 - 600 mg of glycyrrhizin;

As *Succus liquiritiae* :

- 0.5 - 1 g for catarrhs of the upper respiratory tract, 1.5 - 3 g for gastric/duodenal ulcers;
- equivalent preparations.

Mode of Administration

Powdered root, finely cut root or dry extracts for infusions, decoctions, liquid or solid dosage forms for internal use (*Succus liquiritiae*).

Duration of Administration

Not longer than 4 - 6 weeks without medical advice. There is no objection to using licorice root as a flavoring agent up to a maximum daily dosage equivalent to 100 mg glycyrrhizin.

Actions

According to controlled clinical studies, glycyrrhizic acid and the aglycone of glycyrrhizic acid accelerate the healing of gastric ulcers. Secretolytic and expectorant effects have been confirmed in tests on rabbits. In the isolated rabbit ileum, an antispasmodic action has been observed at concentrations of 1:2500 – 1:5000.

HISTORY

Licorice Root is one of those herbs that has been around since ancient times. It was found in great quantities in the tomb of King Tut among his gold, jewelry and art treasures. It was presumed that King Tut wanted to take the root with him on his journey to the next world so that he could make his sweet drink "Mai sus" when he got there. To the Egyptians the sweet tasting Licorice root was a cure-all, much in the same manner that Chinese relate to Ginseng. Remarkably the licorice root was extremely well preserved when it was found by archaeologists, this may be due in part by the unusual preservation qualities the shape of the pyramid has.

Licorice root was used in other areas of the ancient world, the Brahmans of India, the Hindus, Greeks, Romans, Babylonians and Chinese. The ancient Hindus believed it would increase sexual vigor when prepared as a beverage with milk and sugar. The Scythians taught the use of the herb to the Greeks; Theophrastus called it Scythian root, writing in the third century B.C. The Scythians were able to go twelve days without drinking water because they chewed on Licorice root and ate mare's cheese. He also said it was good for coughs and all pectoral diseases. In about 80 AD, Pliny recommended Licorice root to clear the voice and to alleviate thirst and hunger.

Dioscorides, an herbal physician, gave the plant its botanical name (Greek glukos = sweet, riza = root). Dioscorides traveled with the army of Alexander the Great, he told the troops to carry and chew Licorice root in order to allay their thirst when water was scarce and to give them stamina and endurance during their long marches. He also said that it was good for stomach trouble, throat trouble and liver and kidney disorders. It is not known if they had the same trouble that was reported by Napoleon in France; he habitually chewed Licorice root, which eventually blackened his teeth.

During the Middle Ages, Licorice was often taken to alleviate the bad effects of highly spiced and overcooked food, fat and often-contaminated meats, as refrigeration was impossible and most meats were preserved by salting and by packing with aromatic herbs and spices. During this time Licorice extract was said to be equal to that of "grains of paradise", it is not know what that is but it sounds of importance to be documented. To back up the value of licorice, it was reported that a tax was placed on licorice imports to aid in repairing the London Bridge during the reign of Edward I in 1305. About the middle of the fifteenth century, Licorice was named among the wares kept by the Italian apothecaries and it is enumerated in the list of drugs of the City of Frankfurt, written about the year 1450. It was not only important medicinally, but was used as a flavoring agent in sweets and tobacco, and as a foaming agent in fire extinguishers and beers, and used in isolated millboard.

Licorice is imported chiefly from Spain and Italy, the warmer more temperate countries, but cultivation has existed on a small scale in England. Dominican friars introduced licorice to England by bringing it to Yorkshire Dales around the 15th century, where it became famous as an ingredient in Pontefract cakes. In Turner's herbal we learn that the planting and growing of licorice in England began about the first year of Queen Elizabeth, which was in 1558. Culpepper stated, "It is planted in fields and gardens, in divers places of this land and therefore good profit is made." In the 1800's Culpepper included information about Licorice in his famous herbal writings. Southern Europeans drank large amounts of Licorice water (tea) because they believed it to be a blood purifier.

It was the English who introduced the herb to the American Indians, which is strange because it was usually the other way around. John Josselyn of Boston in the sixteenth century lists Licorice as one of the "precious herbs" he brought over from England. He would brew a beer for the Indians when they had a bad cold. It was strongly flavored with elecampane, Licorice, aniseed, sassafras and fennel.

Licorice is official in all pharmacopoeias, which only differ as to which variety is recognized, the botanical name, and whether the accepted root be peeled or unpeeled.

If we look at the use of licorice from a western perspective, we see that its use has changed little over 3,000 years. It is considered demulcent (soothing to irritated membranes), expectorant (loosening and helping to expel congestion in the upper respiratory tract), and stimulates mucous secretions of the trachea. Other well-documented activities include significant anti-inflammatory effects, a protectant effect on the liver against toxic substances and anti-allergic activity.

CHEMICAL CONSTITUENT

The major active component of Licorice is saponin known as glycyrrhizin, also known as glycyrrhizic acid, which is an extremely sweet, foaming triterpene glycoside. It has a similar structure and activity as the adrenal steroids. Glycrrhizin, the potassium and calcium salt of glycyrrhizinic acid, is 50 times sweeter than sucrose and encourages the production of hormones such as hydrocortisone. Diabetic patients can safely take this type of sugar. Glycyrrhiza consists mainly of 20% starch, up to 6.5% glucose, 2 - 4% asparagines, 8% fat, resins, mannitol, gum protein, a trace of tannin, .03% volatile oils, bitter principles and other constituents.

Glycyrrhizin has a cortisone-like effect that raises prostaglandin levels locally, increasing mucous secretion and promoting proliferation of cells in the stomach. The intestinal flora hydrolyzes glycyrrhizin. This action has been found to be useful in the treatment of peptic ulcers and treating Addison's disease. Glycyrrhizin has a similar chemical structure to corticosteroids released by the adrenals, which may aid in relieving withdrawal symptoms from cortical hormones. Licorice has shown estrogenic activity and is anti-inflammatory, antirheumatic, and antibacterial. The flavonoids liquiritin, isoliquiritin, liquiritigenin and isoliquiritigenin found in the root are thought to be responsible for its antiulcer benefits. The flavonoids are also responsible for the yellow color of the root as well as for the health of the arteries.

MEDICINAL QUALITIES

Licorice is one of the more widely consumed herbs in the world. In Traditional Chinese Medicine it occurs in more formulas than any other single herb because it is thought to harmonize the action of all other herbs. Licorice is not only used as a great medicinal herb but Licorice extracts also have uses in such things as candies, chewing gums, flavoring tobacco, liqueurs, cough medication, antismoking preparations, and it is even used to increase the foam in beer. This could be one reason Dr Christopher stressed that we should not procrastinate in obtaining adequate supplies of Licorice root. He stated, "we import tons of it from the Middle East every year for commercial medications and the Licorice candy industry. If there was to be a transportation strike it would cripple the nations economy and people would bemoan the fact that the herb could no longer be obtained". He stated that if we are in the climate to grow it in our yards that we should.

The more popular medicinal actions of Licorice root are as a demulcent, pectoral, emollient and for disguising the taste of nauseous or bitter medicinals (as a flavoring). Some other uses are as an expectorant, anti-spasmodic, anti-inflammatory, laxative, hypertensive, anti-ulcer, estrogenic, emmenagogue, antibacterial, anti-fungal, sialogogue, and immune stimulant.

Licorice is very soothing and softens the mucous membranes of the throat, lungs, stomach, intestines, and at the same time cleanses any inflamed mucous membrane that needs immune system support. This is why Licorice is found in so many cough and sore throat medications. It reduces the irritation in the throat and yet has an expectorant action. It is the saponins (detergent-like action) that loosen the phlegm in the respiratory tract, so that the body can expel the mucus. It is a potent healing agent for tuberculosis, where its effects have been compared to hydrocortisone. For colds and flu, Licorice can be combined with stimulating herbs such as cayenne or ginger to intensify the effect. For sore throat and irritated bronchials, Licorice is more effective when combined with Horehound or Mullein.

Licorice also has a soothing and healing effect on the stomach and digestive tract. It softens, soothes, lubricates and nourishes the entire intestinal tract with a formula as simple as 40% Licorice root and 60% Slippery Elm. The saponin content is effective in soothing various internal pains. Licorice is popularly known for treatment of ulcers of the stomach or duodenem, collective known as peptic ulcer. The glycyrrhetinic acid found in Licorice was the first drug proven to promote healing of gastric and duodenal ulcers. Modern medicines such as antacids, Tagamet and Zantac disrupt the normal digestive process and alter the structure and function of the cells that line the digestive tract and will cause the ulcer to appear again. The cause is not treated. The compounds found in Licorice stimulate the normal defense mechanisms that prevent ulcer formation. These compounds improve both the quality and quantity of the protective substances that line the intestinal tract. It will balance out the production and secretion of hydrochloric acid that is a cause of the formation of a peptic ulcer. The life span of intestinal cells will increase and there will be an improved blood supply to the intestinal lining by using Licorice--it treats the cause.

The 100 Herb List at the School of Natural Healing lists adrenals as the common use for the Licorice. The steroidal (cortisone-like substance) content of Licorice aids in the healing and restoring of the adrenal glands. Glycyrrhizin has a similar chemical structure to corticosteroids released by the adrenals, which helps to stimulate the excretion of cortin hormones by the adrenal cortex. About every five hours, the adrenals need some sort of nourishment in order to continue supplying strength to the body. If the nourishment is not given, the glands go through what is called adrenal exhaustion, or in medical terms hypoglycemia. This exhaustion is also caused by the stresses that life places on us in this fast paced world in which we live. Sugar is often consumed to overcome stress and to get a stimulating lift. This causes more problems and can lead to insulin shock. When a person's adrenal glands become so exhausted that they do not function anymore, they find themselves in a condition called Addison's disease.

Licorice, with its cortisone-type substance, will help the body restore itself to the point where it will produce its own cortisone. It will give the body strength and a stimulating lift without bringing on insulin shock. This will also help the pancreas to function well because of better control of insulin released. The medical profession will prescribe corticosteroid hormones as a replacement drug when the body is fatigued; thus causing a dependency to them. If a person tries to get off these drugs they will go through severe withdrawal symptoms. Licorice begins strengthening and healing the body with as little as two capsules of Licorice each day. As noted by Dr. Christopher, "When people who have been under severe stress, overworking the adrenals and becoming extremely nervous and irritable, begin to take Licorice, they think they have suddenly spiritually arrived. It is my opinion that many who suffer in mental institutions could be helped with this wonderful herb".

The Steroidal content found in Licorice not only helps the adrenal glands but female problems as well. It can trigger higher levels of estrogen in the body, which will aid in the treatment of female infertility, for delayed and irregular menstruation, and in premenstrual syndrome (PMS). It can be used to stabilize the menstrual cycle when coming off of "the Pill." It will help relieve the pain of chronic menstrual cramps as well as premenstrual symptoms such as depression, cravings for sweets, weight gain due to water retention, breast tenderness, etc. Licorice has an alterative action on estrogen metabolism, which means when estrogen levels are too high it will bring them down, and if the levels are too low it will bring them up. This estrogenic action is due to the isoflavone content found in Licorice. Premenstrual syndrome has been attributed to a disruption in the estrogen to progesterone ratio. Licorice helps to bring back the right balance in this ratio, therefore relieving the symptoms that this imbalance causes. If licorice is used, two cups of tea a day, two weeks prior to the onset of menstruation will reduce the symptoms of PMS. After a couple of months the cycle should be improved and no more need to drink the tea. Even though our bodies require a balance of male and female hormones, men who take Licorice don't need to be alarmed about "getting too much" hormone-estrogen properties. Our bodies are a fabulous computer and it selects only what it needs from natural sources such as herbs.

As mentioned previously, Licorice was taken during the middle ages to counter-balance the effects of highly spiced and over cooked food, fat and contaminated meats. Licorice is a highly esteemed herb for the same use today. The root is excellent as a stool softener or mild laxative, especially for children. It doesn't cause the gripping of the intestines that other cathartic herbs are known to do. Licorice also has as anti-inflammatory substance that helps in gastric or bowel irritations and also helps the inflammation caused by hemorrhoids. A looser and softer stool also helps when hemorrhoids are present.

I think the Egyptians may have been on the right track in their thinking that Licorice is a cure-all. A few more uses for Licorice are as a blood cleanser and detoxifier with benefits to the liver. It increases the flow of saliva and alleviates thirst when the root is chewed on and it also makes an excellent natural teething ring for babies to help bring the teeth through. If the baby is a vigorous chewer there may be some purgative or cathartic action as well!

In addition to quenching thirst, Licorice will quench the appetite and reduce the desire to smoke tobacco and consume alcohol. It will increase sexual desire and help a person stay alert (a No-Doz substitute). Mixed with honey it is great for external wounds and skin irritations. Combining Licorice with peppermint, it is great for a singer or a person losing their voice due to laryngitis.

Additional uses from James Duke, in his book "The Green Pharmacy," are preventing tooth decay, treating arthritis, asthma, athlete's foot, baldness, body odor, bursitis, canker sores, chronic fatigue syndrome, colds and flu, cough, dandruff, depression, emphysema, fungal infections, gingivitis, gout, heartburn, HIV infection, liver problems, Lyme disease, menopause, prostate enlargement, psoriasis, shingles, sore throat, tendonitis, tuberculosis, ulcers, viral infections and yeast infections.

I feel the same as this author who wrote on Licorice, "Licorice can be recommended for just about everybody, for male and female alike, young and old, well or sick. It is the grand tonic of the world, in this author's opinion. For that reason, I recommend it as an important tonic in the maintenance of the musculoskeletal system. The amazing anti-inflammatory actions of licorice root extend to the entire surface area of the body, both outside and inside. Not only the skin, but the mucous membranes of the gastrointestinal tract yield to the soothing and healing action of licorice root. The plant reinforces the body's ability to withstand attack from virtually any kind of pathogen, and should therefore be considered a tonic for the musculoskeletal system. If one is looking for a broad-spectrum tonic to protect, maintain health, and heal injuries, there is no herb better than licorice root.".

DOSAGES

Licorice can be found in preparations such as a decoctions, elixir, fluid extract, infusion, powder, syrup, tablets and tincture. Licorice is often used as a sweetening or flavoring agent to mask the bitter taste of other medications. It is very soothing and protecting on inflamed surfaces; therefore licorice can be taken orally as well as applied topically. Often times Licorice is used in combination with other herbs. It is one of the more widely consumed herbs in the world because not only is it used medicinally but also the extract is used to flavor tobacco, chewing gum, confections, soft drinks, liqueurs, ice cream, and baked goods. It can also be found as the foaming agent in beers or fire extinguishers and made into a chemical wood pulp, which is pressed into a board.

<u>Dosage</u>:

Decotion	1 teaspoonful to 1 tablespoonful as required
Fluid extract	½ teaspoonful or 20-60 drops 1-4 times per day
Infusion (tea)	up to 3 cups per day
Powder	½-1 teaspoon
Syrup	1 teaspoonful to 1 tablespoonful as required
Tincture	½-1 teaspoonful

LOBELIA

LATIN NAME Lobelia inflata

Kingdom: Plantae
Clade: Tracheophytes
Clade: Angiosperms
Clade: Eudicots
Clade: Asterids
Order: Asterales
Family: Campanulaceae
Genus: *Lobelia*
Species: **L. inflata**

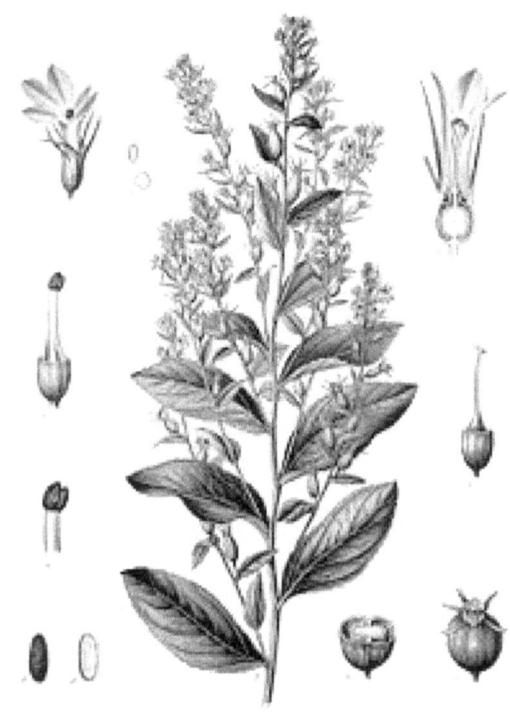

Lobelia inflata, also known as **Indian tobacco** or **puke weed**, is a species of *Lobelia* native to eastern North America, from southeastern Canada (Nova Scotia to southeast Ontario) south through the eastern United States to Alabama and west to Kansas.

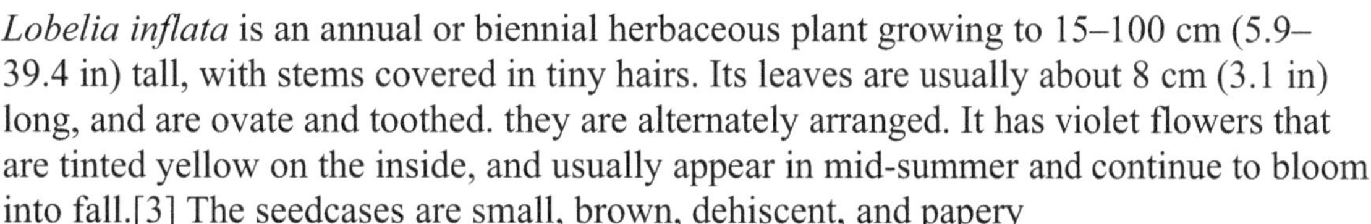

Lobelia inflata is an annual or biennial herbaceous plant growing to 15–100 cm (5.9–39.4 in) tall, with stems covered in tiny hairs. Its leaves are usually about 8 cm (3.1 in) long, and are ovate and toothed. they are alternately arranged. It has violet flowers that are tinted yellow on the inside, and usually appear in mid-summer and continue to bloom into fall.[3] The seedcases are small, brown, dehiscent, and papery

Lobelia inflata has a long use as a medicinal plant, as an entheogenic, emetic, and a dermatological and respiratory aid. Native Americans used it for respiratory and muscle disorders, as a purgative, and as a ceremonial medicine. The leaves were chewed and smoked.[6] The plant was used as a traditional medicinal plant by the Cherokee, Iroquois, Penobscot, and other indigenous peoples. The foliage was burned by the Cherokee as a natural insecticide, to smoke out gnats. It was widely used in the pre-Columbian New England region, long before the time of Samuel Thomson, who was erroneously credited as discovering it.

CHEMICAL CONSTITUENTS OF LOBELIA

Now for the technical part that my puny little brain can barely grasp. Hope I don't get you too confused. The constituents of a plant really are quite interesting, once you get into it. Though the whole plant is responsible for the action, not any single constituent, the constituents are the make up of the plant influencing its action. When we know which constituents are present and what their action is it helps us to understand the action of the whole plant in a clearer way.

Lobelia contains fourteen piperidine-type alkaloids with confusing tongue twister names. Lobeline, lobelanine, and lobelanidine are found in the greatest proportions. Lobelamine, norlobelanine, lelobanidine, norlelobanidine, norlobelanidine, lobinine, norlobeline (=isolobelanine), lelobanidine, lovinine, isolobinine, lobinanidine are present in lesser amounts. How would you like to rattle those names off one after the other? I'm afraid my tongue would get so tangled I wouldn't even be able to say lobelia anymore.

In addition to the alkaloids lobelia also contains a bitter glycoside (lobelacrin), chelidonic acid, lipids (fats), gum, resin, a pungent volatile oil (labelianin), chlorophyll, lignin, salts of lime and
potassium, with ferric oxide. Another constituent of lobelia, beta-amyrin palmitate, has been studied for its antidepressant effects. In one study the in vivo actions of beta-amyrin palmitate on central nervous system activity were compared with those of two antidepressant drugs, mianserin and imipramine with positive results.

The pharmacological effects of lobelia are attributed primarily to the piperidine-type alkaloids, particularily lobeline. Lobelia's alkaloids stimulate the vagus nerve which controls the stomach.

Proctor was the first in 1838 to isolate the liquid alkaloid lobeline which scientists consider to be the active principle of lobelia. Lobeline is found in higher concentrations in the seeds than the rest of the plant. The piperidine alkaloids are closely related to nicotine though less potent and have similar chemical effects on the peripheral and central nervous (CNS) systems.

Other research shows that the principle pharmacological activity of lobeline is not nicotine agonism. Rather, lobeline may affect CNS activity by altering the dopamine chemistry of the brain. Lobeline has been shown to be more potent than d-amphetamine in blocking dopamine uptake into synaptic vesicles. Lobeline induces reflex stimulation of the respiratory center by acting on the chemoreceptors of the glomus caroticus, producing stronger and deeper breathing. This helps to explain why lobelia is useful for respiratory complaints.

 Isolobelanine also called norlobelanine has a balancing effect to lobeline, relaxing the respiratory and neuro-muscular system. Lobeline is a powerful respiratory stimulant, while isolobelanine is an emetic and respiratory relaxant. Can you see how the apparently paradoxical effects of stimulating and relaxing work so well together? Don't worry we'll get more into it when we discuss the medicinal qualities of lobelia.

MEDICINAL QUALITIES OF LOBELIA

The authors of "The Model Botanic Guide to Health" expressed their feelings on the medicinal value of lobelia well when they wrote "/The medical qualities of this invaluable herb are so multifarious that a large treatise might well be written on its curative powers. Suffice it, however, to say that it is a general corrector of the whole system, innocent in its nature, and moving with the general spirits. In healthy systems it will be silent and harmless. It is fully as well calculated to remove the cause of disease as food is to remove hunger; and it clears away all obstructions in the circulation regardless of the nature
of the disease."

Lobelia is most noted for its antispasmodic, emetic, relaxant, stimulant and expectorant actions. Other therapeutic actions attributed to lobelia are: nervine sedative, anti-venomous, counter-irritant, emmenagogue, diaphoretic, diuretic, cathartic, astringent, sialogogue and nauseant. King stated emphatically "It is in no sense a narcotic".

No single constituent of lobelia is responsible for lobelia's healing effects. The whole leaf, as opposed to isolated constituents, is known to be strongly antispasmodic

Lobelia's antispasmodic/relaxing, stimulating (respiratory), emetic/expectorant action makes it valuable for asthma and bronchitis etc. It relaxes the muscles of the smaller bronchial tubes, thus opening
the airways, stimulating breathing, and promoting the coughing up of phlegm, helping prevent spasmodic, nonproductive coughing

Lobelia's actions differ according to the dose used. Small doses tend to have a relaxing effect and large doses a stimulating effect. In moderate doses lobelia stimulates the central nervous system to dilate the bronchioles, increasing respiration. The likelihood that the initial bronchial dilation will be followed by respiratory depression is increased with large doses. The circulation is likewise enfeebled by large doses but strengthened by small doses. Lobelia also affects the vagus nerve which controls the stomach. A small amount of lobelia has the effect of calming the stomach, decreasing nausea, and relieving stomach cramps. Large amounts of lobelia can act as a purgative instead of an emetic, but the end result is the same; emptying the stomach of its contents.

The earliest use of lobelia, that of an emetic, is tightly interwoven with its other therapeutic actions. A large enough dose of lobelia to cause vomiting has a stimulating then general depressing action on the central and autonomic nervous system and on neuromuscular action. Profuse perspiration, nausea, oppressive prostration, relaxation of the muscular system and a languid pulse/rapid heart rate accompany the emetic stage. This is what has scared many people and frightened them into declaring that lobelia is a dangerous herb. The depression, however, is of short duration, and is immediately followed by a sense of extreme satisfaction and wellbeing. Old time doctors used lobelia's effect on the heart to advantage. They felt that "/It makes the pulse fuller and slower in cases of inflammation and fever . . . [and] reduces palpitation of the heart"

When relaxation of the system is required lobelia is invaluable as it is an extremely efficient relaxant, influencing mucous, serous, nervous, and muscular structures. "A Guide to Health" an exposition of the Thomsonian system of practice states "/lobelia is the most powerful, certain, and harmless relaxant that has ever been discovered/". Since Thomsonians believed relaxation was an important indication in the cure of most disease, lobelia was an indispensable article in their materia medica. John King stated in his Dispensatory that "under its action the mental powers are unusually acute, and the muscles are powerfully relaxed."–King's American Dispensatory. For best results the relaxation caused by lobelia should be counteracted by stimulating herbs such as catnip, peppermint, or cayenne. It really works both ways since lobelia increases other herbs effectiveness in cases where relaxation is needed.

What I consider to be the most important property of lobelia can certainly not be attached to any particular constituent of the plant. What makes lobelia great is its ability to go right to where it is needed and carry out the exact action that it should. In conditions that could go either way, this can be a virtual life saver. There are stories of lobelia saving babies when their mothers are miscarrying and other times it did not stop the miscarriage but rather assisted the spontaneous abortion of the dead fetus. In two similar cases of large abscesses, the action of the herb was different, draining internally in a strong and husky boy and externally in the weak and puny boy. It is almost as if lobelia is capable of thinking and because of this has been called the thinking herb. Lobelia even tells you when you have had too much – you will vomit it right back up.

THE BENEFITS OF THE USE OF LOBELIA
IN HERBAL PREPARATIONS

DOSAGES AND APPLICATIONS OF LOBELIA

Lobelia can be used in a large variety of ways. Effective preparations include: decoction, fluid extract, infusion, pills or capsules, poultice, ointment, powdered herb or seed, syrup, and acid tincture.
Lobelia can even be smoked for asthma or used as an enema.

Heat destroys most of the medicinal properties of the lobelia so when making tea an infusion is preferable to a decoction. To make an infusion, pour 1 cup boiling water over ¼ to ½ teaspoons dried leaves; steep 10-15 minutes. Drink 3 times per day. If using the seed it is best to crush them so the medicinal properties can be released into the liquid. A decoction of the herb is still useful as an emetic, the dose is ½ cupful. Tea is not the preferred method because of lobelia's acrid taste.

Tincture, especially the acid tincture made with vinegar is the very best way to use lobelia. It is safer and more effective this way than any other form. The acid tincture is extremely versatile, and with a little creativity is appropriate for most if not all of the conditions that lobelia can be used for. The tincture is especially valuable for croup, asthma, lockjaw, and ringworm. The tincture can be made from the green or dried herb. A tincture made of the seeds is much more potent.

In addition to internal uses the acid tincture and even the alcohol tincture can be used externally as a rub for relaxation, rubbed on the neck and chest and between the shoulders to break up congestion. This is especially good for babies with mucus and spasmodic congestion problems as some feel it is better not to give lobelia internally to infants. It's relaxing effect can be balanced with cayenne, peppermint or other stimulants if desired. Combined with Cayenne or another stimulant it is great for a chest or sinus rub. One other external use is for earache. Place a few drops of warm lobelia tincture in the ear and plug with cotton.

Dosages vary greatly from one herbal to the next often influenced by the author's opinion of the safety or danger of the use of lobelia. Some feel strongly that lobelia is a low dosage botanical and should never be used as an emetic. Others though they realize it must be used wisely, are not afraid of it because they believe an overdose is virtually impossible due to the emetic properties of the herb. It is wise to start with a small dose and increase or repeat doses till the desired results are obtained.

The anticipated results and the condition being treated also affect dosage. A good example of this is in treating asthma and croup. In a crisis situation, such as an asthma attack, relatively large doses are given along with warm herbal tea to encourage vomiting and expelling of mucus. In these situations a teaspoonful dose of the acetic tincture is repeated every 10-30 minutes till vomiting occurs. One man took three tablespoonful doses. Afterwards he said, /". . . My breathing was so difficult that I took a tablespoonful of the acid tincture of lobelia, and in about three or four minutes my breathing was as free as it ever was. I took another in ten minutes, after which I took a third, which I felt through every part of my body, even to the ends of my toes." or a more long range therapeutic approach, working at nourishing and healing over a length of time lesser amounts are used combined with other herbs. Or for the squeamish who are not in a life or death situation, just enough lobelia can be given to gain some decongestant/expectorant action without throwing up. "A Modern Herbal" listed "/5-30 drops every half-hour in elm or flaxseed infusion/" as an expectorant. Given cautiously this seems to be a low enough dosage to avoid vomiting.

Amazingly lobelia is so powerful it has a noticeable effect even in very small amounts such as a dilution of 1:99. Those who feel lobelia is a low-dosage botanical say "5 drops of the acetous tincture taken three times daily (usually in marshmallow tea or with demulcent tinctures) should prove adequate." Lobelia tincture is generally combined with

other tinctures at the rate of 1 part lobelia tincture by volume: 10 parts of a mixture of other tinctures such as mullein, elecampane,
thyme, hyssop, red root, echinacea, etc. by volume). This compound is taken at the basic dosage of one or two droppersful (30-60 drops) 3-5 times daily. Those leery of lobelia's powerful actions give the caution "/Straight lobelia tinctures or compounds containing lobelia should be diluted in at least a full cup of water (240 ml) before ingestion." I found an even stronger warning stating "/A total of 20 mg lobelia per day should not be exceeded. Doses higher than 500 mg are highly toxic and . . . could be fatal.".

Recommended doses for the acetic tincture (1:5) vary greatly from the overly cautious 5 drops three times a day to the more reasonable dose of 1 to 4 ml three times a day. Dr. Christopher suggested ½ to 1 teaspoonful doses (2-4 ml) and he never gave more than 3 doses in succession. "A Modern Herbal" tops them all with a suggested dose of 1 to 4 drachms. Most likely it is supposed to be a maximum daily dosage.

Standard conservative dose for the tincture of lobelia is ½ ml three times per day with a maximum dosage of 2ml a day. The British Pharmaceutical Codex's recommended dose for the tincture (1:8, 60 percent ethanol) is .4 to 1.6 milliliters up to three times a day. The largest suggested dose I found of the U.S.P. tincture was 1 to 4 drachms. That is equivalent to approximately 1/8 to ½ fluid ounce or 14 milliliters.

Recommended doses for the fluid extract (1:1 in 50% alcohol) vary from 0.2 to 0.6 mL (5-15 drops) up to 0.5 to 1.5 ml (10-30 drops) three times per day. The difference in dosage makes sense when you look at the sources. The first source, www.adam.com also said lobelia is a potentially toxic herb, while the last suggested dosage was found in "School of Natural Healing". The dose listed in "A Modern Herbal" is somewhere between the two at 10-20 drops.

The dried herb in powder, capsules, pills, etc. recommended dosages vary as much as the extract and tinctures. According to the British Pharmaceutical Codex, 50-200 milligrams of dried herb three times a day is the recommended dose for asthma, chronic bronchitis, and spastic colon. www.best-home-remedies.com said capsules commonly contain 395 milligrams, tablets 2 milligrams and lozenges 1 milligram.[18] Dr. Christopher's recommended dose of the powdered herb (leaves, stems, flower and/or pods) was 200-650 milligrams. An old home doctoring book gave the dose as 1-5 grains but "A Modern Herbal" gives the dose as 5-60 grains. One grain is equal to 64.8 milligrams so "A Modern Herbal's" dose equals a whopping 3888 milligrams. Really makes me wonder if the 0 is a typo and it should read 5-6 grains which would be 324-388.8 milligrams. All these different dosages can be quite confusing. To simplify things just follow Dr. Christopher's dosage recommendations he used lobelia for years and I'm sure he knew what he was talking about.

For children adjust the recommended adult dose to account for the child's weight. Most herbal dosages for adults are calculated on the basis of a 150 lb (70 kg) adult. Therefore if the child weighs 50 lb (20-25 kg), the appropriate dose of lobelia for this child would be 1/3 of the adult dose.

Doses for four more preparations of lobelia follow. Dosage for syrup of lobelia 1 to 4 teaspoons or 1 to 4 drachms; solid extract 100-300 milligrams or 2 to 4 grains (129 to 259 ml); Etherial tincture, B.P., 5 to 15 drops. The solid extract and etherial tincture are no longer on the market as far as I know. It's a good thing too. Dr. Christopher warned against the latter saying "Do not use lobelia tincture from drug stores, as it is extracted with an etheric menstruum." The solid extracts were inferior as well, being heat evaporated tars with many of their constituents oxidized by heat. The oil of lobelia seed has also faded into history. Dosage was 1 drop rubbed up with 20 grains of ginger or triturated with one scruple of sugar and divided into 6 to 12 doses. This was considered useful as an expectorant, nauseant, sedative, and diaphoretic, when given every one or two hours.

To use lobelia as an enema, also called internal bathing by some, follow these directions "/This herb may be administered by means of the internal bath, namely, taking a solution of one ounce of the powdered lobelia to a quart of water and injecting this solution into the intestines, through the rectum./" Dr. Christopher and Jethro Kloss both recommended adding lobelia to a catnip enema for fever, pneumonia, pleurisy, nephritis, hepatitis, meningitis, etc. The reason for this being "/The bowels are lined with tiny blood vessels which will absorb the herb into the system./" – "Modern Encyclopedia of Herbs"

Lobelia can be made into a poultice for external treatment of bruises, insect bites, sprains, felons, ringworm, erysipelas, and poison ivy irritation. Lobelia plasters and liniments are used to treat sprains, muscle spasms and bruises because of the plant's relaxing and stimulating effect. Dr. Christopher instructed to make a compress or plaster of lobelia for swellings, pneumonia, pleurisy, boils, etc. For any external problems Dr. Christopher said "Apply a poultice consisting of 1 part lobelia and 2 parts slippery elm." I've listed Jethro Kloss's lobelia poultices with the formulas. Please refer to page 61 for information on them.

Here are directions for making your very own lobelia tincture.

First off for a lobelia tincture we use vinegar rather than alcohol. Due to lobelia's unique constituents and properties lobelia extracts made with vinegar are more effective than those made with alcohol and water. We use 4 oz. of the dry herb to 1 quart solvent in this case organic apple cider vinegar. Put the lobelia in a quart jar and cover with the vinegar. Macerate for two weeks. That means shake it every day when you go past. When the 14 days are up, strain the vinegar out of the lobelia. Put the herb in a cheese cloth and squeeze to get as much good out of it as you can. Compost the spent herb and store your lobelia tincture for future use in a dark glass bottle.

MARSHMALLOW

Marshmallow root

LATIN NAME Althaea officinalis

Kingdom: Plantae
Clade: Tracheophytes
Clade: Angiosperms
Clade: Eudicots
Clade: Rosids
Order: Malvales
Family: Malvaceae
Genus: *Althaea*
Species: **A. officinalis**

Althaeae radix
Eibischwurzel

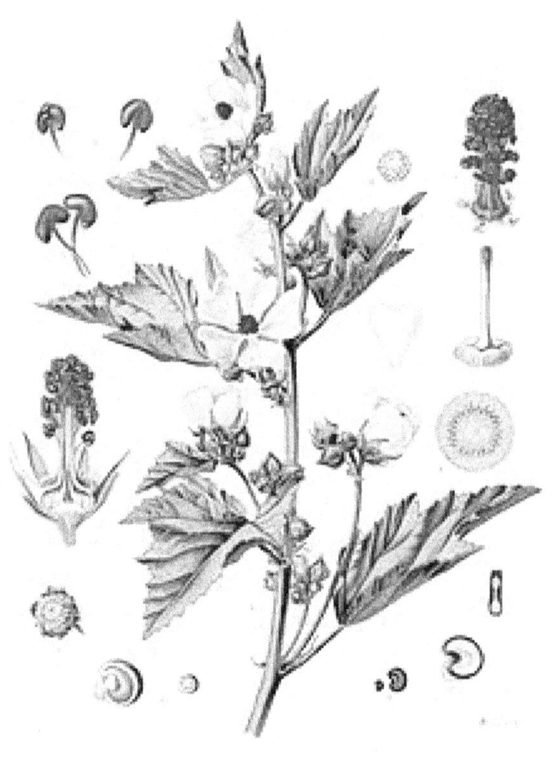

Name of Drug

Althaeae radix, marshmallow root.

Composition of Drug

Marshmallow root consists of the dried root, unpeeled or peeled, of *Althaea officinalis* L. [Fam.Malvaceae], as well as its preparations in effective dosage.

Uses
(a) Irritation of the oral and pharyngeal mucosa and associated dry cough.

(b) Mild inflammation of the gastric mucosa.

Contraindications
None known.

Side Effects
None known.

Interactions with Other Drugs

None known.

Note: The absorption of other drugs taken simultaneously may be delayed.

Dosage

Unless otherwise prescribed:

Daily dosage:

- 6 g of root;
- equivalent preparations.

Marshmallow syrup:

- Single dose: 10 g.

Mode of Administration

Cut or ground root for aqueous extracts as well as other galenical preparations for internal use. Marshmallow syrup to be used only for use (a).

Note: Marshmallow syrup: diabetics need to allow for sugar concentration (according to declaration of manufacturer) percent (equivalent to...bread units).*

Actions

Alleviates local irritation
Inhibits mucociliary activity
Stimulates phagocytosis

*[**Ed. note:** This relates to the need for diabetics to consider and allow for the sugar content of the syrup as stated on the label and is written precisely as it appears in the original German.]

Marshmallow. Just seeing the word brings to mind the fluffy, sugar laden pillows sold so readily in grocery stores. Originally, marshmallows were made from the root of the marshmallow plant, although today they are made from corn syrup, sugar and gelatin. The Marshmallow plant looks nothing like its sugary namesake. In most places, it appears as a virtual mat, hugging the ground. In rich, moist areas it may attain a foot or more in height.

Marshmallow flourishes in the wild and in the garden. Many people struggle vainly against it, trying to remove the "weed" from their garden. Dr. Christopher said that we should be grateful that it comes back, and instead of trying to obliterate it, we should honor and use it. The most common form of Marshmallow is Malva Neglecta. It is also known as cheesies, because of the cheese shaped seeds it produces. Althea officinalis is more commonly seen in England and Europe. Althea officinalis is a taller species with mauve or blue flowers.

Unlike most herbalists, Dr. Christopher used marshmallow to treat gangrene. He had numerous success stories, including several where the medical profession wanted to amputate the gangrenous limbs. The patients would hurry to Dr. Christopher, who would tell them to make a strong decoction of marshmallow root, and use it either in fomentations, or to soak the afflicted limb. He would also tell his patients to drink cups of marshmallow tea.

Marshmallow is also a diuretic and is good for the kidneys. One of Dr. Christopher's students gave her a son a marshmallow root to chew on when he was doubled over in pain from severe kidney pain from being unable to void his urine. Within seconds of chewing the root he was able to void his urine, and received relief from the excruciating pain.

Other uses of Marshmallow include soothing and healing to the inflamed respiratory, alimentary, intestinal, and genitourinary areas. It has been used for mastitis, skin irritations, and in sitz baths to relieve rectal irritations. It is also helpful in dealing with gravel, inflammation of the kidneys, cystitis, and bladder infections. The herb is mainly used internally, especially for bronchial afflictions. It can also be used for constipation.

Historically, Marshmallow has been used by a variety of people for a variety of ailments. Hippocrates felt that it was of immense value in the treatment of wounds. Charlemagne demanded that it be cultivated in his domain. The ancient Arabs used the leaves to suppress inflammation, sores and swelling. The Egyptians ate mallow for food. In France, the tops and tender leaves of Marshmallow were used in spring salads to stimulate the kidneys. Gypsy babies chew Marshmallow roots to help them with their teething.

MILK THISTLE

Milk Thistle fruit

LATIN NAME Silybum marianum

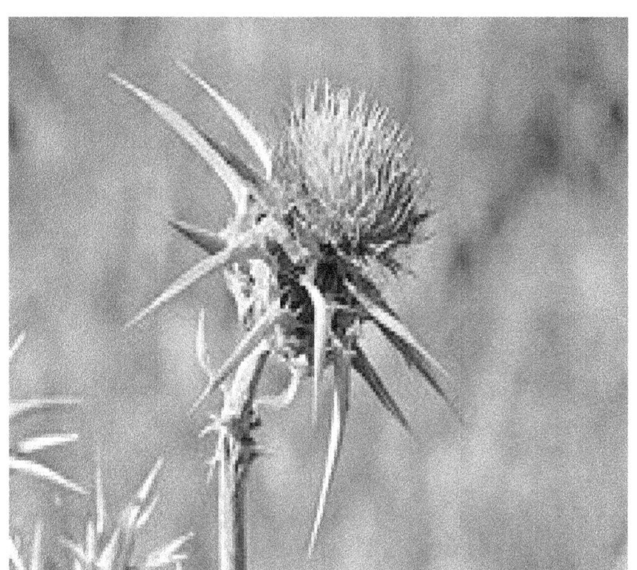

Kingdom: Plantae
Clade: Tracheophytes
Clade: Angiosperms
Clade: Eudicots
Clade: Asterids
Order: Asterales
Family: Asteraceae
Genus: *Silybum*
Species: **S. marianum**

Cardui mariae fructus
Mariendistelfrchte

Name of Drug

Cardui mariae fructus, milk thistle fruit.

Composition of Drug

Milk thistle fruit consists of ripe seed of *Silybum marianum* (L.) Gaertner [Fam. Asteraceae], freed from the pappus, and its preparations in effective dosage.

The drug contains silibinin, silydianin, and silychristin.

Uses
Crude drug:

- Dyspeptic complaints.

Formulations:*

- Toxic liver damage; for supportive treatment in chronic inflammatory liver disease and hepatic cirrhosis.

Contraindications
None known.

Side Effects

Crude drug:

- None known.

Formulations:

- A mild laxative effect has been observed in occasional instances.

Interactions with Other Drugs

None known.

Dosage

Unless otherwise prescribed:

Average daily dose of drug:

- 12 - 15 g;
- Formulations equivalent to 200 - 400 mg of silymarin, calculated as silibinin.

Mode of Administration

Powdered drug for making infusions and other galenical formulations to be taken by mouth.

Actions

Silymarin acts as an antagonist in many experimental liver-damage models: phalloidin and -amanitin (death-cap toxins), lanthanides, carbon tetrachloride, galactosamine, thioacetamide, and the hepatotoxic virus FV3 of cold-blooded vertebrates.

The therapeutic activity of silymarin is based on two sites or mechanisms of action:

(a) it alters the structure of the outer cell membrane of the hepatocytes in such a way as to prevent penetration of the liver toxin into the interior of the cell;

(b) it stimulates the action of nucleolar polymerase A, resulting in an increase in ribosomal protein synthesis, and thus stimulates the regenerative ability of the liver and the formation of new hepatocytes.

HISTORY

Milk Thistle's name.

There seems to be some discretion between writers regarding the Botanical name of Milk thistle, with some saying it is Carduus marianus and others saying it is Silybum marianum. They also suggest that there is some discretion in the use of the common name, with the area where the plant was found and where the individual lived being common factors in the name used. Common names given to the Milk thistle include, Our Lady's thistle, Marian thistle, St Mary's thistle, Sow thistle and Wild artichoke.

Most sources use the botanical name Silybum marianum, with only a few using the name Carduus marianus. Dr Rudolf Weiss, who studied botany and medicine at the University of Berlin comments on the use of the names, "Botanists now classify it as belonging to a genus different from Carduus, but pharmaceutical nomenclature still uses the old name Carduus marianus". David Hoffmann M.N.I.M.H. speaking of both the common name and the botanical name, states "The importance of botanical accuracy is highlighted here. In different places this herb is called Milk Thistle, Mary Thistle and even Sow Thistle. To complicate matters the botanical taxonomists have changed the binomial. Milk Thistle is now correctly called Carduus marianum and not Silybum marianum".

The King's American Dispensatory does not distinguish between the botanical names, Carduus marianus and Silybum marianum, or between the common names of Mary thistle, Milk thistle and St Mary's thistle. Henriette's herbal home page to which the King's American Dispensatory belongs makes mention of this after the title to which it writes it as Carduus marianus - St Mary's thistle, then proceeds, "The seeds of Carduus marianus, Linne (Cnicus marianus, Silybum marianum, Gaertner). Nat. Ord.- Compositae. COMMON NAMES: Mary thistle, Milk thistle, St. Mary's thistle.".

Mrs Grieve refers to the botanical name Carduus marianus as being the seeds of the milk thistle, she writes "The seeds of the Milk Thistle (Carduus Marianus), known also as Silybum Marianum . One of the major suppliers of herbal products in the United Kingdom, Herbal Apothecary of Leicester (www.herbalapothercary.net), list Milk thistle seed as Carduus marianus in their product catalogue.

What seems to be the case is that either of the botanical names refer to the herb Milk thistle, whether it be the seeds or the whole plant. I personally know Milk thistle as Carduus marianus through my dealings with the Herbal Apothecary.

Tradition has it the milky-white veins of the leaves originated from the milk of the virgin Mary which once fell upon a plant of the thistle, hence the names St Mary' thistle and Our Lady's thistle, and also the names marianus and marianum.

.

The Use Of Milk Thistle in History

Milk thistle has been used in traditional herbal medicine for a long time, with references dating back to the first century. It is said that the Roman naturalist, Pliny the Elder (AD. 23-79), wrote about the plant's juice and it's virtues of "carrying of bile", which in his time referred to a general description of any internal fluid. Dioscorides, the Roman army Doctor used the seeds of Milk thistle as a remedy for infants and those bitten by serpents. Mrs Grieve uses Gerard's quotation of Dioscorides use of the herb, she writes " 'Dioscorides affirmed that the seeds being drunke are a remedy for infants that have their sinews drawn together, and for those that be bitten of serpents:' ". Gerard himself used the herb and was of the opinion that it was the best remedy for all melancholy diseases, which physicians at the time considered a liver complaint. Gerard's writing is quoted by Mrs Grieve who writes "Gerard wrote of the Milk Thistle that -
'the root if borne about one doth expel melancholy and remove all diseases connected therewith…. My opinion is that this is the best remedy that grows against all melancholy diseases,' ".

Culpepper, the famous British herbalist who practised half a century later, used the name Our Lady's thistle instead of Milk thistle. He recommended its use in the treatment of disorders affecting the liver and spleen, the kidney's in provoking the flow of urine, to break and expel stones and also to treat dropsy. He considered Milk thistle to be as effective as the Holy thistle, Carduus Benedictus, for agues and the opening of obstructions in the liver, as well as being a excellent blood cleanser. He writes, "It cleanses the blood exceedingly: and in spring, if you please to boil the tender plant (but cut off the prickles unless you have mind to choak yourself) it will change your blood as the season changes, and that is the way to be safe.". Culpepper suggests that thistles in general were under the dominion of Jupiter.

The Milk thistle was also used by the Saxons as a remedy to ward snakes. The seeds were used by the Saxons as a remedy to cure the infectious disease contracted by a man who was bitten by a rabid animal known nowadays as hydrophobia. Mrs Grieve states "we find in a record of old Saxon remedies that 'this wort if hung upon a man's neck it setteth snakes to flight.' ".

On the subject of Milk thistle being as effective as the Holy thistle, it is said that the Milk thistle is a breeder of milk and of help to nursing mothers. Mrs Grieve quotes a John Evelyn who wrote " 'Disarmed of its prickles and boiled, it is worthy of esteem, and thought to be a great breeder of milk and proper diet for women who are nurses.' ".

The leaves and stalks of the Milk thistle were at one time used in salads, soups and pies, with the leaves surpassing the finest of cabbage. The heads were also eaten, in most cases they were boiled and treated like those of the Artichoke.

By the 19th century Milk thistle was recommended and used by German physicians for the treatment of liver and blood problems, as well as for intestinal cleansing. Formerly regarded as a bitter, the herb gained recognition as one of the best remedies for liver complaints. It was the seeds that were found to contain the active principle that has the specific effect on the liver. A German physician of the early 19th century called Rademacher gave his patients a tincture made from the seeds. It was said to be successful with his tincture "Tinctura Cardui Mariae Rademacher" still listed in pharmacopoeias today.

More recently, studies on the Milk thistle have shown that it has a role of protection regarding the liver. Scientists in Germany, where most of the research has been done, noticed that it seemed to protect the livers of animals from poisoning with highly toxic carbon tetrachloride. The particular active ingredient that protects the liver was isolated and its chemical constitution established, a previously unknown flavonol, that was given the name silymarin. No other plant principle has been as extensively investigated in recent years as silmarin, with further studies showing that it is effective in the treatment of a number of disorders affecting the liver. Cirrhosis, deathcap mushroom poisoning, all types of hepatitis, gallstones, occupational toxic chemical exposure and skin disease all showing positive results under tests.

CHEMICAL CONSTITUENTS

Constituents of Milk Thistle.

Milk Thistle contains a bitter principle, antioxidant properties, essential oil, polyacetylenes, tyramine, histamine, and flavolignans collectively referring to Silymarin. These are silybin, silychristin, and silydianin.

How Milk Thistle Affects the Liver.

It is thought that silymarin works in three different ways. Firstly, it strengthens the outer membranes of the liver cells, therefore preventing the penetration of liver damaging poisons and substances. Silymarin is also a powerful antioxidant that offers the liver cells protection against chemicals that are formed by the use of high fat diets, smoking and other substances such as alcohol abuse. It is also thought that the antioxidant affect of the silymarin is ten times more powerful than that of Vitamin E. Michael Castleman in his article entitled "Milk Thistle: Nature's Liver Protector" writes,

"The best known antioxidants are Vitamin A (beta-carotene), Vitamin C, Vitamin E, and the mineral selenium. However, in the liver, silymarin [milk thistle extract] is more than 10 times as potent an antioxidant as Vitamin E." . It is also thought that silymarin inhibits the action of the enzyme largely responsible for causing inflammation in hepatitis. Milk thistle may also have positive effects on the blood and immune system due to it's action of decreasing basophilic histamine release, and increasing of T-lymphocytes as well as reducing immunoglobulins. It is also thought that silymarin may decrease cholesterol and HDL levels.

Milk Thistle and Liver Function Test.

Many studies have shown the qualities of Milk thistle in its use as a medicine, with more recent studies showing how good herbal medicine is when it is compared to the limited medicine of the medical establishment when it comes to treating liver problems. On the one hand, unless your liver function test shows that it is abnormal, they will say that there is nothing wrong with the liver while you are manifesting symptoms such as skin disease, constipation, low blood sugar, heartburn, indigestion and food allergies. On the other hand, the liver function test is showing that it is abnormal, they will tell you they can not do anything for you. This is the wonders of modern medicine.

Milk thistle when used properly is excellent in this situation. The liver, through our lifestyles of stress, drinking of alcohol to the excess, smoking, incorrect diet, and the taking of powerful synthetic medication, gets over worked. The chemical Silymarin counteracts against this helping to produce a normal liver function. Studies have shown that those taking synthetic drugs and also having a abnormal liver function test were helped by taking an extract of Milk thistle. Michael Castleman comments on this stating, "In one study, 66 women taking anticonvulsant or psychiatric medications showed abnormal liver-function tests. They began taking silymarin [milk thistle extract] in addition to their medication, and 52 of them showed significant improvements in liver function.".

Milk Thistle and Carbon Tetrachloride.

A number of studies have shown that Milk thistle is an effective remedy in protecting the liver against hepatotoxins such as carbon tetrachloride, thioacetamide, a-amanitin, and the death cap mushroom Amanita phalloides.

Poisons such as carbon tetrachloride are ingested by over 25,000 children under the age of 5 in the United States, but most of the deaths that occur as a result of accidental poisonings occur in the teenage years. Tests carried out on rats where carbon tetrachloride induced liver damage was present showed that Milk thistle extract had a protective effect.

Of the many symptoms that carbon tetrachloride produces, one is Central Nervous System depression that produces sleep. This is used to assess the extent of the damage to the liver and also the effectiveness of the protection of drugs used to treat the liver. David Hoffmann writes concerning the effect an extract of silymarin has on such subjects, "a reduction of the prolongation of hexobarbital sleeping time produced by carbon tetrachloride. This is a common method for assessing protective effects on the liver against the effects of chemical toxins.". If there is an increase in sleeping time the implication is that the livers ability to metabolize the hexobarbital is somewhat impaired. Tests show that carbon tetrachloride poisoning increases the sleep time, but significantly silymarin reduces this sleep time by up to 60%. suggesting that there is liver protection from the toxin while the Milk thistle is being used. David Hoffmann writes, "When Milk Thistle is added the increase in sleeping time normally produced by the carbon tetrachloride is reduced by up to 60%, suggesting that the herb is protecting liver function from the toxin.".

Other studies have shown that carbon tetrachloride also raises the serum levels of enzymes such as glutamic oxaloacetic transminase (G.O.T), glutamic pyruvic transaminase (G.P.T) and also sorbitol dehyrogenase (S.D.H). It was found that under treatment with silymarin these increases were significantly diminished. Rudolf Weiss comments on the aspect of serum tolerance and transaminase activities in relation to the use of Milk thistle and silymarin, saying,"… and serum tolerance and transaminase activities became normal.".

Milk Thistle and Hepatitis.

Hepatitis is generally put into three categories, A, B, and C, defined by the Merck manual as "An inflammatory process in the liver characterized by diffuse or patchy hepatocellular necrosis affecting all acini." (16). Sometimes these progress to what is known as Chronic Hepatitis lasting for more than six months, defined once again by the Merck manual as, "A spectrum of disorders merging between acute hepatitis and cirrhosis.". This disorder often results in liver failure or cirrhosis, or sometimes it results in both. Modern medicine deals with acute hepatitis by doing nothing at all apart from telling the patient to reduce their alcohol intake and get rest if they feel the need. Chronic hepatitis is treated by the use of corticosteroid therapy, but this can make the situation worse as they are contra-indicated in most types of hepatitis.

Studies show that with taking Milk thistle the affect of hepatitis is greatly reduced and that the affects of the virus are removed much quicker than any thing that modern medicine can do for the disorder. One such study suggests that taking Milk thistle reduced the recovery time by nearly 30% compared to what modern medicine can do. Michael Castleman writes concerning this study, "77 people with hepatitis were divided into two groups, one treated with silymarin [milk thistle extract], the other with a placebo. Average recovery time for the placebo-takers was 43 days, but those who took silymarin [milk thistle extract] recovered in an average of just 29 days." .

Other studies show that in cases of chronic hepatitis of all types, silymarin helps with general symptoms in relation to the gastrointestinal tract, improved appetite, less discomfort and an overall improvement in well being and physical performance. Rudolf Weiss comments on the efficacy of silymarin, "there is an improvement in the general condition within the first two weeks of treatment, particularly where gastrointestinal symptoms are concerned, there being a reduction of meteorism and relief of the tension or pressure felt in the right epigastrium.". Whilst Milk thistle has an affect on the symptoms of hepatitis, it will if given early enough prevent any damage to the liver cells by the virus. This is achieved by the silymarin acting on the membranes of the liver cells in a way that prevents the entry of the virus toxins and other compounds, thus limiting the damage to the cells. Rudolf Weiss makes an excellent point in relation to this and the use of silymarin, "A good result can thus be achieved at the acute stage of hepatitis, preventing necrotic changes and making the condition less severe. This explains why the symptomatic response has always been so good. The protective effect on the cell membranes cannot reverse the whole process in chronic forms of hepatitis caused by toxins, but it can often prevent further deterioration.".

From this we can safely say that in all cases of disease where the liver is involved, whether it be skin disease, cancer, hepatitis or just cleansing the body, Milk thistle will offer protection during the breakdown of toxins present in the liver and the body.

Milk Thistle and Death Cap Mushroom Poisoning.

Death cap mushroom causes many deaths every year with about half of all the reported cases proving fatal. It is hard to distinguish from other such wild mushrooms hence the large number in need for treatment. The standard medical treatment for the poison of this fungus is not particularly effective, with activated charcoal being the main form. It takes only a handful of the mushrooms, around 50 grams, to kill an adult, and even less for a child.

The toxins produced by the fungus have a special affinity with the liver. It manifests itself with symptoms that occur in two separate stages. During the first stage there is nausea, vomiting and abdominal pain which then subside for around 24 hours only for the second stage to bring more serious problems for the liver and kidneys, due to the highly poisonous amatoxins. Help in the form of silymarin can be given in between the two stages after the stomach contents have been emptied, for which, Lobelia tincture will be of great help. According to Rudolf Weiss it is silibinin, the principle component of silymarin that is the effective remedy, with the clinical progress being satisfactory and further liver destruction being prevented. He writes, "The next and crucial step is to make use of the latent period, i.e. temporary improvement after the first stage, to prevent damage to the liver and kidneys. Silibinin, the principal component of silymarin, has proved highly effective for this.". He then proceeds to explain how the silibinin works in the prevention of further damage to the cells of the liver. He writes "It occupies the receptors on the cell membranes preventing amatoxins from entering.".

Treatment for Death cap mushroom poisoning has to be given within 48 hours to stop any damage to the liver and in the case of using silibinin or silymarin administered by the mouth the dose has to be relatively high. Again Rudolf Weiss writes "If silibinin cannot be obtained in time, silymarin is given by mouth in relatively high doses. If silibinin or silymarin is given within 48 hours of the fungus having been ingested, clinical progress may be expected to be satisfactory. If treatment is delayed by more than 48 hours, toxic liver damage leading to coma is highly likely to develop. Even at this stage, silibinin will in most cases prevent further destruction of liver cells and the resulting coma." (23).

In Germany a company called Madaus produces a silymarin product that is in a solution that can be injected into the blood stream to achieve faster results. This is based on the assumption that because flavonoids do not dissolve well in water other means are needed to get at the properties in the Milk thistle. The Flavonoids dissolve well in 75% alcohol, so presumably there was not enough money in producing an alcoholic extract for the purpose of administration by mouth as this is much stronger than a infusion or decoction. Rudolf Weiss states, "Silymarin does not dissolve well in water, but it has now proved possible to make silibinin water-soluble, producing a solution that can be injected, to achieve rapid action (produced by Madaus in ampoules containing 50mg).".

Milk Thistle and Cirrhosis.

In the United States, cirrhosis is the third leading cause of death in the 45 to 65 age group, and in most cases they are secondary to chronic alcohol abuse. In some cases cirrhosis is as a result of chronic hepatitis. As we have seen earlier, Milk thistle is of help in the treatment of hepatitis, but those who are unfortunate to miss out on treatment with Milk thistle and have progressed to cirrhosis there is hope in using an extract of Milk thistle.

In general, modern medical treatment of cirrhosis extends to that of being supportive, the withdrawal of toxic agents and drugs, the attention to nutrition which may involve vitamin and mineral supplements, and the treatment of complications at the time they arise.

In 1989 the Journal of Hepatology published a study carried out on 170 people with advanced alcoholic cirrhosis that is often a fatal condition. The 170 people were separated into two groups, one taking 200 mg three times per day of Milk thistle extract of which 140 mg was of silymarin extract, and the other group received a inactive placebo. Michael Castleman comments on the study, "Both groups were followed for four years. During that time, the death rate in the placebo group was about 60 percent, but among those taking silymarin [milk thistle extract], only 40 percent died, a highly statistically significant difference.".

Other studies in regard to Milk thistle and cirrhosis have shown similar benefits for those who are suffering. Clinical trials have replicated the laboratory studies in that they show the livers ability to reverse many disorders that affect the organ through the stimulation of hepatocytes to replace diseased tissue. David Hoffmann writes, "Milk Thistle arrests the course of these diseases as well as stimulating hepatocyte regeneration. Over time, complete restoration of the liver is possible, with regeneration at four times the normal rate.".

Milk Thistle and Gallstones.

In the United States, 20% of the population over the age 65 have gallstones and of these, over 500,000 undergo a cholecystectomy each year. They occur more in women, those who are obese, and those that have a family history of gallstones or those who follow the typical Western diet. The major component of most gallstones is cholesterol to which a diet high in animal and saturated fats is a major contributor. In most cases the medical professions answer for those who are manifesting symptoms of gallstones is to remove the gallbladder, there is an answer in herbal medicine. Apart from using the gallbladder cleanse of apple juice and olive oil to remove the gallstones, the use of a Milk thistle extract as a preventative is of great help. It is suggested by Michael Castleman that a low fat, low cholesterol diet helps prevent gallstones and so does Milk thistle extract. He writes, "In one study, people with gallstones were given 420 mg of silymarin [milk thistle extract] a day. Without diet changes, after several weeks, they showed significant reductions in the cholesterol concentration of their bile, which minimized the risk of stone formation.".

MEDICINAL QUALITIES

Milk thistle is an effective plant remedy for many types of liver diseases. Laboratory and clinical studies have found that it is a worthy remedy in the treatment of metabolic liver disease, acute viral hepatitis A, B and C, chronic hepatitis, cirrhosis of the liver and also fatty degeneration of the liver. According to David Hoffmann, he suggests that the best results with using Milk thistle are found in toxic metabolic hepatitis and cirrhosis, in that it shortens the length of viral hepatitis, minimizes complications and also protects the liver against problems arising from surgery. He writes, "This all goes to make it an excellent remedy to use in the prevention and treatments of many liver disorders. The earlier treatment is commenced the better the prognosis but effective treatment is possible at virtually every stage.".

Because of the devastating effect of some drugs on the liver, it will be of great benefit if the individual took Milk thistle along with such medications. Because of the ability of Milk thistle to cause cell regeneration it provides the liver and the body with the ability to cope with the harmful effects of daily life and its encounters with air, water and food toxins. David Hoffmann comments, "Using Milk Thistle daily, and combining it with other hepatics, offers an effective and safe approach to liver protection.".

Among other qualities that Milk thistle has is that it is also useful for breaking and expelling gallstones, jaundice, splenic congestion, haemorrhages of the spleen and liver, and also uterine haemorrhage. It has also been used as an anti-cancer agent, digestive tonic, to increase urine flow, dropsy and also melancholy (depression), vomiting of pregnancy, pelvic tension and also amenorrhoea.

DOSAGES

Dosages.

Milk thistle can be taken in the powdered form, also as an infusion, a decoction, glycerine extract, and also alcohol extract, with the alcohol extract being the strongest.

In the powdered form a dosage of two to four grams three times per day is normal. For the infusion use one teaspoonful of the powdered herb to 150 ml of boiling distilled water left to infuse for ten minutes and drink this three times per day. For the decoction use three teaspoonfuls of the seeds to half a pint of distilled water and simmer for about twenty minutes, drink this three times per day. In the case of the glycerine and alcohol extract take 2.5 mls three times per day. In the case of poisoning where there is need to act quickly take 1:1 liquid extract at doses of 10 mls three or more times per day.

Applications.

Milk thistle has been widely used throughout Europe for a long time as a digestive tonic and as a stimulant to help the milk flow in nursing mothers. David Hoffmann writes, "as the name of this herb shows, it is an excellent of milk secretion and is perfectly safe to be used by all breastfeeding mothers.".

This once popular remedy has now a new identity as a remedy for real or perceived liver disorders. This remedy has been introduced into the dispensary of the Herbalist for its use as a liver remedy through the results of laboratory and clinical studies. Simon Mills referring to the Milk thistle comments, "It finds a place in many prescriptions where burdens on the liver are seen to be a dominant feature in the condition treated, especially in the aftermath of a drug-abuse problem, alcoholism or long-term treatment by conventional medicinal drugs ...".

Milk thistle is also used to increase the flow of bile from the liver and gallbladder and in that respect can be used in all problems related to the gallbladder. It was once used in Germany as a popular remedy for curing jaundice and biliary problems. Its action is gentle and protective and can be used in cases because of this where bitter herbs are contra-indicated or it can act as a buffer to their effect. It is in this light that it is used in the treatment of hepatitis A, B and C, cirrhosis of the liver due to alcohol abuse and also toxic poisoning as in the case of Death cap mushroom.

It also has the effect of lowering fat levels in the blood, which has been shown by research. We can also assume that because Milk thistle has an effect on the liver in cleansing and regenerating the liver tissue, it will have an effect on lowering blood cholesterol in the liver. Simon Mills writes, "As the liver is the organ most involved in affecting such levels after the effects of diet and exercise are taken into account, then the connection may not be too tenuous.".

MULLEIN

Mullein flower

LATIN NAME Verbascum thapsus

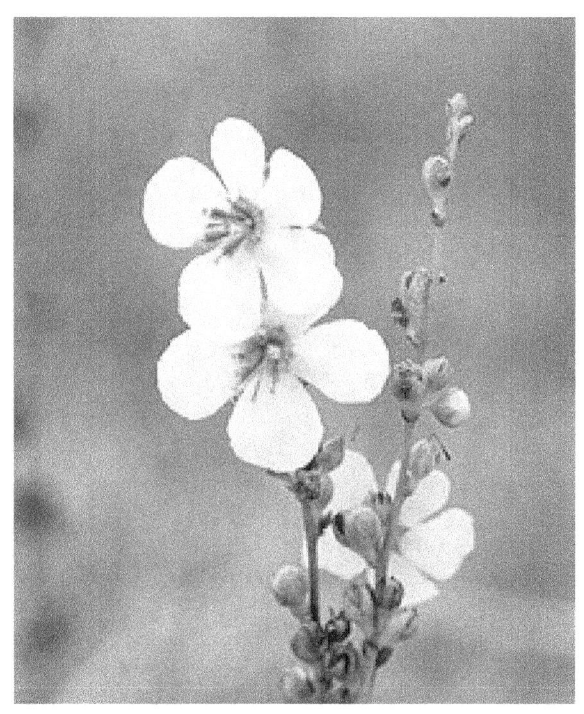

Kingdom: Plantae
Clade: Tracheophytes
Clade: Angiosperms
Clade: Eudicots
Clade: Asterids
Order: Lamiales
Family: Scrophulariaceae
Tribe: Scrophularieae
Genus: *Verbascum* L.

Verbasci flos
Wollblumen

Name of Drug

Verbasci flos, mullein flower.

Composition of Drug

Mullein flower consists of the dried petals of *Verbascum densiflorum* Bertoloni and/or of *V.phlomoides* L. (syn. *V. thapsus* L.) [Fam. Scrophulariaceae], as well as their preparations in effective dosage.

The drug contains saponins and mucopolysaccharides.

Uses
Catarrhs of the respiratory tract.

Contraindications
None known.

Side Effects
None known.

Interactions with Other Drugs

None known.

Dosage

Unless otherwise prescribed:

Daily dosage:

- 3 - 4 g of herb;
- equivalent preparations.

Mode of Administration

Comminuted herb for teas and other galenical preparations for internal use.

Actions

Alleviating irritation
Expectorant

Benefits of Mullein Leaf for the Lungs

This past summer much of the western United States was choking on a constant cloud of thick smoke. Looking at a map of current wildfires made it seem that everything from Montana to California was on fire.

In my own valley, the air quality was often listed as hazardous, with the recommendation to avoid going outside. Local emergency services handed out masks. A friend of mine with a newborn baby rarely left the confines of her house for months.

Not everyone can stay inside, however, and it wasn't long before I started getting calls from folks wondering what they could do to protect their lungs.

Enter mullein.

Mullein leaf has long been loved for soothing the lungs and quelling coughs. It is a mild relaxant to the lungs and also a mild demulcent. It soothes inflammation and dryness – often the causes of irritation for people with smoke exposure. In addition to the leaf, mullein flowers can have an added benefit to these dry irritated conditions. I often combine it with another demulcent such as mallow (*Malva neglecta*) or marshmallow (*Althaea officinalis*). Click here to read Sue Kusch's article and see the Relax and Replenish the Lungs Mullein Tea Recipe.

Mullein is wonderful for coughs and lung inflammation from all kinds of irritants and pathologies, whether it is particulate matter in the air or symptoms from asthma or an upper respiratory infection. Once you experience mullein's ability to soothe the respiratory system, you'll be amazed at the power of this ubiquitous plant. Yet it is a gentle herb that is safe for children and the elderly.

In the herbal world, it won't do to simply call a cough a cough. Instead we need to know the quality of the cough. Is it dry or wet? Is it strong or weak? Here are some specific indications for coughs well suited to mullein:

Mullein is considered a specific in bronchitis where there is a hard cough with soreness. Its anti-inflammatory and demulcent properties indicate its use in inflammation of the trachea. In painful coughing, Mullein leaves combine well with Elder and Red Clover. - Darcey Williamson[1]

Mullein leaf is best when the cough is dry, irritating and unproductive, with a definite lack of mucous production.
- Robert Dale Rogers[2]

[Mullein] is particularly used for dry, irritable, tickly coughs – the tickle sensation is usually evidence of inflammation conjoined with water stuck in the mucosa or skin. It is indicated in old coughs where the velvety carpet of the lungs, the hairs, are inflamed or worn down, so to speak. There may be tightness preventing full inspiration, tightness in the throat or voice box, or tightness in the sinuses and a feeling of tightness in the brain.
- Matthew Wood, Earthwise Herbal (Old World Plants)[3]

As long as the symptom pattern of dry, irritated and inflamed lungs fits, consider mullein for any type of cough, as a tea, tincture, or even inhaled as smoke or vapor.

Benefits of Mullein Leaf to Stop Smoking

Mullein leaf is commonly used by herbalists to aid those who want to quit smoking. It is often recommended to take the tea or tincture internally to support the health of the lungs, while concurrently using it as a smoking herb to assist with the desire to smoke something.

And while it sounds a bit counterintuitive, inhaling mullein smoke is a way to directly get mullein's relaxant qualities to the lungs, to relax constrictions and aid in stopping a cough. Like anything, this method can be overdone, but when you get it just right it can have dramatic and quick results.

Benefits of Mullein Leaf as a Nutritive

Mullein leaf is nutrient dense. When prepared as a nourishing herbal infusion, you can drink it frequently, not only to support lung health, but also to benefit from its high levels of calcium and magnesium[4].

Mullein's roots dig deep into the earth, bringing minerals and metals into its leaves. While this can result in nutritive leaves, mullein also has the ability to uptake heavy metals, which could pose a health hazard for humans if the soil is contaminated but also have positive benefits for the soil.

Mullein Benefits for Soil Remediation

Mullein is a hyperaccumulator of heavy metals. This means it can uptake heavy metals from the earth and store it. This ability has led to some interesting research on using mullein for soil remediation. Researchers in Serbia tested five different plants for cleaning up a heavily contaminated site. Their research concluded, "Because mullein efficiently transported metal pollutants into the above-ground parts and because it fits well the desired characteristics for its use as a biomass, it is our plant of choice for further bioremediation use at the polluted industrial site."

Mullein is generally regarded as safe; however, it always is important to harvest plants from healthy soils and to resist the temptation of the roadside mullein plants.

Benefits of Mullein Leaf Used Topically

Mullein boasts large hairy leaves that can feel like thick dense wool. The complex web of plant fibers covering the leaves protect the plant from the strong rays of the sun. These same plant fibers are a bit irritating to human skin, which can be annoying, medicinal, or both. When processing a lot of mullein leaves you may want to wear gloves.

The action of irritating the skin is called rubefacient. This irritation dilates the capillaries, increasing circulation to the area. This has a wide variety of therapeutic applications.

Used on the chest, mullein leaves can help move stagnancy in the lungs, increasing a healthy thin mucus that can be readily expelled.

Historically, mullein leaves were commonly used topically to address external hemorrhoids and varicose veins. The Eclectic Physicians – Cook, Felter, and Lloyd – all recommend mullein for piles, as did Nicholas Culpepper in the 17th century.[6,7]

Mullein leaf can also be used to address lymphatic stagnancy. It is recommended internally, as a tea or tincture, as well as used externally over the affected area.[8]

And if you are simply interested in seeing a rubefacient work, try rubbing the fresh or dried leaves on your skin to see the results. It was reportedly used as blush substitute in communities where make-up wasn't allowed.

Benefits of Mullein for Joint Pain and Rheumatism

There are many historic references to using mullein leaf externally on painful and rheumatic joints.

More recently, mullein root has become popularized for back pain. Herbalist jim mcdonald says, "Mullein root on its own, though, is also markedly effective. Prepared either as an infusion or taken in small doses as a tincture, it's been a lifesaver for me when working a bit too gung-ho has me wake up the next morning with my back 'kinked' and not quite able to straighten up. I usually take about seven drops of tincture, stretch out a bit, and the kink disappears and I feel perfectly aligned. While the occasions when this has worked are too numerous to recount, it doesn't always work...just most of the time."[9]

Matthew Wood describes his reasoning for mullein's mechanism of action in his book, *The Earthwise Herbal: A Complete Guide to Old World Medicinal Plants*: "It releases synovial fluid into the bursa and disperses internal fluids into the surrounding tissues, lubricating joints, muscles, bones, and ligaments. It is thus a remedy for complex fractures, where the bone needs to be lubricated to be returned to its place. It is also indicated in spinal dryness, inflexibility, and pain, and nerve pain along pinched or irritated nerve tracts."

Benefits of Mullein Root for the Bladder

In addition to back pain, mullein root is also used to address a variety of urinary incontinence issues, including stress incontinence, pregnancy incontinence, menopausal incontinence, and childhood incontinence. It can also be used to assist those with interstitial cystitis and benign prostatic hyperplasia (BPH, enlarged prostate).[11] For more information about mullein root uses for incontinence see Christa Sinadinos' article in the references.

Benefits of Mullein Flowers

Mullein's biggest claim to fame is as an earache remedy. Mullein flower infused oil is commonly found in health food stores and apothecaries. This historic use is backed up by the experiences of countless present-day parents and children. While it is sometimes use as a simple, it is often combined with garlic and/or St. John's Wort in the infused oil. Mullein flower infused oil acts as an anodyne to take away the pain of the earache, while also exerting lymphatic action on the area around the ear to help resolve the infection. A small bottle of the oil can be warmed in a warm water bath until the drops are about body temperature; then a few soothing drops can be placed in one or both ears and guarded with cotton balls.

Benefits of Mullein as an AntiViral?

Michael Moore reports that mullein flower tea has a negative effect on the herpes simplex virus (HSV-1) and seems especially helpful for women and children who have frequent outbreaks around the mouth triggered by sun, food allergies, or estrogen surges before ovulation.[13] Preliminary (in vitro) research shows some antiviral qualities against HSV-1 as well as influenza.[14,15,16]

Benefits of Mullein: The Mullein Plant

Great mullein, *Verbascum thapsus*, is the most common species of mullein that is readily found in North America. There are other species that are used similarly, such as *V. virgatum, V. densiflorum,* and *V. olympicum.* These two latter species have flower stalks that are denser than *V. thapsus*, making for an easier flower harvest. Medicinal seed suppliers often carry these other species.

The following describes *V. thapsus*.

Mullein loves to grow in disturbed soils. It prefers sun and can grow in poor, gravelly soils.

Mullein is a biennial plant, meaning it takes two years for it to complete its life cycle.

In the first year, a large basal rosette of silvery green and hairy leaves appears. By the late summer and fall the leaves can be very erect and easily up to a foot in length.

In the second year, it sends up a long flower stalk. The bottom of the stalk will have leaves growing alternatively and becoming smaller with height. The stalk then transitions to yellow flowers. The height of this stalk can reach two meters or more.

The flowers have five petals and five stamens. They start blossoming at the base of the stalk and then bloom progressively up the stalk.

The flower stalk darkens to brown in the fall and often persists through the winter and even into the next year.

Mullein stalks produce millions of tiny seeds that will persist in the soil for hundreds of years.

The roots are thin, branched taproots with a creamy color.

Benefits of Mullein: Harvesting Tips

The first step to making herbal preparations is harvesting the desired part at the right time. Because mullein is a biennial plant (taking two years to complete its life cycle), leaves and roots can be harvested at the end of the first and beginning of the second year, while flowers can only be harvested from the second year.

Mullein often grows in colonies – where you find one mullein plant you find many! It readily spreads by seed and its many seeds stay viable in the soil for possibly hundreds of years. While mullein is not an endangered plant and it would be difficult to negatively affect a population, I still approach it with admiration and respect.

There have been times when friends have offered to let me weed their garden of mullein; in those cases I harvest the entire plant. However, when harvesting leaves and flowers in the wild, I harvest here and there to ensure a thriving population. If you live in an area where mullein is not abundant, then it will be especially important to harvest in a way that supports further plant growth.

Mullein Leaves

Harvest mullein leaves when they are fresh and vibrant looking, ideally when the leaves are still in a basal rosette. The best times are in the fall of the first year's growth or in the spring of the second year, before the flower stalk starts to grow. In a pinch, the leaves can be harvested from a plant with a flower stalk. When harvesting the leaves, take a few from a single plant, leaving plenty to ensure the continued life of the plant.

Mullein Roots

Harvest the roots during the fall of the first year plant or the spring of the second year plant. It's not ideal to harvest the roots after the plant has gone to flower or seed.

Mullein Flowers

Harvest the flowers one by one as they appear on the flowering stalk, ideally harvesting from a plentiful patch of mullein, taking a couple of flowers from each plant. You may need to visit a mullein plant on numerous occasions to get enough flowers.

Benefits of Mullein: Plant Preparations

Mullein Leaves

Dry the leaves for use in teas, nourishing infusions, or as a smoking or vaporizing herb. Strain teas through a coffee filter to avoid ingesting irritating hairs.

Leaves can be applied topically as a poultice. Whole/flat leaves can be frozen to preserve them as future poultice material.

Fresh or dried leaves can be used in an alcohol extract.

- Fresh Leaf Tincture: 1:2, 50-60% alcohol.
- Dry Leaf Tincture: 1:5, 50-60% alcohol

Suggested dosage for leaves:

- Tea: 10-30 grams per day (more if desired)
- Tincture: 90-120 drops, 3 times a day

Mullein Roots

Chop and dry for use in decoctions.

Chop, dry, and powder for use in capsules.

Fresh or dried root can be used in an alcohol extract.

- Fresh Root Tincture: 1:2, 90% alcohol
- Dried Root Tincture: 1:5, 50-60% alcohol

Suggested dosage for roots:

- Decoction or powder: 15 grams (Michael Moore lists 2-4 ounces for decoction)
- Tincture: 30-60 drops, 1-3 times a day

Mullein Flowers

Dry the flowers for use in teas.

Infuse fresh or freshly dried flowers in a carrier oil for earache remedies (olive oil is nice).

Fresh or dried flowers can be used in an alcohol extract.

- Fresh tincture: 1:2, 90% alcohol
- Dried tincture: 1:5, 60% alcohol

(Note: Because the flowers are so light in weight, it will take a huge quantity to make a few ounces of tincture or oil.)

Suggested dosage for flowers:

- Tea: 5-10 flowers per cup, 3 cups daily
- Tincture: 30-90 drops, 3 times a day

The above dosage suggestions and tincture ratios were compiled from Michael Moore (*Medicinal Plants of the Mountain West*) and Christa Sinadinos.

MISTLETOE

Mistletoe herb

LATIN NAME Viscum album

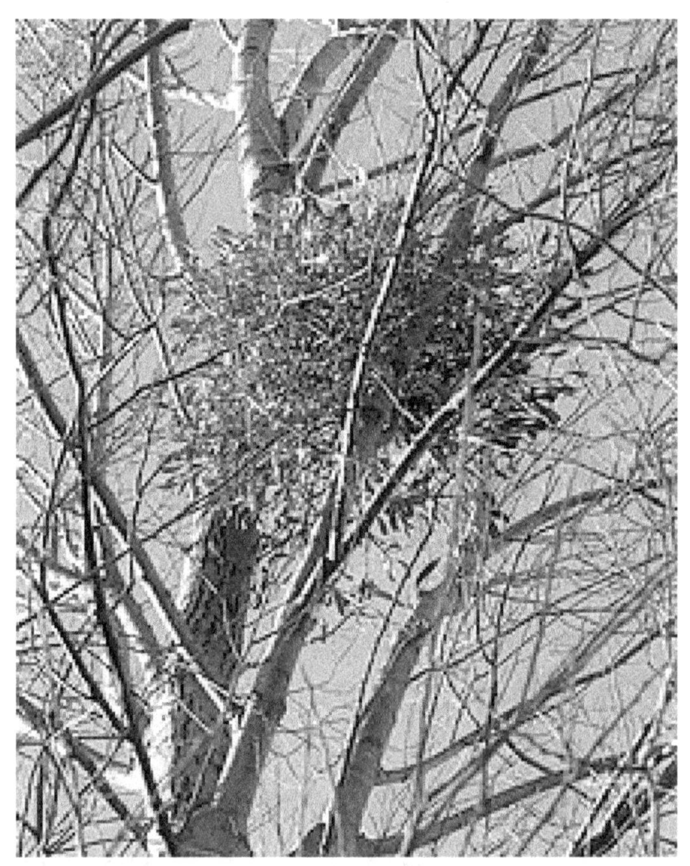

Kingdom: Plantae
Clade: Tracheophytes
Clade: Angiosperms
Clade: Eudicots
Order: Santalales
Family: Santalaceae
Genus: *Viscum*
Species: **V. album**

Visci albi herba
Mistelkraut

Name of Drug

Visci albi herba, mistletoe herb.

Composition of Drug

Mistletoe herb consists of fresh or dried younger branches with flowers and fruits of *Viscum album* L.[Fam.Viscaceae], as well as their preparations in effective dosage.

Uses
For treating degenerative inflammation of the joints by stimulating cuti-visceral reflexes following local inflammation brought about by intradermal injections.

As palliative therapy for malignant tumors through non-specific stimulation.

Contraindications
Protein hypersensitivity, chronic-progressive infections, e.g., tuberculosis.

Side Effects
Chills, high fever, headaches, angina, orthostatic circulatory disturbances and allergic reactions.

Interactions with Other Drugs

None known.

Dosage

Unless otherwise prescribed:

- According to directions of the manufacturer.

Mode of Administration

Fresh plant, cut and powdered herb for the preparation of solutions for injections.

Actions

Intracutaneous injections cause local inflammations which can progress to necrosis.

In animal experiments cytostatic, nonspecific immune stimulation.

Note: The blood pressure-lowering effects and the therapeutic effectiveness for mild forms of hypertonia (borderline hypertonia) need further investigation.

What is Mistletoe?

Nearly everybody associates mistletoe with its Christmas traditions, but did you know that this parasitic herb had a variety of uses beyond stealing a Christmas kiss? **In fact, mistletoe has a number of potential health benefits and a long tradition of use especially in Europe, for its ability to treat epilepsy and other nervous conditions.**

More recently, it has been extensively studied for its anti-cancer uses and its potential to improve lifespan and quality of life following cancer treatment. **Some estimates suggest that mistletoe is used by around 50% of cancer patients in Europe in some form or another.** Aside from cancer, it also may have other potential medical uses ranging from its calming effects to its ability to reduce blood pressure.

Mistletoe is a parasitic shrub that lives and grows on the stems of various other trees especially broad-leaved ones such as lime, apple and poplar trees. There are actually some 900 species of mistletoe overall some of which are known to be toxic. **However, there is a common misunderstanding that all mistletoe is toxic, which is definitely not the case though certain parts of the shrub are toxic especially its berries.**

The European mistletoe known scientifically as Viscum Album L is the species most used in medicine. While mistletoe can be drunk as a tea or used extracted to make tinctures, it is often used medically in inject-able form. The extracts contain a low level of mistletoe lectin which reduces the risk of toxicity.

1) Mistletoe and Cancer

When it comes to the potential health benefits of mistletoe, the one which has been subject to the most studies is its role in cancer therapy. Some studies have focused on its anticancer properties while others have demonstrated its ability to improve quality of life and reduce symptoms during and after chemotherapy. **Mistletoe extract is already widely used in Europe as part of a cancer treatment regimen.**

There is certainly a growing interest in mistletoe's potential to treat cancer and its reputation is continuing to grow. **Because of this, more and more research is being conducted and there is a generally positive trend within the studies conducted so far whether they were in vitro, animal or even clinical studies.**

As well as the promising research, there is a considerable amount of well documented anecdotal evidence regarding the effects of mistletoe on cancer. **An example is the 37 year old mother diagnosed with colon cancer which then spread to the liver and told she had an 8% chance of living more than 2 years.**

The patient requested mistletoe injections having been told about it by another doctor who specialized in complimentary therapies. **Although her regular oncologists knew little about mistletoe treatment, Dr. Diaz from John Hopkins Cancer Center reluctantly began treating her with mistletoe therapy although reluctantly at first.** Dr. Diaz says "I reviewed the literature on mistletoe in other parts of the world and there is some acceptance of it. I was willing to work with her."

According to Dr. Diaz, the response was amazing and the patient improved almost immediately with more energy and the color returning to her face. **The patient has been free of cancer ever since and attributes this to a combination of lifestyle, diet and mistletoe therapy and is trying to raise awareness of mistletoe in the United States.**

Research on Mistletoe and Cancer

A review published in 2009 analyzed 49 clinical studies that had used mistletoe extract or Iscador on cancer survival rates. **While the review acknowledged certain weaknesses in the studies, they concluded that the overall positive effects were impossible to ignore.**

An earlier review conducted in 2003 identified 23 studies conducted on the efficacy of mistletoe in cancer survival and quality of life. **Of the 23 studies, 12 demonstrated more than one statistically significant positive result and a further 7 showed at least one beneficial effect.** The reviewers concluded that the generally positive trend showed sufficient potential for future well designed research.

Mistletoe preparations are used to stimulate the immune system, to kill cancer cells, and to help reduce tumor size. **It may also help improve the quality of life and survival of some cancer patients, especially those using chemo and radiation, and may help reduce pain and side effects of these treatments.**

A major German study conducted over 27 years involving 35,000 patients demonstrated that using mistletoe (Iscador) as an adjunctive cancer treatment could increase the survival time of patients by up to 40%.

2) Mistletoe for Blood pressure

Millions of people are affected by high blood pressure putting them at risk of heart disease and strokes. **While its effects on blood pressure have not been as widely studied as its anticancer potential, there is some evidence that mistletoe can be used to treat hypertension.**
It also has the potential to prevent atherosclerosis or the build-up of plaque in the arteries which can cause many dangerous and life threatening heart conditions.

3) Mistletoe for Inflammation

Mistletoe is believed to have natural anti-inflammatory properties and one of its most common traditional uses was to treat internal and external bouts of inflammation including arthritis and other joint pains.

Arthritis is a very common condition and drinking mistletoe tea may be the perfect remedy to ease your pain and improve your mobility. **Of course, there are no guarantees that it will work for you but because of its anti-inflammatory ability, mistletoe may also be good for easing digestive and gastric conditions.**

4) Mistletoe and Diabetes

The ability of mistletoe to treat diabetes has not been firmly established but it has a long history of use and several animal studies have already demonstrated its anti-diabetic potential. **Research on animals has shown it can reduce blood sugar levels and can regulate the body's insulin levels.**

Mistletoe for Immune System

One of the greatest health benefits that mistletoe has is its effect on the immune system. One of the main reasons that mistletoe is so effective as a complimentary cancer treatment is its ability to bolster immunity and protect against further illness. **A strong**

immune system is absolutely vital to our overall health and mistletoe has the potential to improve our body's natural defenses.

5) Mistletoe Calming effects

Mistletoe was traditionally used for its calming properties and its ability to treat nervous disorders like epilepsy, tremors and tics. **Many people believe that it can be used to treat other nervous conditions like anxiety and stress as well as helping you to sleep better.**

6) Mistletoe for Respiratory Conditions

There is no scientific evidence relating to mistletoe's ability to treat respiratory complaints but according to anecdotal evidence and historical use, it can soothe irritation and distress in the respiratory system. **It can be used to treat coughing, sore throats, bronchitis and chest tightness.** Some believe that it works because it calms the mind and the relationship between physical symptoms of distress and mental anxiety.

7) Mistletoe and Menstrual Pain

If you are unfortunate enough to suffer from very painful menstrual cramps and pain, mistletoe is a potential natural remedy to ease your symptoms. **It can soothe muscular spasms and reduce inflammation as well as having a positive calming impact on your mind.**

MYRRH

LATIN NAME Commiphora myrrha

Kingdom: Plantae
Clade: Tracheophytes
Clade: Angiosperms
Clade: Eudicots
Clade: Rosids
Order: Sapindales
Family: Burseraceae
Genus: *Commiphora*

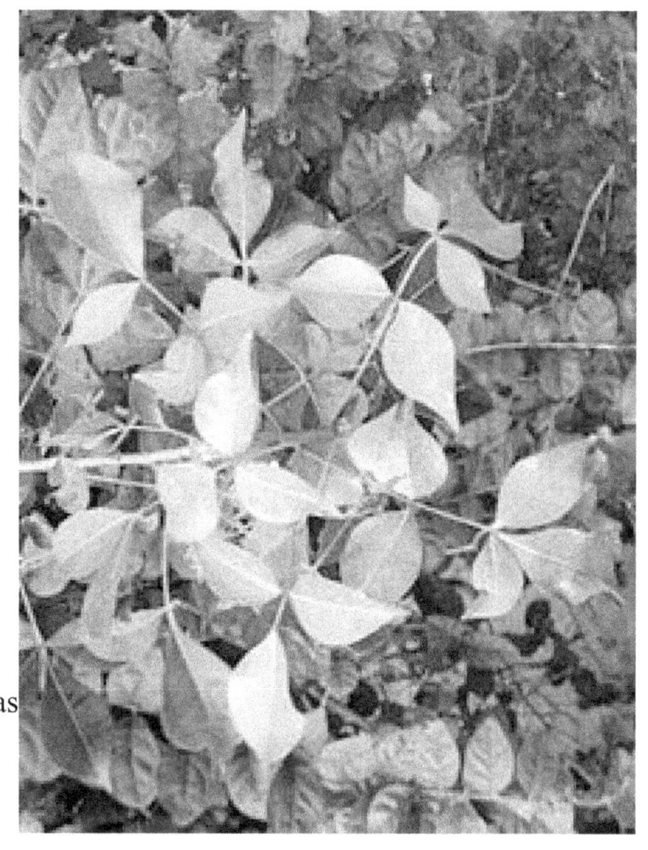

Composition of Drug

Myrrh consists of oleo-gum resin extruded from the stems of *Commiphora molmol* Engler [Fam. Burseraceae], then air-dried, as well as its preparations in effective dosage.

Myrrh can also originate from other *Commiphora* species, if the chemical composition is comparable to the official drug.

Uses
Topical treatment of mild inflammations of the oral and pharyngeal mucosa.

Contraindications
None known.

Side Effects
None known.

Interactions with Other Drugs

None known.

Dosage

Unless otherwise prescribed:

- Myrrh tincture:
  Dab 2 - 3 times daily with undiluted tincture;
- As a rinse or gargle:
  5 - 10 drops in a glass of water.
- In dental powders:
  10 percent of powdered resin.

Mode of Administration

Powdered resin, myrrh tincture and other galenical preparations for topical use.

Action: Astringent

HISTORY

Through the time span of its rich history and usage, myrrh's fragrant and alluring aroma has been an inspiration to writers, poets, aristocrats, merchants, priests and civilizations, and has held an esteemed position in many cultures as an effective medicinal herb. The name myrrh comes from the Arabic word *morr* which means "bitter."

In fifth century B.C., Herodotus noted that the Egyptians used myrrh as an embalming agent. Egyptian women also burned myrrh pellets to rid their homes of fleas as well as to mask the stench of the day due to lack of proper hygiene and sanitary conditions (Innvista).

During the time of Christ, myrrh was one of the most highly valued commodities in trade and was cherished as a precious oil (ABC). It was used by the Hebrew people to anoint the altar and sacred vessels of the Jewish Temple, and was one of the three gifts given by the Wise Men to Jesus Christ when they paid Him tribute (Christopher, <u>SNH</u> 505). Myrrh was used in a purification procedure used to beautify the women who were presented before King Ahasurerus of the Medes and Persians when he was choosing a queen. This is mentioned in Esther 2:12, "…for so were the days of their purifications accomplished, to wit, six months with oil of myrrh, and six months with sweet odors, and with other things for the purifying of the women"(<u>Rainbow Study Bible</u> 636-637).

Myrrh has a long history of therapeutic and medicinal use in Indian Ayurvedic medicine. In this system of medicine, it is currently used internally to treat mouth ulcers, gingivitis, pharyngitis, respiratory conditions, stomatitis (inflammation of the mouth), several female complaints, and topically for ulcers and gum conditions. Sometime during the seventh century A.D., it was introduced into the Chinese and Tibetan systems of medicine. The *Gyu-zhi*, or *Four Tantras*, by Chandranandana, was the earliest Indian medical text to be translated into Tibetan during the eighth century A.D.(ABC). The Chinese call myrrh, mo yao and have used it in Chinese medicine as a wound healer since before the time of the Tang Dynasty (Innvista). In this form of medicine myrrh has been used to treat impact injury, incised wounds, hard to heal wounds, sinew and bone pain, menstrual blockages, and hemorrhoids, as well as pain and stiffness, swelling, bruising, blood stagnation and as a dissolvent for masses and fibroids (ABC)(About).

Myrrh was among the 65 herbs that Samuel Thomson used regularly in his herbal practice. Samuel Thomson was a self-taught American herbalist, who brought an herbal revolution to the United States that angered doctors of his day. Time after time he proved that herbs could be more effective than medicines such as mercury that were being used in the late 1700's. He was particularly fond of myrrh's antiseptic and cleansing properties (Griggs 161). Dr. John R. Christopher, was a Naturopath and Herbalist who practiced and taught herbology in the mid-1900's during a time when herbs were scorned by the medical profession at large. *The School of Natural Healing*, was one of the legacies Dr. Christopher left behind that contains much of his herbal knowledge and experience. In this book, he says, "Myrrh stimulates the flow of blood to the capillaries and gives a warm and pleasant sensation of the stomach. It increases the number of white blood corpuscles up to four times of the original, when there is a need for fighting infection, and quickens the heart action. It enhances the eliminative function of the mucous membranes in the bronchi and genito-urinary tract, at the same time disinfecting those tissues and reducing mucus discharge from those specific areas." Dr. Christopher also included instruction on how to use myrrh various applications. He gave preparations for sore throats, ulceration of the mouth, tongue or throat, chronic diarrhea, skin conditions, bronchitis, bad breath, colic, flatulence, hemorrhoids, diphtheria, shock, congestion, rheumatism, sprains, bruises, and as a treatment for worms (500-504).

Myrrh gum resin and myrrh tincture are both recognized as official in the *German Pharmacopeia*, and approved in the Commission E monographs. The tincture form is official in the Standard License monographs where it is used as a component of many dental remedies, mouthwashes, ointments, herbal paints (an herbal preparation "painted" on the skin), and coated tablets. Bed sores, gingivitis, stomatitis, infant oral *Canadensis* (thrush), and relief of prosthesis pressure marks are some of the ways these preparations are applied. Myrrh was formerly official in the *United States Pharmecopia* and *National Formulary*. In these books, it was indicated as an aromatic, astringent mouthwash. The *British Herbal Compendium* indicates use of this aromatic herb as a gargle to treat pharyngitis, tonsillitis and as a mouthwash for gingivitis and ulcers. Its use is also suggested externally for sinusitis and minor skin inflammations. In France, topical use of myrrh is approved for the treatment of nasal congestion from the common cold, small wounds and as an anodyne to treat infections of the buccal cavity (cavity between the jaws and cheeks), and the oropharnyx (part of the throat at the back of the neck, including the back of the tongue, the soft palate and tonsils). It is also noted in the *Pharmacopia of Austria,* and the *British Herbal Pharmacopoeia* as an antiseptic (ABC).

CHEMICAL CONSTITUENTS

Many of the chemical constituents found in myrrh are currently being studied for their activities on various conditions and diseases. Research on myrrh is just showing that those before us had wisdom in the area of medicine long before we give them credit. Myrrh has several main constituents. These are from about 9 to17% volatile oil, 20 to 40% alcohol-soluble resin, and approximately 30 to 60% water-soluble gum (ABC).

The volatile oil contains heerabolene, acadinene, elemol, eugenol, cuminaldehyde, numerous furanosesquiterpenes including furanodiene, furanodienone, curzerenone, lindestrene, 2-methoxyfuranodiene, and 3-epi-alpha-amyrin and a few other compounds (Hoffmann)(Chromadex). Myrrh is also credited to have myrcene and *a*-camphorene, as well as a few steroids including Z-guggulsterol, and I, II, III guggulsterol. Herbs that contain volatile oils are aromatic and tend to be antimicrobial and disperse congestion (McDonald). Steroids found in plants are known as sterols and resemble human steroids in structure. Modern clinical studies have shown that they play a role as analgesic and anti-inflammatory agents (Singh and Sanhu).

The resin in myrrh is made up of alpha-, beta-, and gamma-commiphoric acids, heeraboresene, alpha-, and beta-heerabomyrrhols and commiferin (Hoffmann). Resins are a diverse group of chemical compounds that share chemical characteristics such as insolubility in water, solubility at room temperature, and lack of a nitrogen group. "Resin compounds formed with sugar are called glycoresins; those formed with oils are called oleoresins" (Isnar). According to the UCLA Biomedical Library, resin does not decay and is found to be bacteriostatic (Darling). Resins are soluble in alcohol or ethanol which is why myrrh is often prepared as a tincture.

The water soluble gum or mucilage content in myrrh is about 30 to 60%. It is "… composed mainly of acidic polysaccharide with galactose, 4-O-methyl-glucuronicacid, and arabinose in a ratio of 8:7:2, with approximately 18 to 20% proteins" (ABC). "Mucilage is a thick, glutinous substance related to the natural gums, comprised usually of protein, polysaccharides, and uranides. It swells but does not dissolve in water" (Columbian Electronic Encyclopedia). Mucilage is often used in emollient or demulcent preparations. This could account for the many uses of myrrh in cosmetic and beautifying preparations that have been used in centuries past as well as the preparations on the market today.

Myrrh also contains ash, salts, sulphates, benzoates, malates, acetates of potassium, formic acid, acetic acid and many more constituents (Chem). Tannins are also found in myrrh. "Several actions have been attributed to tannins including antidysenteric, antimutagenic, antimephritic, antioxidant, antiviral, bactericide, cancer-preventative, hepatoprotective, pesticide, psychotropic, and viricide properties"(Ultimate Water Massage).

According to the *PDR for Herbal Medicines, 2nd Edition*, some of the chief components in myrrh are sesquiterpenes (535). Sesquiterpenes are a large family of C15 -isoprenoid molecules found in plants, microbes, and some marine organisms. Isoprenoids also called terpenoids, are "…unsaturated hydrocarbons found in essential oils and oleoresins of plants…"(American Heritage Dictionary). They are hydrocarbons with 15 carbon atoms and are naturally occurring alcohols that very rarely exist as volatile oils. When distilled from plants, these bitter constituents stimulate the glands and the liver, and have antibacterial, antifungal, anti-allergen, antispasmodic, and anti-inflammatory properties (Natural Healthcare)(Hobbs). The Department of Food Science at Rutgers University, New Brunswick, New Jersey, found that the gum exudates of *Commiphora myrrha* contain six sesquiterpenes including two new furanosesquiterpenes. One of the latter exhibited cytotoxic activity (destroys specific cells) against a MCF-7 breast tumor cell line (Zhu et al 1460-1462). Myrrh oil "…has one of the highest levels of sesquiterpenes, a class of compounds that has direct effects on the hypothalamus, pituitary and amygdale, the seat of our emotions" (Essential Oils Desk Reference).

MEDICINAL QUALITIES

Traditionally, myrrh has been used orally to treat arthritis, digestive complaints, painful menstruation, respiratory infections, leprosy, syphilis, cancers, sore throats, asthma, coughs, and bad breath. Topically, myrrh has been used to treat muscular pains, arthritis, ulcers, sores, wounds, weak gums, loose teeth, bacterial and fungal skin infections and acne (Innvista)(E Drug Digest). Myrrh has often been mixed with golden seal powder and sprinkled on the umbilical chord stumps of newborn babies. This application is still used today. It has also been used in tincture form to treat abscesses (Christopher and Gileadi 68, 158). Traditional Chinese use of myrrh includes treatment for many of these conditions as well as for pain and stiffness, swelling, bruising, blood stagnation, and as a dissolvent for masses and fibroids (ABC). In Ayurvedic medicine, myrrh is used as a blood cleanser and for improving the intellect (Innvista).

Today, use of myrrh is very similar although scientists are discovering a few of the reasons why myrrh works as it does. Myrrh is thought to stimulate the production of white blood cells, making it a possible treatment of conditions where an antimicrobial agent is needed. One source suggests using myrrh as a specific treatment for "infections in the mouth such as mouth ulcers, gingivitis, pyorrhea, as well as the catarrhal problems of pharyngitis and sinusitis. Myrrh may also help with laryngitis and respiratory complaints. Systemically, it is of value in the treatment of boils and similar conditions as well as glandular fever and brucellosis (a widespread infectious febrile disease affecting cattle, swine, and goats and sometimes man). It is often used as part of an approach to the treatment of the common cold. Externally it is healing to the skin and an antiseptic for wounds and abrasions (Hoffmann). Commission E, a body of scientists that set standards for herbal usage in Germany, has endorsed the use of powdered myrrh as a treatment for mild inflammations of the mouth and throat due to myrrh's tannin content (Duke 141).

In a letter to the journal *Nature*, researchers from the University of Florence gave a report on their study of myrrh as an analgesic. They tested its effect on mice that had been set on a hot metal plate to see if their level of pain tolerance increased. Their findings showed that myrrh did have an analgesic affect on the mice. The researchers also isolated three sesquiterpenes from myrrh and tested them on the mice. These sesquiterpenes were: furanoeudesma-1,3-diene, curzarene and furanodiene. They found that furanodiene was not effective, but that furanoeudesma-1,3-diene and curzarene increased the amount of pain tolerance in the mice. Further testing done by these researchers "…suggested that furanoeudesma-1,3-diene may affect opioid receptors in brain membranes, which influence the perception of pain" (Herbalgram). Another research group came up with similar results. In this study, researchers found that when a dose of 500 mg/kg body weight of the petroleum extract of the oleo-gum resin of *Commiphora molmol* was given, carrageenan induced inflammation was significantly reduced. The extract also showed significant antipyretic activity in mice (Tariq M. et al. 381-382).

Research shows that a group of compounds known as sesquiterpene lactones, show strong antibacterial and antifungal activity against *Staphylococcus* (involved with myriad infections, internal and external), *Candida albicans* (commonly responsible for yeast infections), and pathogenic strains of *E. coli* (often involved with food poisoning and diarrhea) (Upton). In an issue of *Planta Medica*, myrrh was studied for its anesthetic, antibacterial and antifungal properties. The researchers reported that after extracting and purifying eight sesquiterpenes from *Commiphora molmol*, they found that a "mixture of furanodiene-6-one and methoxyfuranoguaia-9ene-8-one showed antibacterial and antifungal activity against standard pathogenic strains of *Escherichia coli, Staphylococcus aureus, Pseudomonas aeruginosa* and *Candida   albicans…*" "These compounds also had local anesthetic activity, blocking the inward sodium current of excitable mammalian membranes"(Dolara et al. 356-358).

The Department of Pharmacology in Saudi Arabia reported research which showed that pretreatment with myrrh oleo-gum resin before introducing 80% ethanol, indomethacin, or a mixture of both into the stomach, provided dose-dependent protection against ulcergenic effects. It also protected against depletion of stomach wall mucus, reduction in protein and nucleic acid concentrations and protected against histopathological lesions on the stomach wall lining including necrosis, erosion, congestion, and hemorrhage. The researchers attribute these affects to myrrh's free radical-scavenging, thyroid-stimulating and prostaglandin-inducing properties
(al-Harbi et al., <u>Anti-ulcer</u> 141-150).

Out of six indigenous African plants studied to prevent thrombosis in mice, myrrh exhibited the strongest antithrombotic activity. The other plants screened in this study were *Azadiractha indica, Bridelia ferruginea, Garcinia kola, and Curcuma longa* (Olajide 231-232).

Myrrh and aloe gums were shown to effectively increase glucose tolerance in normal and diabetic rats in a study done with plants that Kuwaiti diabetics use (A-Awadi and Fumaa 37-41).

Schistosomiasis is a parasitic infection of a type of blood fluke that is widespread over Asia, Africa and tropical America. Currently, treatment of schistosomiasis is chemotherapy with the drug praziquantel. Resistance to this drug has now been seen, so researchers are considering alternative drugs. A study was done on 204 patients infected with the disease. All but twelve of the cases had previously been treated with praziquantel. Four of the twelve were unable to undergo the praziquantel treatment due to vomiting immediately after ingesting the drug. Two different types of parasites were found in these cases, *S. haematobium* and *S. mansoni*. Some of the patients were infected with one type of parasite and some had both. Myrrh was given at 10 mg/kg body weight for three days to all the patients, with a cure rate of 91.7%. In the twelve cases that had received no prior chemotherapy treatment, the cure was 100% effective. Re-treatment with the same dose was given to the cases that did not respond from the first treatment with a cure rate of 76.5%, increasing the overall cure rate to 98.09%. The treatment was tolerated well with only mild side effects reported in 11.8% of the cases of which giddiness, somnolence, or mild fatigue were the most common. Twenty healthy patients were also given the same treatment simultaneously with no reported side affects (Sheir et al. 700-704). Another study done at the Cairo University, Egypt, in 2004 consisted of 1019 individuals infected with the same two parasites as the above study, *S. haematobium* and *S. mansoni*. In this pilot study, Mirazid, a drug completely derived from myrrh consisting of 8 parts resin and 3.5 parts volatile oils, was given to all the patients. The dosage was 2 capsules of 600 mg given on an empty stomach an hour before breakfast for six days. Upon examination three months after the treatment, it was found that Mirazid was 97.4% effective on *S. haematobium* and 96.2% effective on *S. mansoni* with no reported side effects. Those that did not respond showed a marked reduction of egg intensity. The researches concluded that Mirazid was a safe and effective treatment (Abo-Madyan, Morsy and Motawea 423-426).

A similar problem today especially in Egypt, is the infection of fascioliasis, a liver fluke which infects sheep, goats and cattle. Humans can become infected by this parasite through eating contaminated meat. Researchers at Cairo University, Egypt, studied myrrh's effect on seven patients infected with this disease. The drug extract Mirazid was given to all the cases in doses of 12 mg/kg body weight per day, for six consecutive days. The patients showed a dramatic drop in fecal egg count at the end of three weeks and had a complete cure with no sign of eggs three months after treatment. The researchers that piloted this study feel that although their study was done on a small scale, they were able to prove that myrrh was an effective treatment for this disorder (Massoud et al. 96-99).

Another study was done on the efficacy of myrrh on the larvae of *S. littoralis*, the cotton leafworm. The results showed that although myrrh is not as effective as the chemical insecticides on the market today, it was effective in killing many of the larvae and when added to the chemical insecticides, it increased their effectiveness (Shonouda, Farrag and Salama 347-356).

Exciting new research on myrrh has been published in the last couple years, supporting ancient use of myrrh as a cancer cure. Co-researcher, Mohamed M. Rafi, Ph.D., is Assistant Professor in the Department of Food Science at Rutgers University in New Brunswick, New Jersey. Rafi and his colleagues believe myrrh works by inactivating a protein called Bcl-2 which is overproduced by cancer cells found particularly in breast and prostate cancers. This action in myrrh may be due to the high number of sesquiterpenes myrrh contains. Rafi reports, "The myrrh compound definitely appears to be unique in this way; it is working where other compounds have failed." "It's a very exciting discovery," says Rafi, "I'm optimistic that this compound can be developed into an anticancer drug." In his laboratory research he also found that the myrrh compound inactivated MCF-7, a protein found in many breast tumor cells that has been resistant to traditional treatment. Although myrrh is estimated to be 100 times less potent as other anticancer drugs such as paclitaxel, vinblastine and vincristine, it seems to be able to kill cancer cells without killing healthy cells, something the other treatments aren't able to accomplish. It also doesn't build up resistance as the other drugs do. Rafi says, "This is very exciting news; the fact that something that is so safe…can actually kill cancer cells - this could be the basis for a very important new treatment." Skeptics are cautious however, and Rafi warns, "The research is still much too new to make any recommendations of any kind about myrrh supplements." Mohamed Rafi's studies were published in the Nov. 26, 2001 issue of the *Journal of Natural Products* (Rutger's News) (Bouchez). Earlier, in 1994 another study showed the anti-carcinogenic potential of *Commiphora molmol*. The study took mice that had Ehrlich-solid-tumors and evaluated the total count and viability of the tumors before and after 25 and 50 days of treatment. 250 and 500 mg/kg body weight per day was given to the mice. The anti-tumor potential of myrrh was found to be comparable to the standard cytotoxic drug cyclophosphamide (al-Harbi et al., <u>Anticarcinogenic 337-347</u>).

"Myrrh oil may help asthma, athlete's foot, *Candida*, coughs, eczema, digestion, fungal infection, gingivitis, gum infections, hemorrhoids, mouth ulcers, ringworm, sore throats, skin conditions (chapped and cracked), wounds and wrinkles." It is also indicated for use in "…bronchitis, diarrhea, dysentery, hypothyroidism, stretch marks, thrush, ulcers, vaginal thrush and viral hepatitis" (<u>Essential Oils Desk Reference</u>). A study done by the Dental Research Center at the College of Dentistry, University of Tennessee, determined that myrrh oil has cytotoxic activity on human gingival fibroblasts and epithelial cells (Tipton et al. 337-347).

DOSAGES

As the resins in myrrh do not readily dissolve in water, the best way to prepare myrrh is in tincture form. Tinctured myrrh is typically made in a 1:5 ratio meaning 1 part myrrh and 5 parts menstrum. The menstrum used in this particular tincture is 90% ethanol alcohol, and 10% water. The tincture preparation of myrrh is indicated for use as a gargle or mouthwash. 5 to 10 drops (one-sixteenth to one-eighth of a teaspoon) added to 8 ounces of water is the standard dosage for both these uses. Myrrh tincture can also be applied straight on sore gums, lip or mouth tissue up to three times daily. The diluted tincture, which can be made or bought

commercially, can be used as a skin wash or as a vaginal douche for thrush. Amounts for these applications vary (E Drug Digest). The tincture of myrrh can also be used for infections, feverish conditions from head colds to glandular fevers, respiratory conditions and as an ingredient in expectorant preparations (Purple Sage). It can also be used undiluted as a paint for ulcers and wounds (Heilpflanzen).

Diluted myrrh essential oil consisting of 10 drops myrrh and 25 ml water, can be applied to wounds and chronic ulcers. It can also be added to a lotion that is used to treat hemorrhoids. 1 ml oil in 15 ml almond or sunflower oil is an excellent chest rub for bronchitis and colds with thick phlegm. A preparation used for vaginal thrush can be made by using 10 drops of the oil and 30 grams of cocoa butter and formed into twenty-four pessaries. An infusion of myrrh can be made by powdering 1 to 2 teaspoons of myrrh, pouring over it a cup of boiled water and letting it steep for 10 to 15 minutes. One cup three times a day would be the optimal dosage for feverish or phlegm conditions or when the immune system is low.

Another way of taking myrrh is in capsule form. One 200 mg capsule can be taken up to five times a day as an alternative to the tincture or infusion for internal usage (Purple Sage). Although it may be more palatable to take myrrh in this form, the benefits of taking any herb are thought to be more effective when the herb is tasted. This is because taste stimulates the glands in the mouth and the herb often diffuses into the blood stream through the capillaries in the mouth.

OAK BARK

LATIN NAME Quercus alba

Kingdom: Plantae
Clade: Tracheophytes
Clade: Angiosperms
Clade: Eudicots
Clade: Rosids
Order: Fagales
Family: Fagaceae
Genus: *Quercus*
Subgenus: *Quercus* subg. *Quercus*
Section: *Quercus* sect. *Quercus*
Species: **Q. alba**

Quercus cortex
Eichenrinde

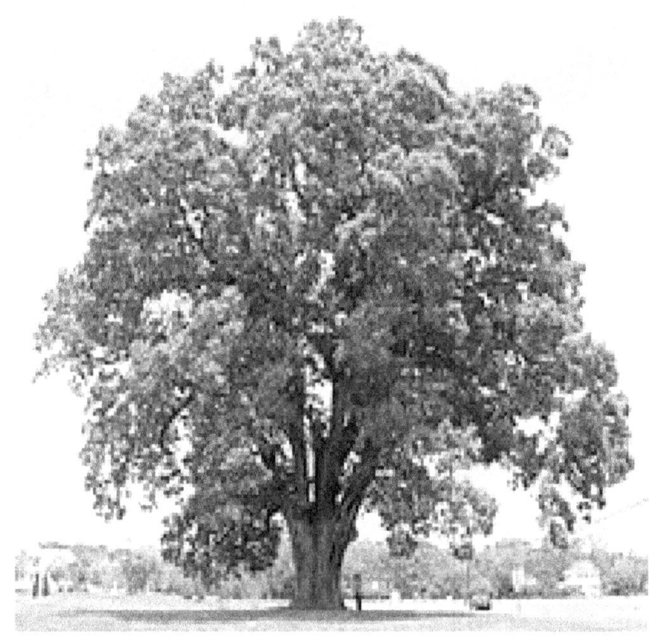

Name of Drug

Quercus cortex, oak bark.

Composition of Drug

Oak bark consists of the dried bark of young branches and saplings of *Quercus robur* L.and/or *Q. petraea* (Mattuschka) Lieblein [Fam.Fagaceae], harvested in the spring, as well as their preparations in effective dosage.

The drug contains tannins.

Uses
External:

- Inflammatory skin diseases.

Internal:

- Nonspecific, acute diarrhea, and local treatment of mild inflammation of the oral cavity and pharyngeal region, as well as genital and anal area.

Contraindications

Internal:

- None known.

External:

- Skin damage over a large area.

Baths:

- Full baths should not be taken, regardless of the active ingredients in the bath, under the following conditions:
    - weeping eczema and skin damage covering a large area; febrile and infectious diseases; cardiac insufficiency stages III and IV (NYHA); hypertonia state IV (WHO).

Side Effects
None known.

Interactions with Other Drugs

External:

- None known.

Internal:

- The absorption of alkaloids and other alkaline drugs may be reduced or inhibited.

Dosage

Unless otherwise prescribed:

Internal:
Daily dosage:

- 3 g of drug;
- equivalent preparations.

For rinses, compresses and gargles:

- 20 g drug per 1 liter of water; equivalent preparations.

For full and partial baths:

- 5 g drug per 1 liter of water; equivalent preparations.

Mode of Administration

Comminuted herb for decoctions and other galenical preparations for internal and topical use.

Duration of Administration

If diarrhea persists longer than 3 - 4 days, a physician must be consulted.

Other areas of application:

- Not more than 2 - 3 weeks.

Actions

Astringent
Virustatic

Health Benefits of White Oak Bark

White oak bark contains numerous nutrients including vitamin B12, iron, and potassium. It also has a **tannin content somewhere between 15 to 20%**. These **tannins** and the nutrients are believed to be responsible for the bark's health benefits.

It is used to treat a range of sicknesses including diarrhea relief, varicose veins, and the cold or flu. **This impressive tree certainly deserves its scientific Latin name of Quercus alba which means 'fine tree'.**

White oak bark is on the GRAS list which means that it is generally recognized to be safe and is available in several different forms. The German Commission E has approved it for use as a treatment for diarrhea and it was listed in the US Pharmacopoeia as long ago as 1916 because of its antiseptic and astringent qualities.

The Native Americans were long aware of the beneficial properties of the bark. They used it for antiseptic, astringent and anti-inflammatory purposes before settlers to North America picked up the mantle and learned how to use it.

Early settlers used the bark to treat numerous illnesses and to help heal wounds and skin problems. While the bark is considered to be the most beneficial part of the tree, the acorns have also been used to make a hot drink that could help control bowel conditions.

1) Astringent Properties

White oak bark has astringent properties because of the high level of tannins present in its bark. **Astringents work by constricting or shrinking the body's tissues on the inside and the outside.** Natural astringents like white oak bark have a variety of therapeutic benefits.

Internally, they can help treat bleeding, varicose veins and reduce diarrhea. They also perform some useful external functions and can help limit bleeding from the skin as well as other skin complaints like burns, bruises, wrinkles, and eczema. **Its anti-inflammatory and antiseptic properties are also excellent for the skin.**

2) Antiseptic Properties

The tannin content of the white oak bark is also responsible for its antiseptic properties which can help to prevent and treat both internal and external infections. **The tannins bind with the proteins present in the tissues which help to stave off harmful pathogens and bacteria.**

White oak bark has been effectively used against urinary tract infections, dysentery, and vaginal infections. To treat any internal problems, you can take white oak bark supplements in capsule, tincture or tea form.

3) For External Use

White oak bark can also be used externally to protect against skin infections and to help treat a number of skin issues. **It has been successfully used to treat poison ivy and to soothe the pain and inflammation from bee stings and bug bites.**

When applied to the skin, it may also help speed up the healing process from minor wounds, cuts, scrapes, and burns. It can even be a helpful natural remedy for mouth ulcers and herpes.

You can apply it directly to your skin or make a cold compress with white oak bark tea or liquid extract. **An alternative is to add a cupful of dried bark to your bathtub and letting your skin soak it up.**

4) Diuretic Properties

White oak bark also has natural diuretic properties meaning that it can help promote both the frequency of urination and the amount of urine you produce. Diuretics like white oak bark are a useful, natural alternative to pharmaceutical diuretic medication for those who would prefer to steer clear of pharmaceuticals.

As a diuretic, white oak bark can help improve the health of your bladder, help treat urinary tract infections and even eliminate kidney stones caused by the build-up of uric acid in the bloodstream.

5) Respiratory Conditions

White oak bark can help to treat infections of the respiratory tract. **Its saponin content means that it might have expectorant properties suitable for getting rid of mucus and phlegm from the respiratory system.**

A tea made from the herb is often used to treat coughs, colds, bronchitis and other respiratory conditions.

6) Oral Health

In the days before dentistry, the native Americans used white oak bark to help treat oral infections and other dental issues like gingivitis and toothache.

The bark contains antibacterial and antiseptic properties which can help prevent and treat oral infections as well as being an astringent that will help oral sores to heal. **You can make a natural mouthwash by boiling up a cup of white oak bark tea and allowing it to cool.**

How to take White Bark

White bark extract is available in several different forms.

- **In capsule form,** the recommended daily dose is around one gram preferably taken with some food.
- **As a liquid extract,** the strength of each product will vary but the dosage range is usually in the region of 30 to 60 drops diluted with water to be taken two or three times each day.

White oak bark can also be applied topically to help with skin conditions and minor wounds. **When applied to the skin, it can help stop bleeding while forming an antiseptic layer that protects the wound and allows for healing to take place with less risk of any infection.**

It can also be used as an antiseptic hemorrhoid wash or douche. Pastes made with oak bark extract, flour and water can also help to draw out stings or splinters because of its astringent qualities.

How to Make White Oak Bark Tincture

As long as you have access tom the tree, it is not hard to make your own white bark tincture. **These are the steps to follow:**

You will need white oak tree twigs, some pruners, a vegetable peeler, a mason jar and some vodka,

- Gather up plenty of white oak tree twigs. (using the bark from the twigs is less likely to damage the tree than using the bark from the trunk)
- Clean any dirt or debris from the twigs.
- Peel the bark from the twigs with your vegetable peeler.
- Put the bark into a mason jar then cover the twigs with your vodka.
- Cover and tore the jar in a dark, cool place and let the mixture sit for at least a few weeks but preferably a month before using it.
- When the extract is ready, strain the mixture into a bowl using a strainer lined with muslin or some other cotton material.
- **Make sure that you squeeze down on the remaining bark with a spoon to extract all the goodness from the bark.**

ONION

LATIN NAME Allium cepa

Kingdom: Plantae
Clade: Tracheophytes
Clade: Angiosperms
Clade: Monocots
Order: Asparagales
Family: Amaryllidaceae
Subfamily: Allioideae
Genus: *Allium*
Species: **A. cepa**

Allii cepae bulbus
Zwiebel

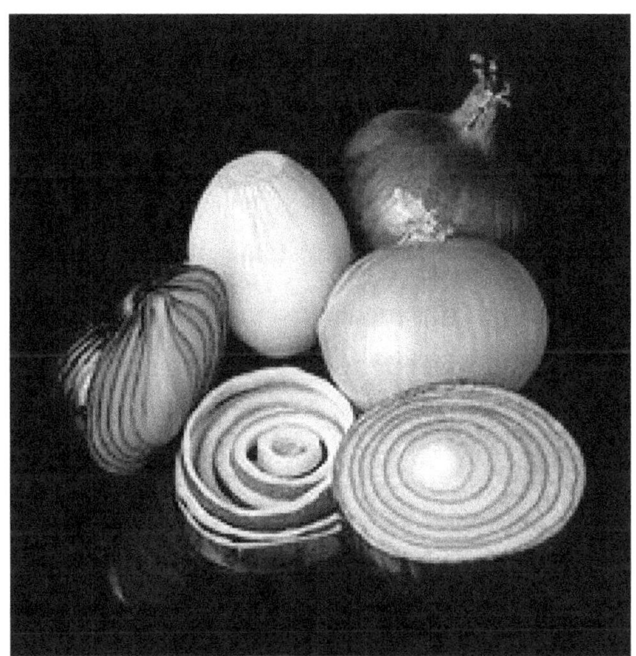

Name of Drug

Allii cepae bulbus, onion.

Composition of Drug

Onion consists of the fresh or dried, thick and fleshy leaf sheaths and stipules of *Allium cepa* L.[Fam.Alliaceae], as well as their preparations in effective dosage.

It contains alliin and similar sulfur compounds, essential oil, peptides and flavonoids.

Uses
Loss of appetite, prevention of atherosclerosis.

Contraindications
None known.

Side Effects
None known.

Interactions with Other Drugs

None known.

Dosage

Unless otherwise prescribed:

Average daily dosage:

- 50 g of fresh onions or 20 g of dried drug;
- equivalent preparations.

Mode of Administration

Cut onions, pressed juice from fresh onions and other oral galenical preparations.

Duration of Administration

Note: If onion preparations are used over several months, the daily maximum amount for diphenylamine is 0.035 g.

Actions

Antibacterial
Lipid and blood pressure-lowering
Inhibition of thrombocyte aggregation

HISTORY

The onion or allium family is a large and diverse one containing over 500 species. It has not one but four possible wild plants it could have evolved from all of which grow in the central Asian region. Because onions are small and their tissues leave little or no trace, there is no conclusive evidence about the exact location and time of their origin. Many archaeologists, botanists and food historians believe onion originated in central Asia.

It is presumed that our predecessors discovered and started eating wild onions very early, long before farming or even writing was invented. Very likely, this humble vegetable was a staple in prehistoric diet.

Most researchers agree that the onion has been cultivated for 5000 years or more and that they were first grown in Iran and West Pakistan. However, the archaeological and literary evidence suggests cultivation probably took place around two thousand years later in ancient Egypt. Since onions grew wild in various regions, they were probably consumed for thousands of years and domesticated simultaneously all over the world. This happened alongside the cultivation of leeks and garlic and it is thought that the "… slaves who built the pyramids were fed radishes and onions".

For over 4000 years, onions have been used for medicinal purposes. Egyptians numbered over 8000 onion alleviated ailments. There is documentation from very early times, which describe the onions importance as a food and its use in art, medicine and mummification.

Egyptians buried onions along with their Pharaohs. The Egyptians saw eternal life in the anatomy of the onion because of its circle-within-a-circle structure. In mummies, onions have frequently been found in the "…pelvic regions of the body, in the thorax, flattened against the ears and in front of the collapsed eyes. Flowering onions have been found in the chest, and onions have been found attached to the soles of the feet and along the legs". King Ramses IV, who died in 1160 B.C., was "…entombed with onions in his eye sockets".

Some Egyptologists theorize that onions may have been used because it was believed that their strong scent and/or magical powers would prompt the dead to breathe again. Other Egyptologists believe it was because onions were known for their strong antiseptic qualities, which were construed as magical, and could be useful in the afterlife.

The onion is mentioned as a funeral offering and onions are depicted on the banquet tables of the great feasts and they were shown upon the altars of the gods. Paintings of onions appear on the inner walls of the pyramids and in the "…tombs of both the Old Kingdom and the New Kingdom". Frequently, a priest is pictured holding onions in his hand or covering an altar with a bundle of their leaves or roots.

Onions grew in Chinese gardens as early as 5000 years ago and they are referenced in some of the oldest Vedic writings from India. There is evidence that the Sumerians were growing onions as early as 2500 B.C. One Sumerian text dated to about 2500 B.C. tells of "…someone plowing over the city governor's onion patch".

Onions may be one of the earliest cultivated crops because they were less perishable than other foods of the time. They were transportable, easy to grow and could be grown in a variety of soils and climates. In addition, the onion was useful for sustaining human life. Onions prevented thirst and could be dried and preserved for later consumption when food might be scarce.

Onions are mentioned to have been eaten by the Israelites in the Bible. In Numbers 11:5 the children of Israel lament the meager desert diet enforced by the Exodus: "We remember the fish, which we did eat in Egypt freely, the cucumbers and the melons and the leeks and the onions and the garlic".

In India as early as the sixth century B.C., the famous medical treatise Charaka - Sanhita celebrates the onion as medicine "…a diuretic, good for digestion, the heart, the eyes and the joints".

It was the Romans who introduced the onion family to Europe. The Romans ate onions regularly and carried them on journeys to their provinces in England and Germany. Pliny the Elder, Roman's observer, wrote of Pompeii's onions and cabbages. Before he was overcome and killed by the volcano's heat and fumes, he catalogued the roman beliefs about the efficacy of the onion to cure vision, induce sleep, heal mouth sores, dog bites, toothaches, dysentery and lumbago. Excavators of the doomed city would later find gardens where, just as Pliny had said, onions had grown. The bulbs had left behind telltale cavities in the ground.

The Roman gourmet Apicius, credited with writing one of the first cookbooks (which dates to the eighth and ninth centuries A.D.), included many references to onions.

The origins of its name are also Roman or at least Latin. The Late Latin name unio was used to describe a species of onion resembling a single white pearl. This was later formed into the basis for the French, "oignon" and then later the English, "Onion".

By the Middle Ages, the three main vegetables of European cooking were beans, cabbage and onions. In addition to serving as a "…food for both the poor and the wealthy…" onions were prescribed to alleviate headaches, snakebites and hair loss. They were also used as rent payments and wedding gifts.

The Greek physician Hippocrates prescribed onions as a diuretic, wound healer and pneumonia fighter. Likewise, Dioscorides, a Greek physician noted several medicinal uses of onions. The Greeks used onions to fortify athletes for the Olympic Games. Before competition, athletes would consume pounds of onions, drink onion juice and rub onions on their bodies.

The first Pilgrims brought onions with them on the Mayflower. However, they found that strains of wild onions already grew throughout North America. Native American Indians used wild onions in a variety of ways, eating them raw or cooked, as a seasoning or as a vegetable. Such onions were also used in syrups, as poultices, as an ingredient in dyes and even as toys. According to diaries of colonists, bulb onions were planted as soon as the Pilgrim farmers could clear the land in 1648.

During World War II the Russian soldiers were so taken with onions ability to prevent infection, that they applied onions to battle wounds as an antiseptic.

And through the ages, there have been countless folk remedies that have ascribed their curative powers to onions, such as putting a sliced onion under your pillow to fight off insomnia.

Yet today, onions are still considered a modern day preventative and healer. These days herbalists use the plant for treating such ailments as earaches, hemorrhoids and high blood pressure. While garlic, another allium, has been highly touted as a cancer preventative, most
people consume far greater quantities of onions.

As Americans search for low-fat, low-salt, and tasty meals, they're eating more Onions …"almost 18 pounds per person per year, which is 50% more than a decade ago". 1 There is great confidence that the onion will be a key in producing long-term health benefit.

CHEMICAL CONSTITUENT

Onions not only provide flavor; they also provide health-promoting phytochemicals as well as nutrients. Onion contains an acrid, volatile principle that stimulates the tear glands and the mucous membranes of the upper respiratory tract.

Of all the healthy compounds contained in onions, two stand out: sulfur and quercetin - both being strong antioxidants. They each have been shown to help neutralize the free radicals in the body, and protect the membranes of the body's cells from damage.

"Antioxidants are compounds that help delay or slow the oxidative damage to cells and tissue of the body. Studies have indicated that quercetin helps to eliminate free radicals in the body, to inhibit low-density lipoprotein oxidation (an important reaction in the atherosclerosis and coronary heart disease), to protect and regenerate vitamin E (a powerful antioxidant) and to inactivate the harmful effects of chelate metal ions".

Major dietary sources of quercetin include tea, onions and apples. Recent studies at Wageningen Agricultural University, the Netherlands, showed that the absorption of quercetin from onions is twice that from tea and more than three times that from apples. Based on studies conducted at The Queen's University at Belfast, Ireland and Wageningen Agricultural University, the "…content of quercetin in onions is estimated to be between 22.40 mg and 51.82 mg per medium-sized onion (100 gram)". Further research at the Agricultural University on Wageningen showed that daily consumption of onions may result in increased accumulation of quercetin in the blood. Studies are in progress to determine whether the increased quercetin accumulation from eating onions translates into significant antioxidant benefit.

White onions contain very little querctin, so it's better to stick with the yellow and red varieties. Most health professionals recommend eating raw onions for maximum benefit, but cooking makes them more versatile and doesn't significantly reduce their potency. In fact, unlike sulfur compounds, quercetin can withstand the heat of cooking as long as it is a low heat.

The strong smell of the onion and its relatives contain thioallyl compound or alliins, and alliins are an amino acid. When cut or crushed, the alliin within the onion is converted by an enzymatic reaction into allicin, this breaks down into sulfide compounds. Sulfide compounds are aromatic and this is what gives the onion, and all the plants in the onion family, their distinctive smell. The cysteine sulphoxides occurring in the genus Allium are precursors for a large number of compounds which are responsible for the typical aroma as well as for the health value of these plants.

Other studies have shown that consumption of onions may be beneficial for reduced risk of certain diseases. Consumption of onions may prevent gastric ulcers by scavenging free radicals and by preventing growth of the ulcer-forming microorganism, Heliobacter pylori.

University of Wisconsin-Madison researchers found that "…the more pungent onions exhibit strong anti-platelet activity. Platelet aggregation is associated with atherosclerosis, cardiovascular disease, heart attack and stroke." A study in progress at the University of Wisconsin is determining the extent to which onion consumption and specific onion compounds affect the in vivo aggregation of blood platelets. "Using an in vivo model, we are beginning to
investigate and, in some cases, confirm the potency of the onion as a blood thinner and platelet inhibitor. Onions may be among the vegetables that will be prized not only for their addition to our cuisine, but for their value-added health characteristics," said Irwin Goldman, Associate Professor of Horticulture, University of Wisconsin-Madison.

A recent study at the University of Bern in Switzerland showed that consumption of 1 g of dry onion per day for 4 weeks increased bone mineral content in rats by more than 17% and mineral density by more than 13% compared to animals fed a controlled diet.

This data suggests onion consumption has the potential to decrease the incidences of osteoporosis. Several studies have shown quercetin to have beneficial effects against many diseases and disorders including cataracts, cardiovascular disease as well as cancer of the breast, colon, ovarian, gastric, lung and bladder.

In addition to quercetin, onions contain the phytochemicals known as disulfides, trisulfides, cepaene, and vinyl dithiins. These compounds have a variety of health-functional properties, including anticancer and antimicrobial activities.

Onions are also a source of vitamin C, potassium, dietary fiber and folic acid. They also contain calcium, iron and have a high protein quality, ratio of mg amino acid/gram protein.

Onions are low in sodium and contain no fat. They are low in calories with only 30 calories per serving, yet add abundant flavor to a wide variety of foods. Onions are also cholesterol free, and provide dietary fiber, vitamin C, vitamin B6, potassium, and other key nutrients.

MEDICINAL QUALITIES

Research shows that onions may help guard against many chronic diseases. That's probably because onions contain generous amounts of the flavonoid quercetin. Studies have shown that quercetin protects against cataracts, cardiovascular disease, and cancer. In addition, onions contain a variety of other naturally occurring chemicals known as organosulfur com-pounds that have been linked to lowering blood pressure and cholesterol levels.7

Onions contain 25 active compounds that appear to inhibit the growth of cancerous cells alliin being the main constituent. Onion has been found to help combat heart disease, inhibit strokes, lower blood pressure and cholesterol, and stimulate the immune system. The potassium salts and the flavonoides that are present perform an anti-inflammatory action. The essential oil is an expectorant, antiseptic, antifungal, anticoagulant, high-blood pressure, antithelmitic, balsamic, rubefciant, and has analgesic properties

In investigating the use of onion in medicinal terms, the onion is found to be a remedy for conditions with symptoms like those which are caused by exposure to onions, such as watering eyes, and a burning and running nose. When looking at the symptoms of cold, it is ironic that we would treat this ailment with an almost like-with-like therapy. Alliums are antibacterial and anti-fungal, so they can help ward off colds and treat colds with sinus congestion that shifts from side to side in the head. Onion will relieve coughs that cause a ripping or tearing pain in the throat or a cough that is merely an irritating dry tickle. The watery and inflamed eyes due to sinus con-gestion and hay fever will be greatly relieved with onion.

The onions ability to relieve congestions especially in the lungs and bronchial tract, is hard to believe until you have actually witnessed the results. The drawing of infection, congestion and colds out of the ear is also remarkable.

The onion will relieve stomach upset and other gastrointestinal disorders and it will also strengthen the appetite.

Onions help prevent thrombosis and reduce hypertension, according to the American Heart Association. 8 The natural constituents of yellow or white onions can "…raise HDL cholesterol by 30% over time", according to Dr. Victor Gurewich of Tufts University.9

The onion is being used for compresses to be applied to the skin for acne, arthritis, and congestion, and used internally for worms. The onion is also known for its diuretic properties.

There have been cases in which the onion has been proven to be so effective as an antiviral that a cut piece of onion placed in a closed off room will prevent the person in the room to be safe from viruses.

Onion will relieve headache centered behind the forehead; earache in children and adults; stuffed up nose with discharge that makes nostrils and upper lip sore or stuffed up nose with discharge from the alternate nostril; toothache, especially in the molar area or the shifting from side to side or from one tooth to another; hoarseness and the early stages of laryngitis; abdominal colic in babies.

Keeping cooler rooms in the home, and getting plenty of fresh air may prevent the symptoms of a stuffy nose and hoarseness.

DOSAGE

Tincture onion using apple cider vinegar. The dosage of this tincture would be 20 to 40 drops 1 to 3 times a day.

Heat 1 -2 medium onions in olive oil for a poultice to be applied to a congested or affected area.

Simmer onion in distilled water for a tea to help with congestion or for a mild diuretic effect.

Powder the onion and place in a 0 or 00 vegetable capsule. Take 1 - 3 capsules 3 times a day.

According to the USDA, to dehydrate onions you need to trim the bulb ends and remove the paper skins. Slice 1/8 to 1/4 inch thick. Onions may be cut into 3/8 to ½ inch dice, but will be slightly less pungent when dried. Dry at 160 degrees Fahrenheit for 1 to 2 hours and then 130 degrees until dry. To tell if they are dry they should feel like paper. Dried onions readily reabsorb moisture, causing deterioration during storage, so they need to be packaged in airtight containers and kept in the freezer.

PARSLEY

Parsley herb and root

LATIN NAME Petroselinum crispum

Kingdom: Plantae
Clade: Tracheophytes
Clade: Angiosperms
Clade: Eudicots
Clade: Asterids
Order: Apiales
Family: Apiaceae
Genus: *Petroselinum*
Species: **P. crispum**

Petroselini herba/radix
Petersilienkraut/wurzel

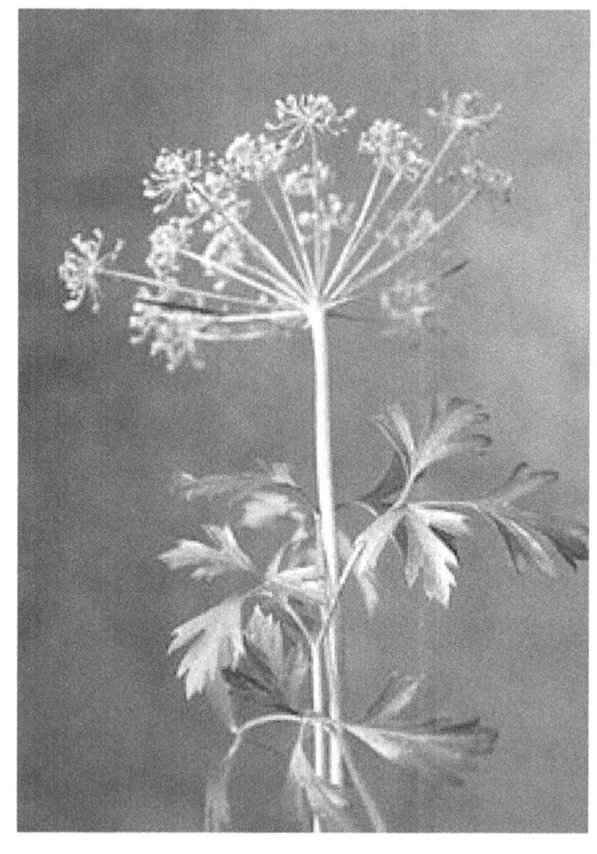

Name of Drug

Petroselini herba, parsley
Petroselini radix, parsley root

Composition of Drug

Parsley, consisting of the fresh or dried plant section of *Petroselinum crispum* (Miller) Nyman ex A. W. Hill [Fam. Apiaceae] and pharmaceutical preparations thereof.

Parsley root, consisting of the dried root of *P.crispum* (Miller) Nyman ex A. W. Hill and pharmaceutical preparations thereof.

Uses
Used in flushing out the efferent urinary tract in disorders of the same and in prevention and treatment of kidney gravel.

Contraindications
Pregnancy; inflammatory kidney conditions.

Irrigation therapy (flushing out treatment) should not be carried out in the case of edema caused by impaired heart or kidney function.

Side Effects

Occasional allergic skin or mucous membrane reactions have been reported.

Interactions with Other Drugs

None known.

Dosage

Unless otherwise prescribed:

Daily dose:

- 6 g of the prepared drug.

Mode of Administration

The crushed drug for infusions as well as other galenical preparations with a comparably small proportion of essential oil to be taken orally.

Warning: The essential oil should not be used in isolation because of its toxicity.

Irrigation Therapy

Large amounts of fluids must be taken.

The leaves, root and seeds of parsley have been used in traditional Greek medicine to treat flatulence, indigestion, spasms and menstrual disorders. Parsley root extract is useful for treating chronic liver and gallbladder diseases because it has diuretic, blood purifying and hepatic qualities. The dried root and essential oil are used in Indian Ayurvedic healing.

Parsley root and parsley are high in vitamins A, C and K and contain copper, iron and iodine. Parsley root is high in sodium, folic acid, potassium, calcium, phosphorus, protein and fiber. It has a substantial amount of flavonoids and is a strong antioxidant.

It is one of the best diuretics I have every used, even in very severe acute situations.

PEPPERMINT

Peppermint leaf

LATIN NAME Mentha × piperita

Kingdom: Plantae
Clade: Tracheophytes
Clade: Angiosperms
Clade: Eudicots
Clade: Asterids
Order: Lamiales
Family: Lamiaceae
Genus: *Mentha*
Species: **M. × piperita**

Menthae piperitae folium
Pfefferminzbltter

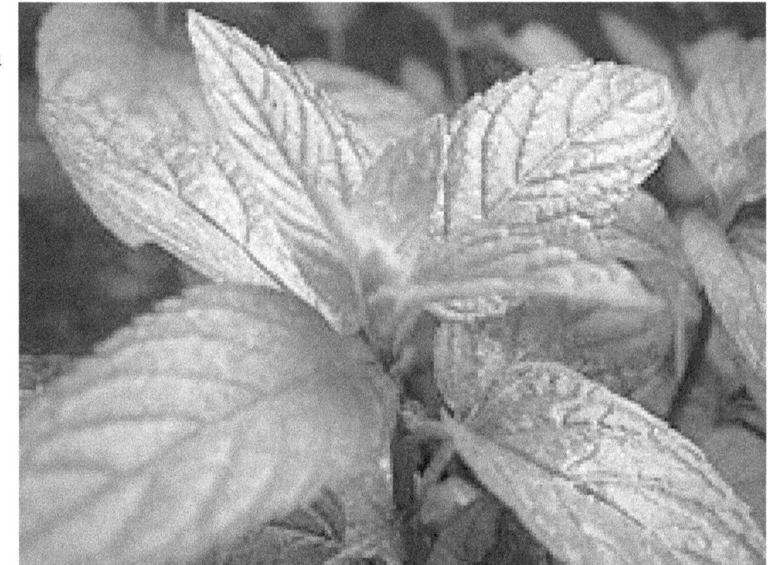

Name of Drug

Menthae piperitae folium, peppermint leaf.

Composition of Drug

Peppermint leaves consist of the fresh or dried leaf of *Mentha* x *piperita* L.
[Fam.Lamiaceae], as well as its preparations in effective dosage.

The herb contains at least 1.2 percent (v/w) essential oil.Other ingredients are tannins
characteristic of *Lamiaceae.*

Uses
Spastic complaints of the gastrointestinal tract as well as gall bladder and bile ducts.

Contraindications
In case of gallstones, use only after consultation with a physician.

Side Effects
None known.

Interactions with Other Drugs

None known.

Dosage

Internal:

- 3 - 6 g of leaf;
- 5 - 15 g of tincture (according to *Erg.B.6*);
- equivalent preparations.

Mode of Administration

Cut herb for infusions, extracts of peppermint leaves for internal use.

Actions

Direct antispasmodic action on the smooth muscle of the digestive tract
Choleretic
Carminative

HISTORY

The value of mint has long been known to mankind. It has been said that the ancient
Assyrians used it in their rituals to their fire god. The Greeks and Romans used mint not
only to flavor their sauces and wines, but also for making crowns to rest on their
noblemen's heads.

According to the Greek philosopher-scientist Theophrastus (300 BC) the botanical name
Mentha was derived from Greek mythology. Mintho was a beautiful nymph who was
loved by Pluto, the god of the underworld. Persephone, who had been abducted by Pluto
to reign with him over his dominion, became very jealous of Mintho and changed her into
a fragrant but lowly plant, the mint.

Biblical mention of this herb states that mint was included among the valuable herbs with
which they paid taxes. It is also speculated that mint was one of the bitter herbs that was
served at The Last Supper.

The Jews of old would strew their synagogue floors with mint leaves so that their
fragrance would scent the air with each footstep. The aromatic fumes that came forth
were supposed to have a sort of sanitizing effect upon the crowded temple gatherings.
This was accomplished by the scent penetrating the lungs and then the bloodstream, like
an airborne antiseptic that would ward off disease.

Mint has even been found in Egyptian tombs dating back to 1,000 BC. They used this
herb to flavor their food and wine. During the Middle Ages, besides a culinary use,

powdered mint leaves were used to whiten their teeth. Chinese medical writings made note of the use of mint since the Tang pen tsao period, which was around 659 AD.

The mint that was written about in all these ancient writings is a forefather of our mint today. In terms of herbal history, peppermint is a fairly new addition to the mint family and herbal medicine.

Peppermint *(Mentha piperita)* is a natural, hybrid cross between watermint *(Mentha aquatica)* and spearmint *(Mentha spicata)* and was first described in 1696 by an English botanist whose name was John Ray (1628-1705). He discovered the pepper flavored mint growing in a field. Its medicinal properties were speedily recognized, and it was admitted into the London Pharmacopoceia in 1721.

Because of the recognition of the importance of this aromatic herb for both culinary and medicinal uses, peppermint was cultivated for commercial purposes. The oldest existing peppermint district is in the neighborhood of Mitcham, in Surrey, where its cultivation from a commercial point of view dates from about 1750, at which period of time only a few acres of ground were devoted to medicinal plants.

One of the main reasons for growing peppermint commercially was to have enough quantity to extract the plant's essential oil which was useful for so many purposes. This oil was in demand not only as a flavoring for cooking, but in flavoring personal care items as well.

The quality of English peppermint oil was superior to other areas of the world where the herb was grown at this time. It had been proven by experience that all parts of the plant do not give the same proportion of oil, and it is more abundant when the plants have been grown in a hot region and have flowered to the best advantage.

At the end of the 18th century, more than 100 acres were growing peppermint. But as late as 1805 there were no stills at Mitcham, to distill the oil, and the herb had to be carried to London for the extraction of its precious oil. By 1850, there were already about 500 acres under cultivation at Mitcham. To this day, the English peppermint plantations are still chiefly located in this district.

The United States, however, is now the most important producer of peppermint oil. Its cultivation was introduced in 1855 to Indiana, Michigan, New York, and Ohio. Thousands of acres were planted with this herb. As of today, this plant grows from

Canada to Florida and everywhere in between. The largest areas of cultivation for the oil is principally done in Indiana, Michigan, Oregon, Washington, and California, with Washington ranking number one in production of the oil.

CHEMICAL CONSTITUENTS

The active constituent of peppermint, found in the leaves and flowering tops, is menthol and is the alcoholic component responsible for the plant's characteristic quality to produce a cooling sensation, as well as its medicinal properties. The presence of various esters, particularly menthyl acetate, impart the familiar minty aroma and flavor so familiar to use.

The quality of peppermint oil is determined by its menthol content, which can vary considerably depending upon the region where it is grown. American peppermint oil contains anywhere from 50 to 78 percent menthol, the English oil from 60 to 70 percent, and the Japanese oil nearly 85 percent.

One source states that there are at least more than one hundred other chemical constituents also present in small amounts in the oil; these include a variety of the compounds known as monoterpenes and the class of chemicals called sesquiterpenes. The exact proportions of these different compounds differ depending on one variety of peppermint to another. Also, the aromatic chemicals in the mint are concentrated when the plant is grown in areas with long, warm, bright summer days.

The book "Healing Herbal Teas" lists these constituents in the peppermint leaf: beta carotene, vitamin B complex, vitamin C, potassium, falconoid (luteolin, rutin), volatile oils (menthol, menthene, methyl acetate, limonene, pulegone) methone, tannins, resin, and romaine acid.

Mrs. Grieve describes peppermint oil as "a colourless, yellowish or greenish liquid, with a peculiar, highly penetrating odour and a burning, camphor scent taste. It thickens and becomes reddish with age, but improves in mellowness, even if kept as long as ten or fourteen years." She ranks it first in importance among essential oils.

MEDICINAL QUALITIES

Peppermint has many medicinal qualities that make it a useful and easy herb to use. One of its paradoxes is that it is both a stimulant and a relaxant. That means that peppermint is predominantly stimulating to the circulation yet soothing to the nerves, thus having both qualities at once. It is possible, however, for one of these qualities to overwhelm the other, depending upon the type of preparation. Peppermint oil is more stimulating and peppermint tea is generally more soothing

Peppermint is well known for its antispasmodic action to relieve nervous irritability and reduce or prevent muscle spasms. This makes it useful when treating Irritable Bowel Syndrome. In a 1996 German double-blind, placebo controlled trial, 45 subjects with IBS were treated with enteric coated peppermint capsules. Pain symptoms, which were reported as being moderate to severe, significantly improved in 89.5 percent of the test group.

Peppermint oil is frequently used as an anodyne or analgesic to ease headaches when applied across the forehead and temples. The first report to suggest that peppermint oil helped to relieve headache was published in the British medical journal Lancet in 1879. But the first double blind, crossover study on the effect of peppermint oil in tension type headache was conducted in Germany in 1996. Researchers analyzed 164 headache attacks of 41 subjects and found that a locally applied ethanol solution of 10 percent peppermint oil significantly reduced pain in the experimental group within 15 minutes, and was as effective in relieving headache as the 1,000 mg. of acetaminophen given to the control group.

Another use of the peppermint herb is to take advantage of its stimulating, stomachic, and carminative properties. Thus the herb is used for the treatment of indigestion, alleviating the symptoms of flatulence and intestinal colic.

A major use of the peppermint herb is as an aid to the process of digestion. The volatile oil content of the herb is the primary agent responsible for this beneficial activity. It increases the flow of all the digestive juices in the stomach and also promotes the flow of bile, at the same time it relaxes the main muscles in the gut. Other digestion benefits lies in its soothing effects upon the lining and muscles of the colon, it alleviates cases of diarrhea and helps relieve a spastic colon.

The production of bile in the liver is increased by peppermint oil as well as the leaf based falconoid to a very significant degree. The traditional use of the herb as a digestive aid is supported to a great extent by this modern evidential confirmation. The peppermint based menthol also results in a lowering of the activity in a liver enzyme known as HMG CoA reductase and this compound may lower the elevated levels of cholesterol.

Used as a rubefacient and applied directly to the skin for various disorders, this remedy helps relieve the pain and reduces sensitivity in the skin arising as a result of external disorders. Used as a chest rub for the treatment of respiratory infections it brings relief. The action of a rubefacient is that upon local application of the herb, it will stimulate capillary dilation and action, and cause skin redness from drawing blood from deeper tissues and organs and thereby relieves congestion and inflammation.

As a sudorific, the essence of peppermint is both a cooling and warming agent. Peppermint will induce the production of heat when it is taken internally and results in an improvement in the circulation within the body. At the same time, the peppermint by dispersing blood to the surface of the body, also induces sweating in the skin. When an herb that is classified as a sudorific is taken cold, it will act as a tonic for the body.

Bitters are defined as herbs having a bitter taste and serving as a stimulant tonic to the gastro mucus membranes. Peppermint derived herbal bitters help in stimulating and cleansing the liver and the gall bladder, and also help in the prevention of gallstone formations.

Emmenagogues are herbs that are corrective to the female reproductive organs that stimulate and promote a normal menstrual function, flow, and discharge. Peppermint is included in this category of medicinal qualities of herbs because it greatly relieves the cramping and pains that accompany this process.

As far as the treatment of chills and fevers, and symptoms of cold and flu, the febrifuge ability of peppermint can be put to very good and effective use. Peppermint possesses strong astringent and decongestant actions, which can help in relieving stuffiness and catarrh in many people who tend to suffer from these illnesses.

Another medicinal application of peppermint is as an antiemetic or to deter nausea. In September of 1997, the Journal of Advanced Nursing reported success with gynecological patients who were given peppermint oil to relieve postoperative nausea. The participating patients experienced less nausea and required less "contemporary" antiemetics.

The aromatic quality of peppermint may be the most famous one of all its many other medicinal qualities. This ability to stimulate the gastrointestinal mucous membranes through its spicy, pungent taste and to relieve headaches and other congestion with its fragrance is usually the first thought that comes to mind when someone mentions peppermint.

The dosage that Dr. Christopher recommends for use of peppermint is: Essence, few drops in water; Extract, 1-2 teaspoons; Infusion, 1 to 2 cupfuls daily between meals (children ¼ to ½ adult dosage); Tincture, ½ to 1 teaspoon.

There are several applications that peppermint can be used for. Baths are a relaxing one. Herbal baths are an opportunity to merge with the herbs of your choice. The herbs constituents are absorbed through the pores of the skin. To prepare a bath with herbal tea, brew a strong blend, using about half a cup of herbs in half a gallon of water. Then strain the tea into the tub. These are my favorite two recipes. Energizing Bath: Use basil, peppermint, rosemary, and thyme. Exact measurements are not necessary. Equal parts work fine, just use whatever you have on hand. Hot Water Bath: Peppermint herb and fresh cut lemon. Pour the tea into the tub.

Facial steams are an excellent application for deep skin cleansing, relaxing facial muscles, and improving circulation. First, wash your face. Then pour 1 quart of boiling water over a handful of herbs in a glass bowl. Tie back your hair. Lean over the bowl and drape a towel over your head. Keep your face about 10 inches away from the water to avoid getting burned. Inhale the sensuous steam for 5 to 7 minutes, lifting the towel to vent the steam if necessary.

Footbaths are a good application for a variety of reasons. Make a gallon of standard herb tea by adding about 16 heaping teaspoons of herb per gallon of water. Strain out the herbs and pour tea into a big basin. Insert your feet and soak until the water cools. Wash your feet with cool water and dry thoroughly.

Mouthwash and gargles are another application. They are made by preparing a standard tea, allowing it to cool and swishing it around in the mouth, or gargling it. Then spit it out.

A steam inhalation is different from a facial steam because it is used for a specific health condition. It can benefit such conditions as asthma, bronchitis, coughs, laryngitis, nasal congestion, and sinus infections. It helps by warming, increasing circulation in, and loosening mucus from the respiratory tract. Bring 1 quart of water to a boil and add 4 heaping teaspoons of herbs. Remove the pot from heat and place it on a heat resistant surface. Lean over the pot, drape a towel over both your head and the pot. Breathe in the steam for about 7 minutes or so. If the water cools enough that the steam starts to dissipate, gently blow into the herb pot and more steam will rise.

Other applications to be used with peppermint would be a fomentation. Make a standard tea and soak a piece of natural cloth in it. Put this cloth onto the affected area and cover with plastic to keep the moisture in. Leave on for as long as necessary.

PINE

LATIN NAME Pinus spp.

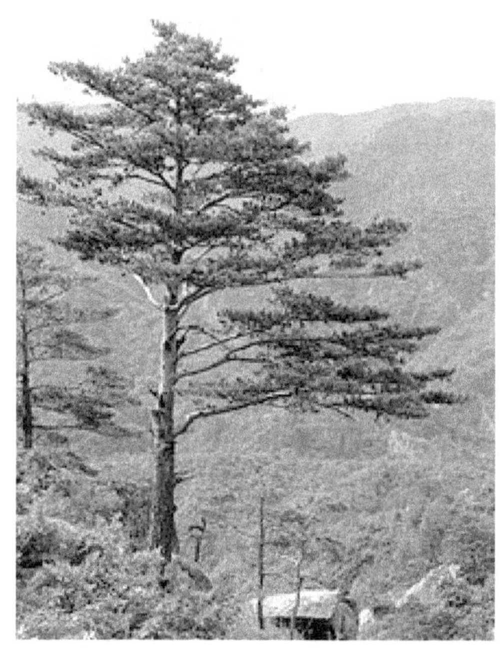

Kingdom: Plantae
Clade: Tracheophytes
Division: Pinophyta
Class: Pinopsida
Order: Pinales
Family: Pinaceae
Subfamily: Pinoideae
Genus: *Pinus*

Overview

Pine needle oil is steam distilled from the fresh needles, branch tips, or the combined fresh branches with needles and branch tips of *Pinus sylvestris* L. (Scots pine or Norway pine) or other essential oil-containing species of *Pinus* (DAB 1997).Scots pine is an evergreen conifer tree native to Eurasia, introduced to North America by European settlers, now cultivated extensively in the eastern United States and Canada. Its natural habitat includes the mountains of Scotland, the Scandinavian peninsulas through central Europe, south to the Mediterranean and east through eastern Siberia. More than 35 different seed sources or varieties of Scots pine are commercially recognized. Pine needle oil is produced in Austria, Russia, and Scandinavia (Leung and Foster, 1996; Koelling, 1999; PFAF, 1997). As a Christmas tree, Scots pine is probably the most cultivated species in the United States (Koelling, 1999).

Pines of all kinds have been used medicinally in many countries from the earliest times (Bown, 1995). Scots pine is the source material of Spirits of Turpentine, B.P. and Russian Turpentine. The young branches of black spruce (*P. nigra*) are the source material for 'essence of spruce,' and the essential oil distilled from the leaves of the dwarf pine (*P. umilio*) is the source material for 'oil of pine' (Grieve, 1979). The topical antieczematic and rubefacient over-the-counter drug Pine Tar USP (syn. *pix liquida*) is obtained from the distillation of the wood of longleaf pine (*P. palustris* Mill.) or other species of pine(Bown, 1995; Budavari, 1996; Taber, 1962). The essential oil distilled from the fresh leaves of *P. pinea* and/or *P. sylvestris* is used in northern India as a component of a compound preparation (oil of pine, magnesii carbonas levis, distilled water) for inhalation to treat chronic laryngitis (Nadkarni, 1976). The steam-distilled essential oil from the balsam of *P. densiflora* Sieb. et Zucc. is official in the Chinese and Japanese pharmacopeias. *Song-jie* (its Chinese name) was first mentioned in Chinese medical literature ca. 500 C.E. as an antiarthritic and analgesic drug. Today, it is used in the traditional medicines of China, Japan, and Korea, administered as a topical paint to treat rheumatism (Bown, 1995; But et al., 1997). The Micmac of Canada prepare an aqueous infusion of the needles and twigs of white pine (*P. strobus* L.) for oral ingestion as a medicine for colds (Lacey, 1993).

In Germany, pine needle oil is official in the *German Pharmacopoeia,* the Standard Licenses for Finished Drugs Monographs, and it is also approved by Commission E. Drops of the essential oil are added to boiling water for inhalation of steam vapor as a supportive treatment for catarrhal diseases of the respiratory tract. The drops are also applied topically by carefully rubbing into the skin for rheumatic complaints (BAnz, 1998; Braun et al., 1997; DAB 1997). The Germans also prepare an aqueous infusion of pine shoots for oral ingestion for the same indications as the oil (Meyer-Buchtela, 1999). In German pediatric medicine, Pumilio pine oil is used as a component of 'Inhalatio composita' formulation (eucalyptus oil 45%, Pumilio pine oil 45%, peppermint oil 10%), intended especially for *coryza* (acute cold and nasal inflammation) and nasal catarrh in children (Schilcher,1997). In the United States, pine needle oil, distilled from the leaves of dwarf pine (*P. mugo* Turra [syn. *P. montana* Mill.] and *P. pumilio* Haenke), is official in the *National Formulary.* It is used as a component in cough and cold medicines, vaporizer fluids, nasal decongestants, and analgesic ointments (Leung and Foster, 1996). The essential oil of Scots pine (*P. sylvestris*)is also used in aromatherapy. This plant is also used in Bach Flower Remedies (homeopathic), available in natural foods stores and herb shops (Bown, 1995; PFAF, 1997).

The approved modern therapeutic applications for pine needle oil are supportable based on its history of use in well established systems of traditional and conventional medicines,and on phytochemical investigations, and pharmacological studies.

German pharmacopeial grade pine needle oil is the steam-distilled essential oil extracted from the fresh needles, branch tips or from the combined fresh branches with needles and branch tips of *P. silvestris* L. or other essential oil-containing species of *Pinus.* Identification is confirmed by thin-layer chromatography (TLC) and organoleptic evaluation. Its relative density must be 0.8550.885, refractive index 1.4701.485, optical rotation 30.0 to +/10.0?, and acid number of maximum 1.0 (DAB 1997). Shelf life is one year when stored and packaged according to the German Standard License monograph requirements (Braun et al., 1997).

Description

The essential oil obtained from fresh needles, tips of the boughs or fresh boughs with needles and tips of *P. sylvestris* L., *P. mugo* species *pumilio* (Haenke) Franco, *P. nigra* Arnold or *P. pinaster* Soland [Fam. Pinaceae] and their preparations in effective dosage.

Chemistry and Pharmacology

Constituents include 5097% monoterpene hydrocarbons, such as *a*-pinene, with lesser amounts of 3-carene, dipentene, *b*-pinen, D-limonene, *a*-terpinene, *g*-terpinene, cis-*b*-ocimene, myrcene, camphene, sabinene, and terpinolene (Schulz et al, 1998). Other constituents include bornyl acetate, borneol, 1,8-cineole, citral terpineol, T-cadinol, T-muurolol, *a*-cadinol, cayophyllene, chamazulen, butyric acid, valeric acid, caproic acid, and isocaproic acid (Leung and Foster, 1996).

The Commission E reported secretolytic, hyperemic, and slight antiseptic activity.

The active principles of some essential oils responsible for the antiviral and antibacterial activities are thought to be limonene, dipentene, and bornyl acetate (Leung and Foster, 1996). Pine needle oil and other essential oils can cause a decongestant effect by stimulating reflex vasoconstriction (Schulz et al., 1998).

Uses

The Commission E approved pine needle oil for catarrhal diseases of the respiratory tract, and externally only for rheumatic and neuralgic ailments. It has been used as a fragrance and flavor component in cough and cold medicines, vaporizer fluids, nasal decongestants, and analgesic ointments (Leung and Foster, 1996).

Contraindications

Bronchial asthma, whooping cough.

Side Effects

Intensified irritation may occur on skin and mucous membranes. Bronchospasms may be intensified.

Use During Pregnancy and Lactation

No restrictions known.

Interactions with Other Drugs

None known.

Dosage and Administration

Internal:

Unless otherwise prescribed:

For inhalation: Add several drops to hot water, inhale vapors.

External:

Apply several drops of liquid and semi-solid preparations, concentrations of 10-50%; rub into affected area.

Ointments: In the form of alcoholic solutions, gels, emulsions, or oils.

PLANTAIN

LATIN NAME Plantago Lanceolata

Kingdom: Plantae
Clade: Tracheophytes
Clade: Angiosperms
Clade: Eudicots
Clade: Asterids
Order: Lamiales
Family: Plantaginaceae
Genus: *Plantago*
Species: **P. lanceolata**

Plantaginis lanceolatae herba
Spitzwegerichkraut

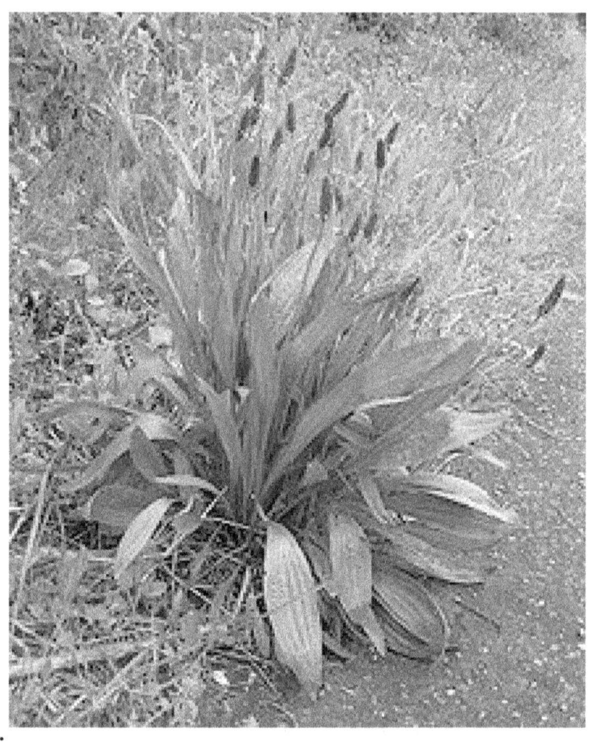

Name of Drug

Plantaginis lanceolatae herba, plantain herb.

Composition of Drug

Plantain herb consists of the fresh or dried above-ground parts of *Plantago lanceolata* L. [Fam. Plantaginaceae], harvested at flowering season, as well as their preparations in effective dosage.

Plantain contains mucilage, iridoid glycosides such as aucubin and catapol, and tannin.

Uses
Internal:

- Catarrhs of the respiratory tract, inflammatory alterations of the oral and pharyngeal mucosa.

External:

- Inflammatory reactions of the skin.

Contraindications
None known.

Side Effects

None known.

Interactions with Other Drugs

None known.

Dosage

Unless otherwise prescribed:

Average daily dosage:

- 3 - 6 g of herb;
- equivalent preparations.

Mode of Administration

Comminuted herb and other galenical preparations for internal and external use.

Actions

Astringent
Antibacterial

HISTORY OF PLANTAIN

"The world is not to be put in order, the world is order incarnate.
It is for us to put ourselves in unison with this order," Henry Miller (Utterback pg 56).

Our idea of what is a weed and what is not needs to be "put in order". We need to understand that a weed is just a plant we don't know how to use or perhaps one growing in the wrong place.

Plantain has been known by many names throughout its history, band aid plant, Breitwegerich (German), broad-leaved plantain, beside cart grass (Chinese in Hawaii), buckhorn plantain, Che Qian Zi (China), common plantain, cuckoo's bread, devil's shoestring, dog's ribs, dooryard plantain, Englishman's foot, hock cockle, kemp (Danish), lance-leaved plantain, Llanten comun and L. major (Spanish), pig's ear, Plantain lanceole (France), plantane (Older English), Podoroshnik (Russian for near or along the road), ribwort, round leafed plantain, rubgrass, slan-lus (Scottish), snakeweed, Spitzwegeric (Germany), Tanchagem-maior (Portuguese), waybread, waybroad, weybroed (Anglo-Saxon), and white man's foot.

Nicholas Culpeper listed plantain in his herbal printed in 1652, *The English Physitian*. Today it is titled *Culpeper's Herbal* and is still among one of the most popular books written in English. Even back at that time plantain was a well-known plant. Culpeper stated, "This groweth so familiarly in meadows and fields, and by pathways, and is so well known that it needeth no description." (Thulesius pg. 51).

Nicholas Culpepper gave this information on plantain.

The clarified juice drank for a few days helps excoriations or pains in the bowels, and distillations, of rheum from the head. It stays all manner of fluxes, even women's courses, when too abundant, and staunches the too free bleeding of wounds.
The seed is profitable against dropsey, falling-sickness, yellow jaundice and stoppings of the liver and reins. The juice, or distilled water, dropped into the eyes cools inflammation in them. The juice mixed with Oil of Roses and the temples and forehead anointed with it, eases pains in the head proceeding from heat. It can also be profitably applied to all hot gouts in the hands and feet. It is also good to apply to bones out of joint, to hinder inflammations, swellings and pains that presently rise thereupon.

The dried and powdered leaves taken in drink kills worms of the belly; boiled in wine, it kills worms which breed in old and foul ulcers. One part of the herb water and two parts of the brine of powdered beef, boiled together and clarified, is a remedy for all scabs and itch in the head and body, tetters, ringworms, shingles and running and fretting sores. All Plantains are good wound-herbs, for wounds and sores, internal and external. (Broad-leaved Plantain, p.2)

Plantain though was in use long before Culpeper's time. The Ancient Persians and the Ancient Arabians used this herb for dysentery. They also favored it for use with all stomach and intestinal problems.

Alexander the Great (356 B.C.-323 B.C.) used plantain to cure his headaches. Pedanius Dioscorides, (40 BC-90BC), was a Greek born in what is today Turkey but at his time it was part of the Roman Empire. He studied medicine in Egypt and was a physician in the Roman Army.

He used plantain for its soothing, cooling, healing and softening properties.

To save someone bitten by a mad dog, Pliny the Roman (23 A.D.-79 A.D.) would use plantain. He also states "on high authority, [that if] it be put into a pot where many pieces of flesh are boiling, it will sodden them together." (Herb a Day, p. 3) Early Christians considered plantain a symbol for the well-trodden path of the multitude who followed Christ.

In ancient India when the mongoose fought against a cobra, it was noticed that if bitten, the mongoose would use plantain to neutralize the venom.

The Anglo-Saxons (450 A.D. to 1066 A.D.) listed plantain as one of their 9 sacred herbs. They considered that it had great healing powers. They used it for ridding their bodies of worms, as a cure for kidney disorders, a diuretic, a laxative and to cure hemorrhoids. They also used it in a salve for "flying venom." The salve included hammer wort, chamomile, plantain, water dock roots, honey and butter.

The *Macer Floridus* (I found 3 possible dates for the writing of it, 9th and 11th century and the 1500's), was read by Douglas Schar who puts it into his words stating:

I noticed that the author rarely has much more than a few words to say on each plant. Plantain is a different matter. According to this volume, the plant can be sued for: wounds of all sorts including dog bites and scorpion stings, black spots, boils, carbuncles, swellings of the lymph gland, epilepsy, excessive bleeding during menstruation, uterine pains, headaches, coughs, fevers, flu, and sore feet. It is also good for the eyes, gums, and bladder. The list goes on, and on, and on. (Schar, p.1)

Desiderius Erasmus, (1466-1536) a classical scholar, stated that plantain was an antidote for the toxins of poisonous spiders. In Ireland plantain is known as the "healing herb" in Gaelic because they used it to heal wounds and bruises. One use of plantain came about because of the way it looked. The flower spikes suggested that it be used for virility.

King Henry the VIII, (1491-1547) was an amateur in medicine and loved to dabble in it, giving advice to others. The British Museum has his collection of 114 favorite recipes, written in his own hand. He used plantain as one of his basic herbs.

Geoffrey Chaucer referenced the healing power of plantain in his works as did William Shakespeare, (1564-1616) who spoke of plantain in his plays, "Love's Labour's Lost" (iii,i), "Two Noble Kinsmen" (I,ii) and "Romeo and Juliet" . From Romeo and Juliet "Radish, Raphanus sativus Romeo. Your Plantain leaf is excellent for that, Benvolio. For what, I pray thee, Romeo? For your broken skin." (American Botanical Council, pp. 11-12) Shenstone also mentions plantain in his play "The Schoolmistress." It goes like this,

"And plantain rubb'd that heals the reaper's wound." (Plantago major, plantain, common p.5)

As 'chemical' surgeons began to come forth in the 1500s they still kept their plants. In fact, they used the plants to counteract the corrosive or irritating effects of their minerals. Plantain was one of the plants that would cool and sooth the system.

Dr. Herman Boerhaave, (1668-1738), a Dutch physician and botanist suggested that plantain leaves bound to your aching feet would relieve their pain and help you endure the fatigue of long hikes. In 1710 Salmon's "Herbal" mentions using plantain for many ailment including the throat, glands and the lungs. It states that it is good for epilepsy, dropsy, jaundice and obstruction of the liver and spleen. It is listed as cooling inflammations in the eyes and reducing the pain in them. It will also ease ear, tooth, and head aches.

Native Americans were already using many herbs to care for themselves when the Europeans arrived. One of their beliefs shares their feelings about being a part of the earth.

The Earth does not
belong to Man.
Man belongs to the Earth.
All things are connected like the blood
which unites a family.
Man does not weave the web of life,
he is only a strand of it.
Whatever happens to the Earth,
happens to all of us.
Whatever Man does to the web of
life on Earth,
He does to himself.
(Dewey,p. 42)

Native Americans embraced this plant after it was brought over by the English. They called it "white man's footsteps" since it seemed to grow wherever the white men went. The Shoshone would mix one part plantain with one part clematis bracts for wounds, bruises, boils and to reduce the swelling of rheumatic pains. They would also heat the leaves and place them on wounds. Plantain was also used with yarrow to stop hemorrhages of the lungs and bowels. The story has come down that the Assembly of South Carolina gave a reward to the Native American who discovered that plantain would cure the bite of a rattlesnake.

The Native Americans chewed the roots of plantain to ease the pain of toothaches. The Cherokee also used plantain. They gave it to children who were learning to walk to strengthen them. The Delawares used it for the "summer complaint" or diarrhea. Native Americans used a combination of yellow dock, cramp bark, yarrow, milkweed, plantain, organic tobacco and tansy in a tea. A second tea used with it was made from alfalfa seed, blessed thistle and golden seal root. These were used as a four day diet for hard and fungus tumors.

Henry Wadsworth Longfellow, (1807-1882) wrote about plantain in "Hiawatha". In fact chapter 21 is titled "White Man's Foot" a section goes like this:

Gitche Manito, the Mighty, The Great Spirit, the Creator, Sends them hither on his errand. Sends them to us with his message. Wheresoe'er they move, before them Swarms the stinging fly, the Ahmo, Swarms the bee, the honey-maker; Wheresoe'er they tread, beneath them Springs a flower unknown among us, Springs the White-man's Foot in blossom. Let us welcome, then, the strangers, Hail them as our friends and brothers, And the heart's right hand of friendship Give them when they come to see us. Gitche Manito, the Mighty, Said this to me in my vision. (Longfellow p.6)

An interesting side note is that the natives of New Zealand came up with a name that was almost the same, "Englishman's foot". They used the boiled leaves for ulcers. The upper side was used to draw the wound and they used the lower side to aid in the healing. Nothing was wasted. The water that the plantain was boiled in was used for scalds and burns. They also drank it as a uterine stimulant.

In China the plant has been used for rheumatism, diarrhea, infertility and urinary tract infections. They feel that it helps with problem deliveries and also with a healthier childbirth in general. In the *Materia Medica* it mentions a study in China of women who fetuses were not positioned correctly for birth. The use of plantain reversed the position 90% of these fetuses for correct delivery. (Schar, p. 3)

The juice of plantain was used to soothe abused feet, lessen the pain of hemorrhoids and insect bites by the Pennsylvania Dutch. They also discovered it was good for getting rid of worms in the intenstines. In the bayou of Louisiana plantain was used to help sores heal. Dried leaves were in linen closets to perfume the linens (although dried plantain doesn't smell bad I haven't noticed a perfume like smell). It also was suppose to keep insects out of the linens.

In 1903 Lady Northcote mentioned in her book, "The Book of Herbs" that an old woman had an ointment that was often used. It included plantain leaves, Southernwood, black currant leaves, elder buds, angelica and parsley. They were chopped and pounded then simmered with clarified butter. She used it for people who had burns or raw surfaces. Lady Northcote also included her own recipe with Celandine, Elder buds, houseleek and plantain. Many of the old remedies included plantain. Ones for kidney disorders, splitting of blood and for piles. It was used in diuretics and to destroy worms.

Plantain used to be used commonly in the United States but during the switch over from rural to urban life most Americans forgot about it. It only took three generations for this wonderful herb to be lost. Rural Americans turned to doctors and their "miracle cures" instead. Many people step on it or over it or even curse it, not understanding it is loaded with nutrition and is important medically.

In 1958 the Food Additives amendment was passed and many additives and ingredients were exempt from the new testing requirements because of their history of long, safe use. Many herbs made this list, Generally Recognized as Safe or GRAS, but plantain did not and so was not supposed to be sold for food or drug use. Americans stepped up to the bat and today the use of herbs is on a more solid footing, but herbal practitioners are bucking big business and must be ever vigilant.

Dr. John Christopher, (1909-1983), chose plantain to represent the Alterative Herb group in his newsletter, volume 1 number 3. In his book "School of Natural Healing" he states that plantain is the best herb for blood poisoning.

Today researchers have proven that many of the old uses of plantain have a good scientific base. Germany's official herbal "FDA" organization is the German Commission E. This group provides research on many herbs. Plantain research shows that it is a good choice for wound healing and as a treatment for lung conditions, including bronchitis, asthma, coughs, mucous membrane irritations, upper respiratory infections. Research has also shown that it is valuable used topically for skin problems.

The Chinese have also done research on plantain. Their studies show that plantain does stop diarrhea in children. The research also shows that this herb is helpful for some of the areas they use it for, including childbirth. Research has also been done by another Asian country, Burma. The Burmese use it to treat blood pressure, sores and fevers for the tropics. Their research shows that plantain in water or alcohol extracts drops arterial pressure in dogs and treats stomach problems. Their research points toward its use with ulcers and increasing the secretion of gastric juices. It also reduces intestinal contractions.

CHEMICAL CONSTITUENTS OF PLANTAIN

Plantain contains many biologically active compounds. The plantain fruit stimulates gastric mucus secretion and growth of the gastric mucosal cells. Plantain's flavonoids can increase the thickness of this layer. The lectins in plantain seem to bind some mannose oligosaccharides that are on some bacteria which help them attach to the gastric and intestinal linings.

The tannins (astringent), allantoin (promotes wound healing, speeds up cell regrowth/healing and softens skin), apigenin (anti-inflammatory flavonoid), aucubin (a glycoside, a powerful anti-toxin, increases uric acid excretioin by the kidneys), baicalein, linoleic acid, oleanolic acid, sorbitol and iridoid glycosides in plantain are considered the major factors in making it a mild anti-inflammatory, as well as an antimicrobial, antihemorrhagic and an expectorant. Aucubin is another glycoside in plantain. It acts as a sedative, anaesthetic, alterative, antiseptic, anti-viral, anti-toxic ,anti-histamin, anti-inflammatory, anti-rheumatic, anti-tumor, anti-cancer, anti-carcinogenic, a diuretic an expectorant, a hypotensive and an organoleptic. This glycoside has been studied numerous times.

Plantain contain high levels of beta carotene (A). It also has ascorbic acid (vitamin C) and vitamin K. Plantain also contains silca which makes plantain high in calcium. This herb is high in mucilage especially the seeds.

Also active in plantains are monoterpene alkaloids, triterpenes, phenois, sugars and the flavonoids lutelin, scutellarin, baicalein, nepetin, hispidulin, plantagoside, and acteoside plantamajoside. Plantain also contains other plant acids such as chlorogenic, citric, ferulic, neochlorogenic, fumaric, hydroxycinnamic, salicylic, ursolic, and benzoic acids. Catalpol stimulates the production of adrenal cortical hormones. This increased the production of adrenal gland androgens, has an anti-inflammatory ability, seems to help in wound healing and increases the production of sex hormones.

James Duke list 39 active chemicals in *Dr. Duke's Phytochemical and Ethnobotanical Databases* as well as 509 distinct activities for Plantago major. One interesting note on his research is the calcium in Plantago major is 23,400 ppm while for horsetail it is only 1550 ppm. A.B. Samuelsen, Department of Pharmacognosy, School of Pharmacy, University of Oslo, states, "A range of biological activities has been found from plant extracts including wound healing activity, anti-inflammatory, analgesic, antioxidant, weak antibiotic, immuno modulating and antiulcerogenic activity."

MEDICINAL QUALITIES OF PLANTAIN

Plantain is an Alterative meaning that it is one of about 100 plants that clean and correct impure conditions of the blood and the eliminative tissues and organs. Dr. John R. Christopher explains that although many herbs might work fast on a given organ to relieve engorgement to really be an Alterative herb it must do the job slowly but surely, toning the organs as well as cleaning the blood. This herb does that and can be used completely. The roots, leaves, flowers and seeds can be used internally or externally.

Plantain is #1 in the field of blood poisoning treatment. You can see the healing at work. Swelling goes down and the "red" line recedes. Limbs poisoned can be saved using this herb. It is used as a poultice on the outside and taken as a tea on the inside. Michael Tierra, L.Ac., O.M.D. states that plantain is an herb that will "dry excess moisture and remove excess fat where toxins are retained." (Tierra, p. 13)

Plantain is also a diuretic so is useful for kidney and bladder problems. It is taken throughout the day as a tea to help the kidneys and bladder. It is used in bed-wetting challenges. It also helps dropsy and water retention. Sometimes diuretics should be teamed with a demulcent herb to buffer the effects on the kidneys. There is no research or recommendations that taking plantain tea requires ones. Actually, plantain itself is a demulcent also.

As a styptic it can be chewed or pounded into a paste and applied to a wound to stop minor bleeding. It is very soothing and cooling as it heals. Taken as a tea or in soup it soothes irritated mucous membranes. It will stop the bleeding of minor cuts and when taken internally, ulcers. Although Mrs. M. Grieve, author of *A Modern Herbal*, disagrees with that stating that they are not useful in internal bleeding although historically it had been used for such. It will slow the flow in excessive menstrual cycles. It also is used for bloody urine.

This herb is used as a vulnerary to heal wounds, cuts and scratches. Because it is found in high traffic areas around playgrounds, baseball fields and parks it is easy to grab, crush and use. Since it contains epidermal growth factor, it can be used in place of comfrey to repair damaged tissue, treat bruises and broken bones.

Plantain is also used as an antivenomous herb in its role as a blood cleanser. Terry Willard, author of *Edible and Medicinal Plants of the Rocky Mountains and Neighbouring Territories*, states that it is good to draw out the poison of snake bites. It is an excellent choice for poisonous bites and stings of scorpions and insects. It does a good job in easing the pain of poison ivy. "I don't know of any itch that can stand up to plantain," states Susan Weed, director of the Wise Woman Center in Woodstock, New York. (Mandile, p. 27)

Plantain is used to treat many skin disorders. Christopher Hobbs educates us on skin problems. "It is often said that you can't judge a book by its cover, but what about the human 'cover', your skin? Doctors recognize many varieties of problems and diseases of the skin. Although we can visualize the skin (in contrast to, say the liver), it is often difficult to determine whether a problem is due to attack from various fungi and bacteria or to an internal process such as psoriasis or eczema, or from factors within and without such as an allergic reaction to an ingredient in your soap.

"I have come to the conclusion that even when the skin is seemingly attacked by an external pathogenic (disease-causing) agent such as a fungus, this is usually preceded by an internal process of imbalance. For example, 'liver heat,' or inflammation due to chronic doses of sapirin, chronic stress, overuse of alcohol, and immune weakness because of improper nutrition can all contribute to a major outbreak of athlete's foot." (Hobbs, p. 28) Christopher Hobbs goes on to say that you have to treat the whole patient and locate the root of the problem. He lists topical herbs for skin problems in the following order: plantain, aloe, calendula, Gotu kola, Oregon grape root, St. Johns wort, chamomile and lavender.

Plantain made the top 25 list of 175 herbs checked for most frequently mentioned as an herbal remedy for Toxicodendron dermatitis. This study checked over 300 print and Internet resources. They then took the top 25 and checked for scientific verification. Nine of those were unproved (no scientific studies at all) and one was disproved. Plantain made the proved list with the qualification that further studies are needed. (Senchina, p. 40)

Plantain tea or juice will heal sunburn, burns, mild ulcers and scalds. James Duke in his book "The Green Pharmacy" explains that plantain has been one of the most popular folk remedies for burns in the United States of America. It doesn't have the research backing that Aloe vera has for this task but appears to be a good substitute when Aloe is not available.

Plantain does an excellent job as a deobstruent. Removing foreign objects and particles from the body. Teamed up with cayenne the unwanted items work their way out even faster. Plantain's refrigerant qualities soothe and cool sores and ulcers. It is excellent to ease and heal hemorrhoids as a tea injected after each bowel movement and applied externally.

Although many people consider this herb a weed it is truly a miracle medicinal herb. Even web sites on how to poison weeds toll the virtues of Plantain while telling you how to kill it.

Plantain is used in tuberculosis and syphilis, again both internally and externally. Rosemary Gladstar states that "This herb is also very effective for treating liver sluggishness and inflammation of the digestive tract." (Gladstar p.357) It is also used for scrofula and specific or non-specific glandular diseases as well as mercurial poisoning.

Plantain roots are powdered to use on toothaches. No powder? Just dig and chew a root for relief. Plantain is an anthelminitic or vermicide and taken as a tea it will kill worms internally in the stomach and the intestines. Plantain is an antiseptic used to clean cuts and wounds. It heals boils and other sores

Plantain decoction is used as an antifungal on ringworm. Apply the decoction then cover with bruised leaves. Wrap with cotton gauze to keep the decoction in place. It has also been used to help with loss of voice.

It is also a safe and effective astringent, antibacterial soother for the throat and for laryngitis. It is anti-inflammatory and antimicrobial. This herb is approved by Commission E for its role in coughs and bronchitis as well as the fore mentioned problems. For colds and flu taking the tea throughout the day assists the body in its fight.

Plantain soothes the cough reflex. It is used for asthma, lung infections, and hay fever relief. It is effective for hoarseness, and bronchial infections. It is also used for respiratory problems that involve mucous congestion. This herb depresses the secretion of mucous, especially in the respiratory system.

Russian scientists have discovered that Plantain and its cousin psyllium are both useful for weight loss. Those taking 3 grams of plantain with water 30 minutes before eating lost more weight than women not using this herb. Plantain contains mucilage which acts as an appetite suppressant while reducing the intestinal absorption of fat and bile. It also lowers LDL cholesterol and the triglyceride levels in blood. Plantain usually lowers blood sugar.

A douche is used to treat infections of the vagina or for cleansing. They should not be used often because it will upset the balance of the natural bacteria that are in the vagina. Repeated infections mean that you need to look at diet and lowered resistance in the body, repair that and the infections will clear up. But for use until that clicks in a strong plantain tea can be used. It can be mixed with goldenseal, uva ursi, comfrey, white oak bark or yellow dock.

When plantain tea is taken internally it is effective for gastritis, diarrhea, dysentery, irritable bowel syndrome and other intestinal problems. Plantain tea is also used for an eye wash for red, irritated or light sensitive eyes. One or two teaspoons of the seeds soaked in two cups of distilled water will offer a milk laxative effect like it's cousin, psyllium.

Karta Khalsa uses plantain in his 7-day cleansing plan to detox the body in the treatment of chronic, degenerative diseases. Karta mentions that cleansing is not a magic bullet, after cleansing you need to address the root problem. Don't be fanatical with a cleanse you can scour yourself raw! He likes fresh plantain juice for its demulcent and cooling attributes.

Plantain is also listed as a way to quit the tobacco habit. It is supposed to help you stop smoking by creating an aversion to tobacco. Instead of lighting up, chew a plantain leaf! It is worth a try, at least you will get a fresher breath. Chewing a plantain leaf before that kiss or important meeting is recommended.

Plantain is definitely an all around herb. Not only can you find it everywhere but it is used in a wide variety of treatments. It soothes the skin and when used in a facial steam will help with acne. It is wonderful in herbal baths to help with any itchy places. It works well as a massage oil and a hair rinse. The leaves put inside your socks on the soles of your feet help protect against sore feet and prevent blisters.

"The Complete Herbal Handbook for Farm and Stable" lists plantain as an important plant for farmers to be familiar with. For goats, sheep and poultry it is a forage plant (seeds and leaves) but its main function is medicinal. Farmers can use this soothing mucilage herb internally and externally on all farm animals. It is used to treat the very same problems that it is used for with humans. Cows and horses do not usually take it on their own but it can be used internally and externally with them.

DOSAGES & APPLICATIONS OF PLANTAIN

The German Commission E recommends the following:

1. 1/4 to ½ tsp (1-3 grams) of the leaf daily as a tea and taking 3 cups a day.
2. The fresh leaves can be used directly on minor injuries, dermatitis and insect stings three or 4 times a day.
3. Syrups or tinctures 3 times a day, about ½ tsp (2-3 ml) each time.
4. ½ to 1 1/4 tsp. (2-6 grams) of fresh plant juice taken in three evenly spaced oral doses.

Dr. John R. Christopher recommends the following doses: Fluid extract of ½ to 1 teaspoon; Infusion of 2 fluid ounces 3 to 4 times daily; powder 1-3 grams; tincture ½ to 1 fluid teaspoon.

1. For anal dosing use a strong tea (1 oz. powdered plantain steeped in one pint of boiled water for 20-30 minutes then cooled). Inject 1 TBSP, three to four times daily. If necessary it can be done more often. Especially inject after each bowel movement. Use for diarrhea, hemorrhoids and piles. Dr. Christopher's piles ointment can be used as needed.

2. For oral dosing the tea can be taken 4 to 5 times a day until relief. Use the tea for blood poisoning, diarrhea, kidney and bladder problems, lumbago, scanty urine and bed-wetting. For dropsy, drink the tea made from the seeds. For scrofula and syphilis use as a tea and as an external application. With thrush or frog make a decoction by simmering one ounce of seeds in 3 cups of water and letting it reduce to 2 cups; sweeten with honey and give one tablespoonful three or four times daily.

3. External dosing
a. Poultices of fresh, bruised or mashed leaves are applied to the damaged area for the bleeding of minor wounds such as cuts, scratches and bruises. You can also drink the tea.
b. For stings and bites of poisonous insects, plants, animals and for boils, carbuncles and tumors: bruise the fresh leaves and apply to needed area; cover them and keep moist by adding the juice of the plantain leaves; change the poultice before it dries out.
c. For malignant or bleeding ulcers apply the infusion with glycerine. Use 100% cotton well soaked with the infusion. Cover it and change as needed.
d. For toothache just apply the fine powder to the roots of the aching tooth.
e. For burns, scalds and erysipelas use the strong tea formula (found under anal doses) and wash frequently. Drink the infusion.
f. For inflamed eyes make the tea in distilled water and be sure to strain it well. Use as an eye wash.
g. For itching, ringworm, running sores or old wounds make the strong tea using equal parts of plantain with yellow dock (Rumex crispus). Bathe the affected area often with the tea.
h. For blood-poisoning: make a fomentation or poultice for the affected area and increase the normal internal dosage.

4. Vaginally for leucorrhea or menorrhagia use a strong tea as an injection or douche. Drink the tea internally as well.

Alma Hutchens Snake Bite Dosage
Take 1 TBSP of plantain leaf juice every hour. Also apply the bruised leaves to the wound.

POKE ROOT

LATIN NAME Phytolacco americana

Kingdom: Plantae
Clade: Tracheophytes
Clade: Angiosperms
Clade: Eudicots
Order: Caryophyllales
Family: Phytolaccaceae
Genus: *Phytolacca*
Species: ***P. americana***

Common Names
Poke Root , American nightshade
Botanical Name
Phytolacca decandra
Syn. *Phytolacca americana*
Family Phytolaccaceae

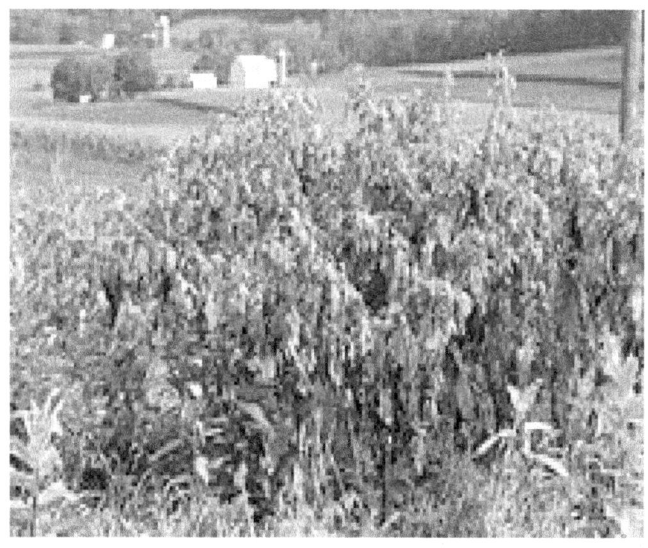

In herbal medicine we use the roots of 'Poke'; an impressive looking plant reaching 4 meters in height and having strong purple-green stems that support flourishes of drooping flowers eventually giving way to large clusters of purple berries.

Poke Root is regarded as one of the most important of the American indigenous plants and one of the most striking in appearance. M. Grieves writes *headaches of many sources are benefited by it... the extract has been used in chronic rheumatism and it is also stated to be of undoubted value as an internal remedy in cancer of the breast.* As with all herbal authors on Poke Root Grieve emphasises the need for caution describing its potential action in higher doses as *a slow emetic and purgative with narcotic properties.*

Poke Root is a powerful cleansing remedy, used to help especially when the lymphatic system has become congested. This may show up in the early stages as being chronically tired with slightly swollen glands but by the time the lymph has really sludged up things may have gone all the way down to advanced rheumatism, respiratory disease or auto-immunity issues; conditions that Poke Root has traditionally been used to treat.

The following is an excerpt from a detailed description of the actions and indications by one of the great Eclectic physicians of the late 19th century; H Felter
Actions: *'Physiologically, phytolacca acts upon the skin, the glandular structures,*

especially those of the mouth, throat, sexual system, and very markedly upon the mammary glands; also upon the fibrous and serous tissues, and mucous membranes of the digestive and urinary tracts. It is principally eliminated by the kidneys. Applied to the skin, either in the form of juice, strong decoction, or poultice of the root, it produces an erythematous, sometimes pustular, eruption. The powdered root when inhaled is very irritating to the respiratory passages, and often produces a severe coryza, with headache and prostration, pain in chest, back, and abdomen, conjunctival injection and ocular irritation, and occasionally causes violent emeto-catharsis. Upon the gastro-intestinal tract doses of from 10 to 30 grains of it act as an emetic and drastic cathartic, producing nausea which comes on slowly, amounting almost to anguish, finally after an hour or so resulting in emesis. It then continues to act upon the bowels, the purging being prolonged for a considerable length of time. Large doses produce powerful emeto-catharsis, with loss of muscular power -occasionally spasmodic action takes place, and frequently a tingling or prickling sensation over the whole surface. Dimness of vision, diplopia, vertigo, and drowsiness are occasioned by large doses not sufficient to produce death. Phytolacca slows the heart's action, reduces the force of the pulse, and lessens the respiratory movements. It is a paralyzer of the spinal cord, acting In poisoning by this agent tetanic convulsions may ensue. The treatment of poisoning by phytolacca is that of gastro-enteritis'

Internal Use: *'Medicines which act directly upon the glandular structures are not numerous. Among those that do so act, none is more direct than phytolacca. The experience of many years with phytolacca with success in what has been understood to be alterative effects, is a matter of Eclectic record. That it powerfully impresses the glands of the skin, lymphatic system, buccal, nasal, and sexual systems, and particularly the tonsils, ovaries, testicles, and mammary glands, we are certain.*

Phytolacca is pre-eminently a remedy for swollen or engorged glands and adenitis. Without phytolacca we should be at a loss to know how to treat glandular affections undergoing swelling or inflammation. Its most direct indication is hard, painful enlargement of the glands with associated pallid mucous membranes. It is not so direct a remedy for suppurating glands. It is of signal value in mumps, and inflammation of cervical, axillary, and inguinal glands, when not due to tuberculosis. Even then its influence is often shown by its power to reduce the glands more or less, but exceedingly slowly; while in those enlargements due to syphilis its effects are more prompt and decided. Its beneficial control over tonsillitis and swelling of the submaxillary glands is well known. In acute mastitis phytolacca is by far our best remedy. This treatment, with mechanical support, gentle withdrawal of the milk, if possible, or sometimes strapping of the gland with adhesive plaster may avert suppuration. After surgical measures for the liberation of pus the use of phytolacca should be continued to reduce any remaining engorgement of the organ. Sore nipples and mammary tenderness, and morbid sensitiveness of the breasts during menstruation are relieved by phytolacca, and it is decidedly useful in the mammary swelling which sometimes occurs in infants. Though its action upon the reproductive glands is less decided than upon other specialized glands and upon the lymphatic nodes, it is not without value sometimes in orchitis and ovaritis. It is most effectual in the former when the inflammation is occasioned by the metastasis of mumps.

Phytolacca is important in dermatological practice.The condition which calls for it internally in skin diseases is one of indolent action of the skin, usually associated with vitiated blood and hard glandular enlargements. There may be scaly, vesicular, pustular, or tuberculous eruptions, and lymphatic enlargements with pain. The skin may be inflamed, but does not itch because there is not activity enough in the part. It is often indicated in chronic eczema, syphilitic eruptions, psoriasis, tinea capitis, favus, and varicose and other ulcers of the leg'

From earlier in the 20th century another great Eclectic physician, Finlay Ellingwood, writes the following on Poke Root *'this agent must now have especial attention in its influence in the treatment of acute inflammations of the throat. It makes but little difference what forms of throat disease we have, from the simplest forms of pharyngitis, through all the variations of tonsillitis, to the extreme forms of diphtheria, this remedy may be given in conjunction with other indicated agents. But few of our physicians neglect its administration in these cases, and they are unitedly profuse in their praises of its influence. If there be an infection of the local glands of the neck, from the throat disease, the agent should be applied externally, as well as administered internally. In the treatment of goitre there is a consensus of opinion concerning the value of this remedy, but it is almost universally administered in these cases, with other more direct remedies. Dr. J. V. Stevens is enthusiastic in his opinion that adenitis needs no other remedy than phytolacca americana. Whatever the cause of the disease or of however long standing, he saturates the system with this remedy, and persists in it, applies it externally and claims to cure his cases. He has used it for many years with success. Others combine other active alteratives as general conditions demand.*
Too much cannot be said of its very positive and invariable influence in the treatment of acute inflammations of the breast during or preceding lactation. It should be given every two hours at least in doses of perhaps ten drops in extreme cases, or five drops in the incipiency of the disease, or mild cases.
The writer has, through a long experience, gotten into the habit of adding this remedy to alterative compounds. This is especially true of those prescribed for children's glandular and skin disorders. It is an efficacious remedy in any of the forms of skin disease, common to childhood. Given in the incipiency of eczema and in some forms of chronic

eczema, especially that of a dry character, where there are cracks or fissures in the skin, these promptly yield to the internal administration of this remedy'

King's Dispensatory writes *'Physiologically, Poke Root acts upon the skin, the glandular structures, especially those of the buccal cavity, throat, sexual system, and very markedly upon the mammary glands. It further acts upon the fibrous and serous tissues, and mucous membranes of the digestive and urinary tracts. In certain conditions of the system which might come under the head of dyscrasia (bad blood), it proves a most valuable alterative. Scrofulous, syphilitic, and rheumatic conditions are invariably benefited by it. It is best suited to chronic rheumatism, and syphilitic and rheumatic joint affections. The condition which calls for it is one of indolent action of the skin; it is often indicated in chronic eczema, syphilitic eruptions, psoriasis, tinea capitis, favus, and varicose and other ulcers of the leg. In diseases of the mouth and throat it is highly esteemed. It is useful in acute and chronic mucous affections, as in tracheitis, laryngitis, influenza, catarrh, and especially in those affections where there is a tendency to the formation of catarrh and phlegm'*

The British Herbal Pharmacopoeia (BHP) describes Poke Root's actions as *antirheumatic, anticatarrhal, mild anodyne, emetic & purgative in large doses,* and says it is indicated for *chronic rheumatism, chronic respiratory catarrh, tonsillitis, laryngitis, adenitis, mastitis & mumps* and specifically indicated for *inflammatory conditions of the upper respiratory tract, lymphatic adenitis.* The BHP suggests a dose of 0.03 - 0.3 gms or by decoction and recommends a tincture in the ratio of 1:10 in 45% ethanol with a dose of 0.2-0.6mls (approx 4-12 drops)

Thomas Bartram describes Poke Root's actions as *'lymphatic, alterative, anti-neoplastic, parasiticide, anti-rheumatic & anti-inflammatory'.* He gives many potential uses for it, including *'swollen glands and lymph nodes, mumps, tonsillitis, sore throat, inflammation of prostate gland, ovaries or testicles. Chronic irritative skin disorders, ringworm, eczema, psoriasis, pityriasis, acne & lupus. Ulceration, internal or external, polymyalgia, rheumatism, arthritis. Breasts; mastitis, mammary abscess, fissured nipples, fibrotic nodules and hard lumps that have been diagnosed benign. Chronic fatigue syndrome. Obesity; eliminating excess fat in fatty degeneration. Mercurial poisoning from dental amalgam in teeth fillings. Lipoma with persistent use. Some forms of cancer spread via the lymphatic system for which Poke Root has an inhibitory effect'.* Bartram suggests a dose of not more than 8mls in a week.

How to use Poke Root

First day - use 2-4 drops (not droppersful, but **DROPS**) in a small amount of water and drink. If this dose is taken during the day, it may be repeated at night before bed. If the infection or soreness is still present the next day, repeat this dose in the morning and again that night. Then use the 2-4 drops in a small amount of water once a day until the infection or soreness is completely gone. This usually doesn't take more than a day or two. This same procedure is recommended for sore throats with swollen lymph glands in the neck. (Poke Root will do nothing for sore throats that do not involve the lymph glands.)

<u>Another suggestion:</u>

Warm a pot of water. Put 4-6 droppersful (not drops) into the pot of water. A dropperful is the amount that is drawn up into the glass pipette when the droppertop bulb is squeezed. It will usually fill it about 1/2 way. Soak a clean white cloth in the Poke Root water, squeeze out the excess, and apply to the sore or plugged area of the breast. Make it warm, but be careful not to burn the skin. This method, known as a compress, works extremely well in cases of plugged ducts, even if it hasn't become an actual breast infection. Continue to re-soak and re-apply this compress for 20-30 minutes. You may briefly re-heat the Poke Root water on the stove if needed (do not boil or microwave it). Repeat this 3-4 times a day or as desired.

<u>One important note</u>: Poke Root is an extremely powerful herb. If too much is taken, nausea and vomiting may occur. Poke Root may be taken while nursing, as the dose required and suggested above is extremely low. Use only when necessary and for no longer than five days at a time. If symptoms persist or worsen, see your medical professional.

RED RASPBERRY

Raspberry leaf

LATIN NAME Rubus idaeus

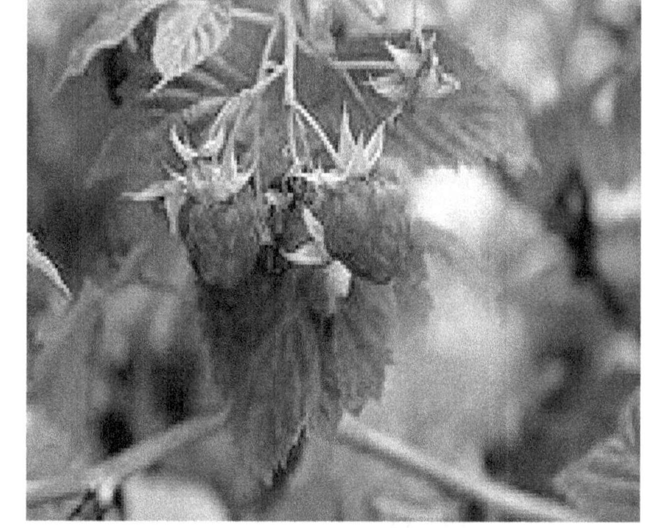

Kingdom: Plantae
Clade: Tracheophytes
Clade: Angiosperms
Clade: Eudicots
Clade: Rosids
Order: Rosales
Family: Rosaceae
Genus: *Rubus*
Subgenus: *Idaeobatus*
Species: **R. idaeus**

Rubi idaei folium
Himbeerbltter

Name of Drug

Rubi idaei folium, raspberry leaf.

Composition of Drug

Raspberry leaf consists of the leaf of *Rubus idaeus* L.[Fam.Rosaceae], as well as preparations thereof.

Uses

Raspberry leaf is used for disorders of the gastrointestinal tract, the respiratory tract, the cardiovascular system, and the mouth and throat, and also for skin rashes and inflammation, influenza, fever, menstrual problems, diabetes, vitamin deficiency, as a diaphoretic, diuretic, and choleretic, and also to "purify the skin and blood."

The effectiveness of raspberry leaves for the foregoing indications has not been documented.

Risks

None known.

HISTORY

Rubus idaeus is the scientific name for red raspberry. The name comes from the Latin word "rubus" which means red and the Latin word "ida," which is the name of a mountain in Phrygia where the plant grew abundantly. Raspberry is a member of the Rosaceae family and is often listed with other species of Rubus in herbals and botany books.   In fact, raspberry was used interchangeably with blackberry by the Greeks, Chinese, Ayurvedics, and American Indians to heal complaints such as diarrhea, dysentery, and the healing of wounds.[1] Rubus idaeus was native to Turkey and was used by the people of Troy. Archeological findings show that the Romans spread the raspberry seed throughout their empire including up into England.[2] Red raspberry has been used for many years throughout the world both as food and medicine.

Raspberry is a valuable food source. The fruit is a popular fruit eaten in the summer months and sometimes into the fall. The fruit has also been used for mild drinks. It was also used as a dye. In England, the roots were boiled and eaten like turnips.

All parts of the raspberry plants were used for their many medicinal properties. A decoction of the flowers has been used for pimples, hemorrhoids, malaria, and as a poultice for eye inflammation, as well as to reduce fevers. [3] The fruit used to be widely used to flavor other unpleasant tasting preparations. Raspberry vinegars have been used for sore throats and coughs. In large quantities, the berries have been used as a laxative and diaphoretic. They have also been used to ease rheumatism and indigestion. The juice from the berries was used for fevers, childhood illnesses, and cystitis. According to MDidea.com, "Gerard believed 'the fruit is good to be given to those what have weake and queasie stomackes'." Historically, a cordial of the juice has been used for gastroenteritis in humans, pet birds, and livestock in Australia. The fruit has also been used for anemia, gum disease, reducing a fever, easing digestion, sobering drunkenness, and stomachaches.[4] The leaves have been used for diarrhea, to wash the eyes, and for a female tonic, especially in pregnancy. Many midwives have used red raspberry leaf to prevent miscarriages and to assist in achieving pregnancy. Midwives have also used the leaves to prevent postpartum hemorrhage. The leaves were used for stomach complaints in children and to prevent morning sickness.   Historically, it was used as a mouthwash to heal canker sores, cold sores, and gingivitis.[5] The leaves, combined with slippery elm, have been used to cleanse wounds and burns, and promote healing. In Tibetan medicine, the leaves are used to cure emotional disturbances, exhaustion, irritability, and chronic infections.[6] The root, like blackberry roots, also in the Rubus genus, has been used for diarrhea.

Red raspberry was used by many different Native American tribes for a wide variety of complaints. The Algonquin used the root for diarrhea while the Cherokee used the root for coughs and toothache. A tea was made for menstrual problems as well as parturition. Both the Chippewa and Pottawatomie used the root bark for the eyes.[7] The Chippewa made a tea of the root bark and washed the eyes three times per day for cataracts.[8] The Chippewa also used red raspberry for dysentery and measles. The Ojibwa used a decoction of the root for bowel complaints in children.

The Iroquois had many uses for red raspberry. They made a tea of the young twigs. The leaves were for kidney complaints. Red raspberry was combined with snakeroot for "ladies who are run down because of sickness of period."[9] The root tips were boiled into a concentrated decoction to be used as a blood purifier and to lower or raise blood pressure.

[1] Opening Our Wild Hearts to the Healing Herbs page 160
[2] Nursery at TyTy
[3] Natural Standard
[4] Natural Standard
[5] Mountain Rose Herbs contemporary information.
[6] Natural Standard
[7] Handbook of Northeastern Indian Medicinal Plants
[8] Opening Our Wild Hearts to the Healing Herbs page 160
[9] Iroquois Medical Botany

CHEMICAL CONSTITUENTS

All plants contain constituents. These may include vitamins, minerals, proteins, fiber, fats, sugars, tannins, and phytosterols. The specific composition of each plant is different from plant to plant and species to species. It is these chemical constituents that give a plant its medicinal and nutritive properties. Raspberry is no different. James Duke lists over 80 constituents found in the leaves, plants, and fruits.[1] Many plants are known for a primary constituent or "active ingredient," however; raspberry is not like these plants because a primary constituent has not been isolated. As a result, raspberry is not generally standardized.[2] This is not necessarily a bad thing. The tendency of modern medicine to standardize herbs to a given constituent renders a drug rather than an herbal medicine. The variation in constituents is part of what makes herbs work effectively. Furthermore, in herbal medicine, the whole is better than the sum of the parts because the constituents work together synergistically to create the medicine. One constituent may be the "active ingredient," but the remaining constituents are the catalysts and protective factors to render the herb safe.

According to the Natural Medicine Comprehensive Database, "Red raspberry contains anthocyanidins, ellagitannins, flavonols such as quercetin and kaempferol, catechins, and phenolic acids. Other constituents include ascorbic acid, beta-carotene, chlorogenic acid, glutathione, and alpha-tocopherol."[3] Both the leaves and berries contain iron citrate. The leaves also contain pectin, malic acid, calcium chloride, potassium chloride, and potassium sulfate. The fruit contains iron, potassium, calcium salts, malic and tartaric acids. The leaves also contain fragrine, which has an affect on the female organs.[4]

Nutritional Profile of Red Raspberry Leaf in 100 grams of dried leaves

Nutrient	Amount	Relative Quantity of Source
Aluminum	39.2 mg	High
Ash	8.00%	Average
Calcium	1210 mg	High
Calories	.55/gram	Average
Carbohydrates	79.00%	Average
Chromium	.13 mg	Average
Cobalt	.34 mg	Low
Crude Fiber	8.20%	Low
Dietary Fiber	32.30%	Average
Fat	1.70%	Average
Iron	10.1mg	Very High
Magnesium	319 mg	High
Manganese	14.6 mg	Very High
Niacin	38.2 mg	Very High
Phosphorus	234 mg	Average
Potassium	1340 mg	Average
Protein	11.30%	Average
Riboflavin	Trace	Very Low
Selenium	.25 mg	High
Silicon	.13 mg	Low
Sodium	7.7 mg	Low
Thiamine	.34 mg	Average
Tin	2.3 mg	High
Vitamin A	18963 IU	High
Vitamin C	967 mg	High
Zinc	Trace	Very Low

The leaves contain 83.1% water when fresh, 6.7% water when dried, and 6% sugars in the forms of sucrose, fructose, and glucose.[5] Although raspberry has a high aluminum content, this is not the same inorganic aluminum that has been linked to Alzheimer's. The aluminum present in raspberry is organic and easily assimilated by the body rather than accepted and stored, which leads to disease.

[1] Dr. Duke's Phytochemical and Ethnobotanical Databases. Scientific name search Rubus idaeus.
[2] Natural Standard
[3] Natural Medicine Comprehensive Database
[4] Hygieia: A Woman's Herbal
[5] Nutritional Herbology page 146

MEDICINAL QUALITIES

Red raspberry fruit is sweet and tart. The edible fruit is laxative and refrigerant[1] as well as, antacid, and parturient.[2]

Red raspberry is astringent, tonic, hemostatic, antiseptic, antiabortient, parturient, antigonorrheal, antileucorrheal, and antimalarial[3] as well as stimulant, alterative, stomachic, anti-emetic, and cathartic.[4] There are some constituents, especially the ellagalic acid, which is an isolate of ellagitannins, in raspberry that have been shown in studies to be anti-carcinogenic, especially in the cervix, colon, mouth, and esophagus[5] as well as the prostate, pancreas, breast, and skin cancers.[6] The quantity of ellagitannins found in raspberry has been studied and, when compared to other plants like strawberries and walnuts, which are known to contain ellagitannins, it seems to be more bioavailable. This could be due to lack of study in the other plants or the fact that they contain smaller quantities of the ellagic acid than raspberries. The other possibility is that those plants, which contain a similar quantity of ellagitannins, have their own unique mix of these tannins. As a result, they might produce a slightly different effect on the body. [7] One animal study showed a tendency of raspberry to reduce blood glucose levels; therefore, it may be beneficial in diabetes.[8]

Raspberry is specific for colds and flu. It cleanses mucus membranes and thins mucus secretions.

[1] American Indian Medicine
[2] The School of Natural Healing. Chapter 4 page 156
[3] Advanced Treatise in Herbology page 113
[4] The School of Natural Healing. Chapter 4 page 156

[5] Handbook of Northeastern Indian Medicinal Plants
[6] MDidea.com
[7] MDidea.com
[8] Opening Our Wild Hearts to the Healing Herbs page 160
DOSAGES

Pedersen suggests a daily dosage of red raspberry leaf as follows:

" Fresh leaf: ¼- ½ cup, Dried leaf: 6-12 gm, Extract: 9 gm dried leaf, 45 ml alcohol, 45 ml water."[1]

Dr. Christopher recommends 1-2 teaspoonfuls of fluid extraction of the leaves, 1 teacupful at mealtimes three times per day either hot or cold of the infusion, 1-2 grams of the powder, and ½-1 teaspoon of the tincture.[2]

Many midwives recommend raspberry for good reason. Its leaf is beneficial to women, especially those who are pregnant. A hot infusion of the leaves balances hormones. It has been shown to relax the smooth muscle of the uterus as well as to contract the uterus when relaxed.[3] Willa Shafer says, "When first pregnant, ladies need this herb above all others. In my experience this herb has been one of the best for preventing birth defects in the newborn. Red Raspberry prevents morning sickness and helps to strengthen the uterus. In most cases, Red Raspberry will prevent miscarriage. Red Raspberry makes delivery faster and prevents tearing of the cervix."[4] There have been several studies conducted on raspberry leaf taken in pregnancy. Most commentary on these studies state that no harm is done by taking raspberry leaf tea in pregnancy, but it doesn't significantly help either. However, the actual results of the studies suggest the opposite. In one study, mothers who consumed raspberry leaf had a shorter labor and their babies were less likely to be delivered by forceps. A study published by the Australian College of Midwives Journal stated, "The findings also suggest ingestion of the drug might decrease the likelihood of pre and post-term gestation. An unexpected finding in this study seems to indicate that women who ingest raspberry leaf might be less likely to receive an artificial rupture of their membranes, or require a caesarean section, forceps or vacuum birth than the women in the control group." [5] Clearly raspberry leaf does have an effect on pregnancy and parturition. There is no definitive dosage on the appropriate dosage in pregnancy. Some midwives recommend 1 cup per trimester per day, with the third trimester being 3 or more cups per day. Some midwives recommend 1 quart per day throughout pregnancy.

Jeannine Parvati states, "It is also helpful against sterility and prized for helping infertile women and men conceive."[6] This may be due to the balancing action on the sex hormones. In rat studies, gonadotropin was given in large doses to the female rats in order to increase the weight of the ovaries and uterus. A water extract of raspberry leaf was then given to the rats. The raspberry leaf extract significantly inhibited the affects of the gonadotropin but did not abolish it.[7] Excess gonadotropin can result in infertility problems. Edwards recommends combining raspberry with red clover blossoms, lady's mantle, or wild grape to enhance fertility.[8]

Cold infusions are antidiarrheal. Mowrey attributes this to the astringent properties due to the tannic acids present. Furthermore, these astringent properties are used in dysentery, internal bleeding, ulcers, and chronic skin diseases.

Dr. Christopher used raspberry for constipation, nausea, diarrhea, dysentery, diabetes, pregnancy, uterine hemorrhage, parturition, uterine cramps, labor pains, cholera infantum, leucorrhea, prolapsus uteri, prolapsed anus, hemorrhoids, dyspepsia, vomiting, colds, fevers, intestinal flu, bowel complaint, thrush, relaxed sore throat, opthalmia, sore mouth, sore throat, spongy gums, ulcers, wounds, and gonorrhea. The formulas mentioned before, found in the School of Natural Healing, should be administered as follows: the eyewash should be used to bathe the eyes freely; the formula for excessive menstruation should be taken ½-1 cupful 3 to 4 times per day; for an inflamed uterus ½ of the inflammation of the uterus formula should be injected into the womb every other day to soothe and tone the uterus; in addition to addressing the glandular toxicity in mumps, 2 fluid ounces of the mumps formula should be taken 3 to 4 times per day; the piles formula should be used externally as needed; and the dosage for the parturition tea is 1 teacupful every hour during labor or as needed.[9]

Raspberry leaf also cleanses mucus membranes and thins excess mucus secretions. This may be one reason, in addition to the antiviral and antibacterial properties, that it is helpful for colds and flu. To aid in this process, Marin's Lung Support Tea should be taken in a dose of one cup every 6-8 hours or as needed. Marisa's Lung Support Formula can be taken to strengthen the lungs and aid in healing the damaged lungs. This should be taken in a dose of 1 dropper 2-3 times per day.

Raspberry contains ellagitannins. One cup per day of raspberries, 40 mg of ellagitannins, has been shown to prevent the growth of abnormal cells. In lower doses they slow the growth of the cells, but in high doses, they instruct the cancer cells to kill themselves. This has been shown in cancers of the colon, breast, prostate, esophagus, pancreas, and skin. Ellagitannins also break down leukemia cells. Another way that raspberries protect against cancer is by preventing cell mutation. Ellagitannins also protect against cancer by binding to cancer causing agents, be it petroleum byproducts, food additives, or tobacco smoke, and rendering them neutral. The ellagitannins also prevent bacteria from mutating, and protect DNA from carcinogens by blocking the carcinogens from binding to the DNA. The ellagitannins in red raspberry have also been shown to lower birth defects, promote wounds to heal, reduce heart disease, and may reverse liver fibrosis caused by chemicals.[10]

[1] Nutritional Herbology
[2] The School of Natural Healing. Chapter 4 page 157
[3] Herbal Tonic Therapies- Remedies from nature's own pharmacy to strengthen & support each vital body system
[4] Midwifery & Herbs page 6
[5] Raspberry leaf and its effect on labour: safety and efficacy
[6] Hygieia: A Woman's Herbal page 44
[7] Herbal Tonic Therapies- Remedies from nature's own pharmacy to strengthen & support each vital body system
[8] Healing our Wild Hearts to the Healing Herbs page 159
[9] The School of Natural Healing chapter 4 page 156-167
[10] MDidea.com

SAGE

Sage leaf

LATIN NAME Salvia officinalis

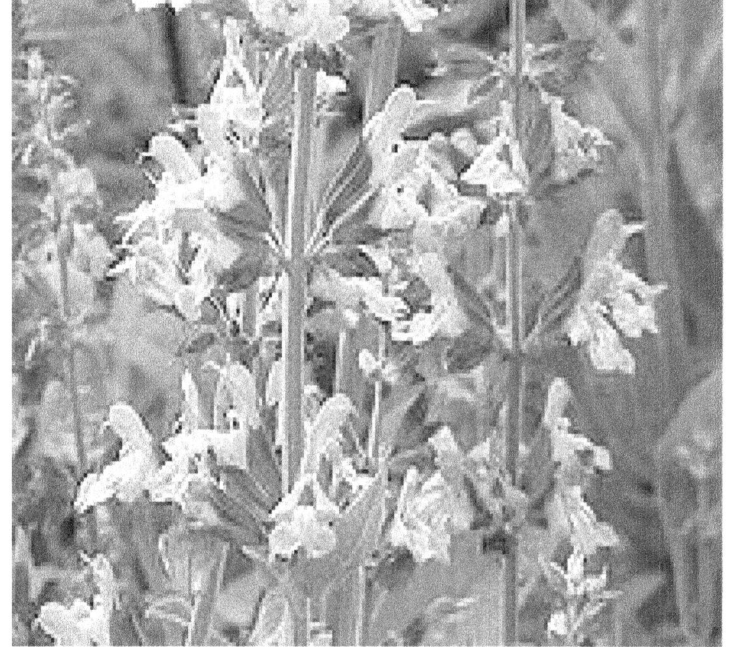

Kingdom: Plantae
Clade: Tracheophytes
Clade: Angiosperms
Clade: Eudicots
Clade: Asterids
Order: Lamiales
Family: Lamiaceae
Genus: *Salvia*
Species: **S. officinalis**

Name of Drug

Salviae folium, sage leaf.

Composition of Drug

Sage leaf consists of the fresh or dried leaf of *Salvia officinalis* L.[Fam.Lamiaceae], and preparations thereof in effective dosage. The leaves contain at least 1.5 percent (v/w) thujone-rich essential oil, based on the dried herb.

Principal components of the essential oil, in addition to thujone, are cineol and camphor. In addition, the leaves contain tannins, diterpene bitter principles, triterpenes, steroids, flavones, and flavonoid glycosides.

Uses
External:

- Inflammations of the mucous membranes of nose and throat.

Internal:

- Dyspeptic symptoms, excessive perspiration.

Contraindications
The pure essential oil and alcoholic extracts should not be used internally during pregnancy.

Side Effects

After prolonged ingestion of alcohol extracts or of the pure essential oil, epileptiform convulsions can occur.

Interactions with Other Drugs

None known.

Dosage

Unless otherwise prescribed:

Internal:
Daily dosage:

- 4 - 6 g of herb;
- 0.1 - 0.3 g of essential oil;
- 2.5 - 7.5 g of tincture (according to *Erg.B.6*);
- 1.5 - 3 g fluidextract (according to *Erg.B.6*).

For gargles and rinses:

- 2.5 g of herb or 2 - 3 drops of essential oil in 100 ml of water as infusion or 5 g of alcoholic extract in 1 glass water.

External:

- Undiluted alcohol extract.

Mode of Administration

Cut herb for infusions, alcoholic extracts and distillates for gargles, rinses and other topical applications, as well as for internal use. Also pressed juice of fresh plants.

Actions

Antibacterial
Fungistatic
Virustatic
Astringent
Secretion-promoing
Perspiration-inhibiting

ST. JOHN'S WORT

LATIN NAME Hypericum perforatum

Kingdom: Plantae
Clade: Tracheophytes
Clade: Angiosperms
Clade: Eudicots
Clade: Rosids
Order: Malpighiales
Family: Hypericaceae
Genus: *Hypericum*
Section: *Hypericum* sect. *Hypericum*
Species: **H. perforatum**

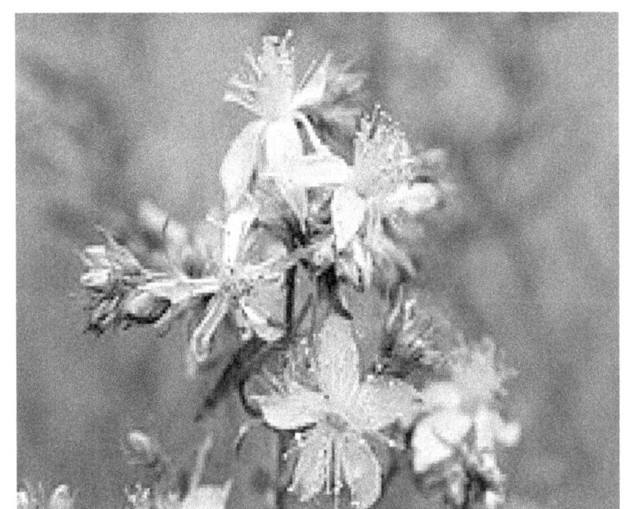

Name of Drug

Hyperici herba, St.John's Wort.

Composition of Drug

St.John's Wort consists of the dried, above-ground parts of *Hypericum perforatum* L. [Fam.Hypericaceae], gathered during flowering season, as well as their preparations in effective dosage.

Uses
Internal:

- Psychovegetative disturbances, depressive moods, anxiety and/or nervous unrest. Oily hypericum preparations for dyspeptic complaints.

External:

- Oily hypericum preparations for treatment and post-therapy of acute and contused injuries, myalgia and first-degree burns.

Contraindications
None known.

Side Effects
Photosensitization is possible, especially in fair-skinned individuals

Interactions with Other Drugs

None known.

Dosage

Unless otherwise prescribed:

Average daily dosage for internal use:

- 2 - 4 g of drug or 0.2 - 1 mg of total hypericin in other forms of drug application.

Mode of Administration

Chopped herb, herb powder, liquid and solid preparations for internal use. Liquid and semi-solid preparations for external use. Preparations made with fatty oils for external and internal use.

Actions

A mild antidepressant action of the herb and its preparations has been observed and reported by numerous physicians. According to experimental observation, hypericin can be categorized among the MAO inhibitors. Oily hypericum preparations demonstrate an antiinflammatory action.

[**Ed. note:**The research suggesting MAO activity was experimental and not conducted in animal systems. Subsequent research has indicated either no or very slight MAO activity in St. John's Wort or its preparations.]

HISTORY

Appropriately dubbed by many as a magical plant, St. John's Wort (*hypericum perforatum)* carries a rich history, full of cultural nuances and mystical legends. Dr. Jonathan Zuess, in his book , "The Natural Prozac Program," eloquently captures the emotion and quintessence of St. John's Wort in his opening statement: "In the crumbling pages of ancient texts on healing, hidden amongst the dusty basement shelves of a neglected Old World library, there are stories of a flower whose tears are magical." Many of these stories, passed through the generations, paint a colorful picture of a multifaceted plant used in a variety of applications, some were even used for supernatural or spiritual purposes because of their "magical" results.

The botanical name for St. John's Wort, *hypericum perforatum,* has several noted origins, all having similar meanings or references. *Hypericum* comes from the Greek word "hyperikon" which is broken down into hyper, meaning "over," and eikon, meaning "image or apparition," a reference to the belief that the herb was so obnoxious to evil spirits that even a whiff of it would cause them to disseminate. Another translation, "almost over ghosts," confirms the mystical beliefs expressed during the Medieval period. The true origins of "eikon" are not fully known due to the cross-pollination of the medicinal and mystical uses of St. John's Wort.

The name *perforatum* is translated as "punctured," and refers to the many tiny dots found on the leaves and flowers of St. John's Wort, which at first glance seem to be small perforations or holes. These small, black, translucent dots are not actually holes but tiny glands which, when pressed, release the essential plant oils and resins.

Legend tells us that in the first century, early Christians were credited for naming St. John's Wort after their beloved John the Baptist as the brightly colored flowers will usually expose themselves on or before June 24th which is celebrated as his birthday. The striking arrangement of its five yellow petals resembles a halo, and when picked exudes a crimson red liquid which was believed by some to symbolize the spilled blood of their beloved John. Many historical authorities have questioned whether the infamous Rose of Sharon as mentioned in the Bible is really St. John's Wort although botanists have confirmed they are two distinct plants but abide in the same family. Wort is simply an Old English word for a plant or an herb.

Of additional spiritual significance, St. John's day is also when daylight is the longest in Europe and is known as the Summer Solstice, an important planting time that is historically rich with pagan, native and early religious rituals. This became a perfect environment for the mystical shroud surrounding St. John's Wort to be unveiled, exposing its supposed spiritual powers which could chase away demons and any other troublesome spirits. A poem from a manuscript dating back to 1400 declared:

St. John's wort doth charm all witches away
If gathered at midnight on the saint's holy day.
Any devils and witches have no power to harm
Those that gather the plant for a charm:
Rub the lintels and post with that red juicy flower
No thunder nor tempest will then have the power
To hurt or hinder your houses: and bind
Round your neck a charm of similar kind.

Historical information dating back to 400 B.C. tells the story of *hypericum* and its medicinal and spiritual evolution. The ancient Greeks and Romans noted that St. John's Wort was used for such things as snake or reptile bites, menstrual cramping, gastrointestinal distress, ulcers, depression or melancholy, superficial wounds, or sciatica. Other noted uses of the herb extended into the spiritual or mystical realm as they believed the odor alone would surely drive off evil spirits, offering protection against the devil's temptations.

Welsh families frequently used St. John's Wort to judge the relative life span of family members. A sprig of the herb was given to each family member and then hung from the rafters during the night. In the morning, depending on how shriveled each person's sprig was, the length of each individual's life was then determined. It was believed that use of St. John's Wort could make a witch powerless and strip her of her will. Sir Walter Scott in his poem, "The Nativity Chant," wrote the following:

Trefoil, vervain, John's Wort, dill,
Hinders witches of their will.

During the Burning Times, a handful of St. John's Wort was often stuffed into an accused witch's mouth to force her to confess.

In an attempt to confer protection to an individual household, St. John's Wort was frequently woven into wreaths in order to keep the devil away. Today, many cultures continue to
use St. John's Wort as an exorcist for demons or ghosts. It was even supposed that St. John himself would appear in a dream, bringing a blessing, if a small sprig of the plant was placed under the pillow before retiring.

Columba, a Celtic saint devoted to John the Baptist, was said to carry a sprig of St. John's Wort with him on his long and dangerous travels in honor of the martyred saint but in all practicality, he may have carried it with him for spiritual protection during his many missionary journeys to the Celtic tribes. The German translation for St. John's Wort is *Johanniskraut*, or "John's plant" and in China, where it has been listed for thousands of years in that country's highly esteemed herbal pharmacopoeia, it is known as *Qian Ceng Lou.* In the American West, St. John's Wort has not been given such a place of honor. Most consider it a troublesome weed also known as Klamath weed or Goat weed.

Many of the Greeks and Romans used St. John's Wort as more of a spiritual herb, by placing sprigs of the plant on the statues of their gods in order to ward off evil spirits. The first written record of St. John's Wort during the first century AD is reportedly found in Pliny the Elder's famous book on natural healing, referring to *hypericum* in a physical application, noting that "The seed is of a bracing quality, checks diarrhea, promotes urine. It is taken with wine for bladder troubles."

First century Greek physicians, Galen and Dioscorides, recommended its use as a diuretic, a wound healing herb and as a treatment for menstrual disorders. As a Roman army surgeon, Dioscorides noted in his medical writings that when the herb was placed in special liquids, it "…expels many cholerick excrement, but it must be given continuously, until they be cured, and being smeared on it is good for ambusta (burns)."

Paracelcus, suggested that St. John's Wort flowers should be picked at sunrise in order to capture the active constituents. The bright, ray-like petals release their precious red liquid most efficiently when soaked in olive oil and left out in the sun for several days. This produces a beautiful, thick, red liquid which can then be applied externally on wounds, sprains, bruises and varicose veins. This oil was commonly referred to as the "blood of Christ".

The Saltenitan drug list, a thirteenth century document, refers to St. John's Wort as "herba demonis fuga," or the herb that chases away the devil. Several hundred years later, medical books still referred to St. John's Wort as "fuga demonum" or devil's scourge, confirming the widespread belief that St. John's Wort could rid a person of the demons haunting them. During this time, the "wise women" and midwives kept both the mystical and practical legends of St. John's Wort alive by passing their knowledge down through the generations as they rendered medical care for their families. Agelo Sala noted that St. John's Wort was highly regarded in treating anxiety, illnesses of the imagination, melancholia and disturbances of understanding.

The ancient belief that St. John's Wort conferred protection against evil spirits may have risen in part due to its use by traditional healers as a treatment for "melancholia" or what was known at that time as "troubled spirits." It was assumed that when the overall disposition or mood of a person was downcast, sad or unsettled, this was the work of evil forces or demons. St. John's Wort was not initially used to treat what we now know as depression or anxiety but, fortunately, this hidden benefit was eventually realized while doctors and herbalists were treating wounds, burns and other injuries.

When an injury was sustained, the individual often felt some measure of anxiety or emotional upset. Upon administering an infusion (tea made from steaming the leaves and flowers) of St. John's Wort orally or applying the infused oil directly to the wound, a calming or sedating effect was noticed. St. John's Wort then began gaining a reputation for bringing clarity, saneness or a sense of calm instead of demonic torment as was previously believed. The natural conclusion was that St. John's Wort carried a measure of spiritual power which was able to protect individuals from the torment of these evil spirits.

Writings during the 19th century continued to incorporate *hypericum* for the treatment of melancholia or as we know it today, depression. Some of these reported medicinal actions of St. John's Wort have now been scientifically verified by double-blind studies, only to prove what the ancients knew all along.

CHEMICAL CONSTITUENTS

Without much difficulty, scientists have been able to determine many of the chemical constituents contained within St. John's Wort. There are, however, many other compounds that have not yet been discovered which will ultimately shed even more light on the use and application of St. John's Wort. To date, current research has identified at least ten groups of components thought to contribute to the pharmacological effects of St. John's Wort. Of these, two primary classes are thought to be the most active: naphthodianthrones and flavanoids. These have been touted as being the primary players in the therapeutic and medicinal action of St. John's Wort; however, there are many more compounds which act in a complementary role, bringing synergy to the plant as a whole. Depending on what part of the plant is used and when it is harvested or picked, chemical constituents can be found in greater concentrations, boosting their specific therapeutic benefits.

The first class - naphthodianthrones - is the umbrella for a class of chemical constituents called quinones, which contain two of the most studied chemicals thought to be responsible for the anti-depressive action of St. John's Wort: hypericin and pseudohypericin. When used for
scientific testing, these compounds are chemically extracted and isolated out of the whole plant, and prepared in a laboratory under strict scientific guidelines in order to obtain a new, standardized extract, typically set at 0.3 percent hypericin or 30 percent.

This extraction is said to be necessary in order to accurately measure dosages for purposes of scientifically testing the medicinal effects of St. John's Wort. Herbalists and many natural practitioners contend that by using just one isolated compound such as hypericin, test results will not be accurate as the complimentary action of all the chemical constituents would not have been taken into account.

These quinones are a type of alkaloid that contain naturally occurring compounds which are easy to spot in plants that display red, yellow or orange pigments. Therefore, the quinines hypericin and pseudohyperidin are found in the greatest concentration in the flower petals and buds of St. John's Wort. Historical documents record that when cattle and other pasture fed animals have been exposed to large amounts of St. John's Wort and allowed to eat freely, they experienced heightened sun sensitivity. In rare cases, this has resulted in severe sunburn or even death.

It has been reported that both of these chemicals, when tested on human subjects using a standardized extract, do contain photosensitive properties. However, if a whole plant preparation is used in moderation, there is no indication of any side effects. Based on experimental studies, it would take approximately 30-50 times the recommended daily dose of 900 mg, using the standardized extract, to produce severe phototoxic effects in humans.

The second class of active compounds are known as flavanoids, a large group of biologically active molecules that fall under the umbrella of polyphenols. The flavanoids present in St. John's Wort include proanthocyanidin, hyperin, biflavone, amentoflavone and quercetin among others. Flavanoids are found in the highest concentrations in the hypericum flowers.

Other chemical compounds that have been identified include terpenoids, which contain essential or volatile oils, xanthones and coumarins. Many of these compounds, found primarily in the leaves and flowers, are minor chemical components providing balance and completeness that otherwise would be lacking.

Another compound found in St. John's Wort are tannins, a subgroup of the large phenol class. These tannins are responsible for much of the medicinal action relating to superficial wound or injury care. The greatest concentrations of these chemicals are also found in the leaves and flowers.

Much extensive research has been completed in an attempt to list all the known chemicals found in St. John's Wort. Scientists have worked diligently, compiling a comprehensive list of these compounds and their estimated percentages.

MEDICINAL QUALITIES

History has long told the tale of the various medicinal uses of St. John's Wort. Until recently, this historical information had to suffice regarding the use and application of

this
multifaceted herb. Science has now 'proven' many of these claims by mapping out a
large number of active compounds and their relative actions.

The most notable action attributed to St. John's Wort through standardized scientific
testing is its effect on mild to moderate depression. Certainly, there are many variables
and inconsistencies in the testing models as well as lack of definitive outcomes, but
historical accounts combined with actual clinical experiences of hundreds, if not
thousands of individuals, can attest to the overwhelming benefit of St. John's Wort in
cases of depression, sadness, decreased energy, fatigue, restlessness, insomnia, irritability
or melancholy. This extraordinary plant acts in harmony with the brain's sleep-inducing
mechanism, enhancing its action instead of overriding it.

Although the primary focus of modern science has been directed at the specific chemical
action of hypericin and pseudohypericin, more recent studies have revealed that these
constituents may not be the primary source of its anti-depressive action. Current research
has suggested that the mood enhancing action of St. John's Wort is improved by a lesser
known compound called hyperforin. This chemical is thought to stimulate the immune
system as well, aiding the body's overall defense mechanisms.

Dr. Walter E. Mueller, head of the department of pharmacology at the University of
Frankfurt is a leading clinical researcher of St. John's Wort. In tests performed by Dr.
Mueller and his colleagues, hypericum extract was found beneficial in reducing the
effects of depression, restoring brain function to normal.

Laboratory testing has shown both hypericin and psuedohpericin as having powerful
antiviral effects on the herpes simplex viruses I and II, Epstein-Barr, influenza A and B,
and
other more specific viruses. Current research is being directed toward combating
hepatitis, obesity, tuberculosis and HIV using St. John's Wort.

PMS or menopause are other conditions for which St. Johns Wort is useful. This is not
surprising as many of the same symptoms experienced with PMS are also seen with
individuals suffering from depression. Childhood enuresis, ADD/ADHD, gastrointestinal
upset related to alcoholism, weight loss, arthritis, sciatica, nerve damage, urinary tract
infections and dysbiosis due to excessive antibiotic or steroid use have also responded
favorably to the use of St. John's Wort.

Positive studies have shown St. John's Wort as a dominant player against breast cancer, several types of skin cancers and gliomas, the most commonly occurring form of brain cancer. It was reported that at low doses it inhibited the growth of new cancer cells and at high doses it actually killed the cancer cells. The immune boosting properties of St. John's Wort are an added benefit in these cases.

The flavanoid content in St. John's Wort is now known to play a crucial role in its antidepressive actions and research is underway to try and determine to what extent. Many of these flavanoids have similar healing properties, but yet each one a unique fingerprint of action. Proanthocyanidins, a common group of flavanoids, are known to have antioxidant, antiviral and antibacterial properties as well as having a positive effect on the heart and related cardiovascular disorders. Quercetin, also found in onions, is known to be a potent anti-inflammatory chemical as well as being a MAO (monoamine oxidase) inhibitor which helps with states of depression.

Hyperin and biflavone have been identified for their effectiveness as sedatives and the compound amentoflavone acts as an anti-inflammatory, a sedative and as an inhibitor of ulcer development. The flavanoids found in St. John's Wort can also have diuretic effects, inhibit tumor growth, strengthen capillaries, dilate the coronary artery, and act as antispasmodics and antifungals. Essential oils, a valuable part of the chemical makeup of St. John's Wort, have been found to have both sedating and antifungal properties.

Tannins, astringent by nature, are responsible for St. John's Wort wound healing ability as these compounds dry and tighten or bind the skin. They are especially beneficial for burn or wound healing and reducing inflammation. Internally, they can stop diarrhea and internal bleeding.

Additional studies have shown that xanthones may also have a strong effect on the antidepressive activity of St. John's Wort, along with the quinones hypericin and pseudohypericin.

The class of chemicals called alkaloids has been reported to have a positive effect on the nervous system by enhancing or retarding the transmission of nerve impulses. Alkaloids are traditionally known for their antiseptic, antibacterial, antiviral, anti-inflammatory and analgesic actions.

DOSAGE

As previously noted, many St. John's Wort preparations are taken internally or applied externally to a wound or site of pain. Much of the dosage information available is related to the use of standardized extracts which, because of their chemical extraction, are measured in milligrams. Herbal preparations, however, are taken either in capsule form, as an infusion or tea, as an external ointment or olive oil preparation, or as an alcohol or glycerin based tincture.

Most bottles of St. John's Wort sold to the general public are standardized at a 0.3 percent hypericin content or 30 percent. This isolated compound has been used almost exclusively for double-blind and placebo controlled testing, but is not necessarily the most beneficial source of the herb. Under these conditions, the typical dosage is 300 mg taken three times each day.

If using the whole plant (which may include using just the leaves and flowers), typical dosages are as follows:

Capsules - 1 capsule 3 times per day

Herbal Extract (alcohol or glycerin) - ½ teaspoon taken three times per day in water or juice. (This tincture is typically made with 250-350 grams of herb steeped in one liter of alcohol or glycerin/water mixture)

Herbal Fluid Extract (1:1) - 10-15 drops taken three times each day in water or juice. (This form of the herb is prepared with 1 liter of alcohol to 1 kilo of the herb)

These dosages are considered to be average and should be adjusted according to the situational need. When working with an herbalist or other healthcare practitioner, the determination will be made as to the best dosage for each individual.

SHEPARD'S PURSE

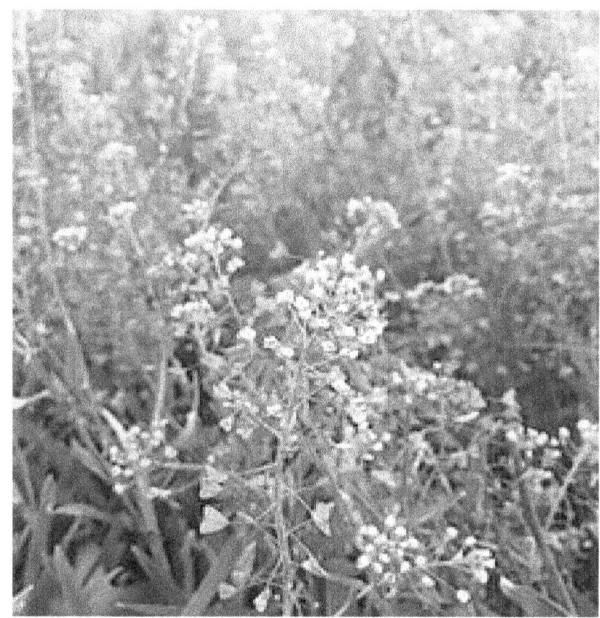

LATIN NAME Capsella *bursa-pastoris*

Kingdom:	Plantae
Clade:	Tracheophytes
Clade:	Angiosperms
Clade:	Eudicots
Clade:	Rosids
Order:	Brassicales
Family:	Brassicaceae
Genus:	*Capsella*
Species:	***C. bursa-pastoris***

Bursae pastoris herba
Hirtentschelkraut

Name of Drug

Bursae pastoris herba, shepherd's purse herb.

Composition of Drug

Shepherd's purse herb consists of the fresh or dried, above-ground parts of *Capsella bursa pastoris* (L.) Medikus [Fam.Brassicaceae], as well as its preparations in effective dosage.

Uses
Internal:

- Symptomatic treatment of mild menorrhagia and metrorrhagia, topical application for nose bleeds.

External:

- Superficial, bleeding skin injuries.

Contraindications
None known.

Side Effects
None known.

Interactions with Other Drugs

None known.

Dosage

Unless otherwise prescribed:

Average daily dosage:

- 10 - 15 g of drug;
- equivalent preparations.

Topical use:

- 3 - 5 g of herb per cup of water as tea.

Fluidextract (according to *Erg.B.6*):

- Daily dosage: 5 - 8 g.

Mode of Administration

Comminuted drug for tea and other galenical preparations for internal use and external application.

Actions

Parenteral application only:

- Muscarine-like effects with dose-dependent lowering and elevation of blood pressure;
- Positive inotropic and chronotropic cardiac effects;
- Increased uterine contraction.

HISTORY

Shepherd's Purse has been known by several other interesting common names over the centuries. Some have called it Witches' Pouches, Poverty Weed, Blind Weed, Beggar Tick, Mother's Heart, or Poor Man's Pharmacy. Other common names used have been Shepherd's Sprout, Case Wort, Cocowort, Shepherd's Heart, Toy Wort, Pick Purse, Pickooker, Pick-Pocket, St. James' Weed, St. James' Wort, St. Anthony's Fire, Pepper Grass, Permacety, and Poor Man's Parmacettie. Additionally, it has been called Shepherd's Bag, Shepherd's Scrip, Lady's Purse, Rattle Pouches, Case Weed, Shovel Weed, Pepper-and-Salt, and Sanguinary. The Irish name, Clappedepouch came into being because the seed pods resembled the bell or clapper the lepers would ring in Ireland as they would beg for alms, offering a cup attached to the end of a long pole in which to receive the alms. The name Shepherd's Purse "Comes from the association with the shape of the purse carried by the shepherd's of Bethlehem. The Poor Man's Pharmacy refers to its past medicinal use and inexpensive availability." In the French language is it called Bourse de Pasteur or Capselle; in German it has been called Hirtentasche, Hirtentaschelkraut, and Taschenkraut. In Russian it is reported to be called Pastushya Sumka which means the same thing as Shepherd's Purse. By this author, it has been called, My Best Friend and a Life Saver!

The Latin name "Capsella means "little box," referring to the fruit, as does bursa pastoris ("purse of the shepherd")."

According to Bown, "Archaeobotanical remains containing Shepherd's Purse seeds were recovered during excavation of the Catal Huyuk site in Turkey (ca. 5950 B.C.E.). Seeds were also recovered from the stomach of the Tollund man (ca. 500 B.C.E.-400 C.E.) (Bown, 1995)."
Shepherd's Purse was well known and used as a medicine in ancient Roman and Greek times, and it retained its popularity all over Europe into the Middle Ages. About 1615, Gervase Markham's book, "The English Housewife," listed a recipe for dysentery or diarrhea that included Shepherd's Purse as one of its ingredients. And in John Josselyn's "Herbal," there is mention that Shepherd's Purse was considered to have been unknown in America prior to the landing of the Pilgrims, and it later was carried as far as ". . . the Heartland between 1826 and 1859." The Chippewa Indians used Shepherd's Purse as an infusion for treating diarrhea, dysentery and for stomach cramps. The Mohegan Indians used the seed pods for relieving stomach aches and for expelling worms. Hutchens mentions that the American Indians roasted Shepherd's Purse seeds and added them to other meals to make pinole bread, which is a meal ground from plant seeds, and then roasted. The leaves were also used cooked or raw, like spinach.

In Philadelphia, the leaves were sold as greens and it was reported in at least two publications to affect cow's milk. If the cows are allowed to eat freely of Shepherd's Purse, it will taint the flavor, yet it was used in England to stop the diarrhea which occurs in calves, in modern days, called scours. Perhaps they should have just given the cows Shepherd's Purse and then allowed the calves to cure themselves of the scours from their own mother's udders! It was used among the common, nonprofessional people in England in the early times as an astringent for diarrhea in humans too.
A fresh decoction was used in hematuria (blood in the urine), hemorrhoids, chronic diarrhea and dysentery. The juice would be put into the ear for earaches, and onto cotton which would then be inserted into the nostrils for nosebleeds. A tincture would work for these purposes too. Shepherd's Purse was used for uterine hemorrhages, with or without cramping.   This author, in fact, has used it personally for uterine hemorrhages with great success. Details of these experiences will be given in Chapter H of this work. It was used for colic, rheumatic afflictions, and hemorrhages from parts of the body other than the uterus. It was highly favored to deal with catarrh of the bladder and ureter, and with ulcerated or abscessed bladder, especially when white mucus is voided with the urine.

Shepherd's Purse increased the flow of urine and gave quick relief. Therefore, it was used for kidney ailments and dropsy, and was combined with herbs such as Couch Grass (Agropyrum repens), or other stimulating diuretics. Dr. Ellingwood found it valuable and soothing for hematuria. He also found it to be a permanent cure for uncomplicated chronic menorrhagia (excessive menstruation), especially with cases that were persistent. Shepherd's Purse was also helpful in cases where the urinary tract would be irritated by such things as uric acid (many times caused by eating meat), insoluble phosphates, or carbonates.

Shepherd's Purse has been used externally as a bruised-plant poultice on Rheumatic joints, skin that oozes blood (ecchymosis), bruises, strained parts, and extravasations (leakage into the surrounding skin and tissue of fluids from an intra venous infusion).

In the 1700's, Culpeper mentioned that it helped bleeding from internal and external wounds. He further stated: "If bound to the wrists or the soles of the feet, it helps the jaundice. The herb made into poultices, helps inflammation and St. Anthony's Fire. The juice dropped into the ears, heals the pains, noise and matterings thereof. A good ointment may be made of it for all wounds, especially wounds in the head." Parkinson also stated, "Some do hold that the green herb bruised and bound to the wrists of the hands and the soles of the feet will help yellow jaundice."

As one contemplates Shepherd's Purse being 'bound to the wrists or the souls of the feet', one is reminded how well fresh poultices can affect healing, as the medicinal properties can be absorbed right through the skin, into the bloodstream. One should further, remember that 'fresh is best', <u>especially</u> with Shepherd's Purse. Another important point that is well worth remembering is that putting Shepherd's Purse on the souls of the feet would be of great benefit from a foot reflexology point of view, since nerve endings for all the parts of the whole body end in the feet, and can be affected by herbs being applied there as well as massage. Moreover, in the case of jaundice, helping the other major organs at the same time as the liver via the soles of the feet would of course, help the liver heal quicker since all of the major organs affect each other.
In Russian folk medicine, it was used for stomach troubles, such as diarrhea, dysentery, gastritis, gall bladder, kidney and bladder trouble, liver colics, disturbed metabolism, venereal disease, lung tuberculosis, bleeding lungs, and malaria. For stomach ulcers, bleeding ulcers and typhus it is used in a vodka menstruum. In Russia, it is clinically used for female bleeding, bloody urine and bleeding from the stomach. During World War One, when the Russians were unable to import Canadian Golden Seal (Hydrastis canadensis), interest was renewed in Shepherd's Purse. This herb has played a prominent role since then in folk medicine and clinical use. The leaves were used in soups and salads, and the seeds were used instead of mustard.

Mrs. Grieve felt it to be one of the most important medicinal herbs from the Cruciferous family because it is the best at stopping hemorrhages from the stomach, lungs, uterus and especially from the kidneys. Its ". . . haemostyptic . . ." qualities were thought to be equal to those of ergot and hydrastis. Then, during World War One, when ergot and hydrastis were no longer available to the German people, they resorted to a liquid extract of Shepherd's Purse made by extracting it with boiling water. During this time, Bomelon used one to two teaspoons of the liquid extract for ". . . bleedings and floodings . . .". Although Mrs. Grieve felt that the odor of Shepherd's Purse was ". . . peculiar and rather unpleasant, though more cress-like than pungent.", she was aware that small, wild birds would love to eat the seeds of Shepherd's Purse, and that the seeds were considered a valuable component of feed for caged birds. She also shared that after poultry has eaten of Shepherd's Purse in the spring, it has been found to turn the egg yolks darker in color, even to a greenish-brown or olive color. The flavor of the eggs becomes stronger too. I wonder what, if anything, it would do to the flavor and color of the meat if eaten? Regarding poultry and Shepherd's Purse, Dr. John Raymond Christopher expressed his opinion: "Poultry seek it eagerly, and people who must raise chickens in confinement would do well to pull handfuls of this herb, as well as of wild lettuce, comfrey, plantain, purslane and other succulent wild greens, to give to their poultry in cages. You will be amazed at how eagerly the chickens devour this wild food and how the quality of their eggs vastly improves with this simple addition to their diet. To let your chickens run free and find the greens themselves is of course a better alternative." This author wholeheartedly agrees, with Dr. Christopher's sentiment and further adds that the health of the chickens will be better from the healthy 'live' food and the sunshine and exercise!

A technique used by the French gypsies, was to bathe a wound in a strong infusion of Shepherd's Purse, then fill the wound with clean cobwebs! The poor Chinese cultivate it, and the seed pods are even eaten. The Chinese characters representing the Shepherd's Purse plant represent the meaning ". . . protecting life plant . . . ", because it was reported to repel night insects such as mosquitos. The roots and leaves are used for stomach and liver ailments. It was surprising to discover that the ashes are used for bleeding and for treatment of sore eyes! If used for an extended period of time, the seed pods will aid vision. The flowers are reported to destroy some parasitic worms and to control dysentery.

In addition to China as mentioned in the previous paragraph, "Shepherd's Purse is cultivated in India and other temperate and warm regions around the world. The material of commerce is collected mainly from wild plants in southeastern Europe, particularly from Bulgaria, Hungary, former Yugoslavia, and the former U.S.S.R."

Dr. Christopher considered Shepherd's Purse to be a good plant to include in a diet, because it is a good general tonic and a wonderful digestive tonic. Plant extracts have been proven in laboratory tests to prevent duodenal ulcers in rats that were put purposefully under stress. Using a variety of test conditions with animals, Shepherd's Purse extracts have proven to have anti-inflammatory and anti-tumor properties. However, the extracts do not inhibit bacterial growth like garlic and cayenne. Although many authors have expressed a dislike for Shepherd's Purse's flavor as a pot herb, especially in its raw state, this author found it tasting like broccoli when eaten raw.

LeArta Moulton expressed her opinion this way: "The plant has been used as a substitute for spinach and is very good when blanched. It has a good flavor of cabbage which makes it a nice addition to fresh salads." A few comments found by other authors were also positive regarding its taste, like this one from Deb Schwartz: "When harvesting the plant, you may notice a distinctive and not quite pleasant odor. Don't worry, it doesn't taste like that." She went on to comment about eating Shepherd's Purse roots in this manner: "The young roots are also edible, but I either haven't developed a taste for them yet or haven't stumbled upon the proper method of preparation. I have read that the seed pods can be used for a peppery seasoning, but the one's I've tried had no flavor. The seeds themselves can be ground into meal or used as is." Her recipe and instructions for preparing Shepherd's Purse is listed in Chapter G of this work.

Many garden plants' flavor or hotness varies in strength due to the volume of water and various nutrients the plant has received. Radishes, for example, can be quite hot or cooler to the taste when harvested, depending on the amount of water it has received. Perhaps, therefore, the reason some people find Shepherd's Purse peppery or strong in flavor, while others find it tastes more like cabbage or broccoli, might be due in part to these factors. Two other factors might be the time of year it is harvested, or whether one is in need of the nutrients or healing powers of the plant.   Many times one likes something more that contains nutrients the body is lacking. When this author was hemorrhaging, the plant tasted delicious. Another time, it did not taste quite as wonderful.

Shepherd's Purse must, indeed, be a very well known and popular plant. It must be so, since a poem has even been written in modern times about it:

"SHEPHERD'S PURSE
By John Haines

Poverty Weed or Beggar Tick,
some days in the field
are leaner than others.

Let the stalk be strong,
the flower head high
and the seedbox full–

November like a tax collector
will come to the poor,
the cut and the shaken,

with nothing to save
but their paper mittens
and a straw whistle.

In a time of hard money
keep a small purse,
spend little.

Be sure to have more
than one heart,
and you may survive.

The last entry in this chapter is a touching story that needs to be told in its entirety shared with the author by a dear friend when requesting information and experiences with Shepherd's Purse: "Shepherd's Purse is like a long lost friend to me. When I was in the fourth to sixth grade my twin and I had an interesting experience with the plant. My mom divorced my dad when we were three and had no where to go with no money. She went on welfare but I'm not sure what benefits they gave her, but I don't think it was enough. We were always skimping to find food. We'd go to food pantries and W.I.C. I remember we got our school lunches free and I would think it was a "King's Feast" and would eat everything on my tray and I still felt like I was starving. I could never understand why other children would leave half of their food on their tray and complain that it was awful. Whatever was going on with me and my twin I don't know, but one day in the fourth grade we were walking home taking our time walking in the tall weeds trying to find paper to eat. I know that sounds strange, but my twin would look for old paper to eat off the ground. But as we were thus doing I noticed little white flowers on the tips of these "fun to explore through" weeds. I all of the sudden got the inclination to eat it. So I did. I tell you it was the most delicious thing I've ever tasted. I had my sister taste it. It immediately took our attention away from eating paper and satisfied us, after eating a fourth of a street block, from our hunger. Every day we'd run home to that big patch of Shepherd's Purse. Each day we'd eat less, feeling more and more satisfied. We got our younger brother to start eating it. After two years our hunger pains were nearly gone. They were still there a little though because of our poor diet at home, but every time we felt unsatisfied with food we'd run over to the big patch.

We usually only would have to eat a big handful to feel satisfied. In the 8th grade my mother remarried and we moved away. Every chance I saw the plant I'd eat it. It wasn't until four years ago I learned what the plant was. In 1996 my husband and I moved into a trailer on one acre of mud! Yuck! We didn't have money to plant grass so the next year the good Mother earth brought up thousands of Shepherd's Purse plants. My old friend was back! We had lots of other "weeds" too. I studied what they were and shared them with my husband and children. It was fun. I found out though that by late summer they start to mold her in Illinois. I guess from the humidity. The third year only little patches of the plant came up and the fourth year none came up. I've looked for them in other fields and they are rare here. They seem to come up well when they are not crowded out by more dominating herbs and plants. I've gone back to the big patch of Shepherd's Purse of my youth and they were no longer there also. They may lay dormant until a certain time they decide to come up. Perhaps." Carmela Hearle. In a phone conversation after this communication, Carmela was asked what the Shepherd's Purse tasted like to her and her siblings. She reported that it tasted like broccoli to them.

CHEMICAL CONSTITUENTS

It is nice to see that there has been improvement in the amount of information available, and the testing that has been done on Shepherd's Purse and its constituents in the past 70 years or so. Back in 1931, when Grieve originally published "A Modern Herbal", this is what she had to say about Shepherd's Purse's chemical constituents:

"Several partial analyses have been made of it, but no characteristic principle has been definitely separated. The active constituent is said to be an organic acid, which Bombelon, a French chemist, termed bursinic acid. He also found a tannate and an alkaloid, Bursine, which resembles sulphocyansinapine. A peculiar sulphuretted volatile oil, closely similar to, if not identical with oil of mustard, as well as a fixed oil, have been determined and 6 per cent. of a soft resin."

Then approximately 30 to 40 years later, although some laboratory analyses showed Shepherd's Purse to be low in Vitamin C, it had been used as an antiscorbutic (anti scurvy). Dr. Christopher's thoughts regarding this topic were: "It may be, however, that through transformation in the digestive tract the combinations of materials in the plant might help prevent scurvy."

As time has progressed on through the 1960's and into the 1970's, 80's and 90's, an overwhelming amount of information has turned up about the constituents of Shepherd's Purse, due to more laboratory research having been done, and the climate in Europe being so open and accepting to herbs as alternatives to prescription pharmaceutical drugs. This seems overwhelming mostly, due to the fact that this author is not a chemist! Thankfully, as the chemical constituents are known, it will further the knowledge of how Shepherd's Purse can be used.

As a result of modern research, we have learned that "Shepherd's Purse contains the active components saponin, mustard oil, the alkaloid bursine, the flavonoid glycoside diasmium, organic acids, tannin, large quantities of vitamin C and K and the amines choline, acetylcholine and tyramine."   It seems there is no doubt now about the mustard oil nor the vitamin C. We have also learned that "The herb must be free of the parasitic fungus Cystopus candidins."

There is lots more information on the nutrients in Shepherd's Purse than before. Schwartz informs us that "The leaves are very high in thiamin (B-1), choline, inositol, and fumaric acid. They are a good source of ascorbic acid (C), riboflavin (B-2), calcium, potassium, and phosphorus. They also provide beta carotene (A), vitamin K, niacin, iron and rutin. It also contains compounds (such as fumaric acid), which are known to have anti-cancer effects."

We also now know that "Efforts to determine a bioactive hemostatic principle in Shepherd's Purse point to an unspecified peptide" and that it ". . . contains flavonoids, including luteolin and quercetin 7-retinosides and luteolin 7-galactoside; glucosinolates (e.g., sinigrin) (Iurisson, 1973; Wichtl and Bisset, 1994); . . ." and "approximately 0.02% volatile oil . . .". Lastly, it seems that there is some controversy regarding Shepherd's Purse because "The previously reported occurrence of biogenetic amines and saponins is disputed (Wichtl, 1996)."

Hopefully, as the present proceeds into the future, researchers, practitioners and the general public will come to realize that the Good Lord meant for these chemicals to be left intact and together in the plant, and used as a whole plant, the way God intended.

MEDICINAL QUALITIES

Most herbalists agree on most of the medicinal qualities of Shepherd's Purse, they being astringent, styptic, diuretic, anti-scorbutic, vasoconstrictor and blood coagulant, which therefore makes it anti-hemorrhagic (or hemostatic). Additionally, Kloss listed it as having detergent and vulnerary qualities, Grieve said it was anti-diarrheal, Duke mentioned its antioxidant qualities and Schwartz claimed it to be anti-inflammatory. Moore got more specific, mentioning that Shepherd's Purse uses were: "Urinary tract astringent, uric acid diuretic for hyperuricemia; hemostatic for hematuria, excess menses, and so forth; and an oxytocin agonist for postpartum bleeding or difficult placenta delivery."

Weed and Schwartz both mentioned that fresh is best with Shepherd's Purse since the dry loses its medicinal power quite quickly. Since Shepherd's Purse quickly loses its power, tinctures are usually prepared with the fresh plant while available, to have on hand when it is not. Karen Erickson, a Naturopath Doctor and Lay Midwife, shared, "It is very temperamental in terms of its preparation and has only a very short shelf life preserved as a tincture (less than one year). For this reason I use it combined with other herbs (Achillea, Geranium, etc.) and carefully date the bottle."

Christopher reported that Shepherd's Purse can raise blood pressure by constricting blood vessels, and can also normalize the blood and heart action whether too high or low. Schwartz, on the other hand, was less sure when she stated, "It constricts the blood vessels (usually), lowers blood pressure (usually), and contracts the uterus. It is used during or after childbirth and to ease difficult menstruation." Lust mentioned that it promotes bowel movements in the same manner that it will promote uterine contractions during labor.

"Intraperitoneal administration of Shepherd's Purse extract to rats blocked the formation of stress induced ulcers and reduced recovery time (Kuroda and Takagi, 1969). Anti-neoplastic, central nervous system-depressant, and hypotensive effects have also been observed, and in vitro tests have shown smooth-muscle stimulant effects. Cardiac activity includes increased coronary blood flow, negative chronotropic effects, positive inotropic effects, and coronary vasodilation in laboratory animals (Kuroda and Takagi, 1969; Iurisson, 1971)."

DOSAGES

Generally, dosages would be as follows although dosages may need to be changed to fit the situation. "Decoction, 2 fluid ounces 3 times daily between meals. Fluid extract, 1 teaspoonful (1/8 of decoction). Infusion, 1 cupful. Powder, 1-4 grams. Tincture, ½ -1 fluid teaspoon (30-60 drops)."

The most commonly known use for Shepherd's Purse has been for bleeding in general and uterine hemorrhage postpartum specifically, as it constricts blood vessels. It is usually used in conjunction with other anti-hemorrhagic herbs such as cayenne, mistletoe, yarrow etc., along with lobelia. Weed feels, that the dosage to control bleeding after completing a miscarriage, should be 10-20 drops of the tincture, and 20-40 drops for postpartum hemorrhage. With the fresh plant tincture being better and stronger, she says that if the dried plant extract or tincture is all you have available, try 1 teaspoon, (150 drops) under the tongue and repeat every minute or as needed.

King suggests having Shepherd's Purse powder or tincture ready during labor, 'just in case'. He mentioned that it can be used to regulate excessive menstrual flow, and that a tincture or fomentation of Shepherd's Purse can be rubbed into the abdomen for prolapsed uterus, starting with the vagina and working upward. He also suggested 2 C daily of the tea for menstrual cramps. King said it can be used as a douche for fibroid tumors of the uterus. Moore mentions "Trillium . . . works remarkably well for fibroid (myomas and fibromyomas) bleeding combined with 30 drops of Shepherd's Purse." And "For mid-cycle spotting, especially during ovulation, use the same approach, taking the Trillium and Shepherd's Purse doses for at least a couple of days." (Regarding Trillium, that is Trillium ovatum.) It is also a "hemostatic for hematuria, excess menses and so forth; oxytocin agonist for postpartum bleeding or difficult placenta delivery." Shepherd's Purse in extract form ". . . is found in a few anti-dysmenorrhea drugs (Wichtl and Bisset, 1994)."

Davis said, that for a slow trickle of blood after delivery of the placenta ". . . give several droppersful of shepherd's purse and blue cohosh tinctures." Erickson, said that due to Shepherd's Purse being ". . . very temperamental in terms of its preparation . . ." and having ". . . only a very short shelf life preserved as a tincture (less than 1 year)", she uses it ". . . combined with other herbs (Achillea, Geranium, etc.) . . .". She also said, "For postpartum hemorrhage specifically, I try to use capsella and another anti-hemorrhagic in equal parts. If I have time I may add capsicum, zingibir, etc. in small amounts. I use high doses because I need it to work; usually several ml as a loading dose, than 1 ml or so every 5-15 minutes depending on action. I have never used it for more than an hour!" Among all her many references to using Shepherd's Purse for various situations during labor, birth and postpartum where bleeding may occur, Block is clear to mention that the Shepherd's Purse must be used cold. Hutchens shared further that Shepherd's Purse is indicated in cases of excessive menstruation.

This author has also happily learned that Shepherd's Purse is good for constant menstruation (metrorrhagia). A dear long time friend shared the following story with us: "Due to a hormone imbalance, I suffered from constant menstrual bleeding for 16 years. I tried medical intervention, but that only served to mask the symptoms for a time and the bleeding would always return. An herbalist I spoke to advised me to try fresh Shepherd's Purse. I picked a bag full and every day for 2 weeks blended up one quart of the herb with canned pineapple juice and drank it. After 2 weeks the bleeding stopped. Then one or two weeks later I had my first normal 5-day period in 16 years. This was seven years ago, and I have been regular every month since." The mixture of herbs blended with the pineapple juice is commonly called a 'green drink' and can include any herbs. The herbs can be left in and drunk or strained out before drinking.

Shepherd's Purse has a variety of other applications. It can be used alone or in conjunction with other herbs for equalizing blood pressure, and can be an alternative herb for use with hypothermia. The plant pulp can be bruised or chewed and inserted into the nostril for nosebleeds, and can be used instead of Cayenne for nosebleeds with children.

The pressed juice from Shepherd's Purse can be dropped into the ear for earaches, can be used as a tea to increase bodily circulation with gangrene, and can be used with nettle for shock. Shepherd's Purse can be used in conjunction with other herbs as a poultice for mastitis or bleeding wounds.

Shepherd's Purse acts on the kidney and bladder, as a stimulant and moderate tonic for catarrh of the urinary tract indicated by much mucus in the urine. It is also good for internal bleeding of the lungs and colon, diarrhea and intermittent fever. When combined with Agrimony (Agrimony eupatoria), it is good for bed-wetting. Moore adds that it is good as a uric acid diuretic, can be combined with Bidens (Bidens frondosa, b. pilosa, B. pinnata) for this purpose, and is helpful for prostate problems. It is helpful for glaucoma, hemorrhoids, is a tonic when cold and a diaphoretic when hot.

"In China, a decoction of the dried whole plant is used . . . as a hemostatic agent for treatment of chyluria (fat globules in the urine) and hematuria (Huang, 1999). "In India, it is applied topically to injured varicose veins as an antihemorrhagic agent (Karnick, 1994).

Shepherd's Purse has applications as a food as evidenced by the wonderful story in Chapter A, History of Shepherd's Purse, pages thirteen and fourteen. It is used by many as a salad: "Shepherd's Purse grows like crazy in my back yard, and I use it as a salad green all summer, the seed pods and the leaf." Schwartz shares, "So far my favorite way to cook the greens is to put them in a loosely covered dish with a little water, some mushrooms, and a sprig or two of thyme, microwave it on high for 4 minutes, and serve with butter. They are also very good to mix with other greens. The roots are also edible, but I either haven't developed a taste for them yet or haven't stumbled upon the proper method of preparation."

Surprising as it may seem, Shepherd's Purse even has some unusual applications! "The seeds, aside from sticking to insects, are also reported to be toxic to mosquito larvae, and, when put in the water, may possibly help control mosquitos. Shepherd's Purse will also absorb excessive salts from the soil, and may be planted for that purpose." "Most recently, Shepherd's Purse has been investigated for its possible use as a biomonitor of heavy metals contamination in the environment. The authors of this study reported that it may become a particularly useful plant for monitoring short-term changes in pollution levels in urban areas (Aksoy et al.,1999).

SLIPPERY ELM

LATIN NAME Ulmus rubra

Kingdom: Plantae
Clade: Tracheophytes
Clade: Angiosperms
Clade: Eudicots
Clade: Rosids
Order: Rosales
Family: Ulmaceae
Genus: *Ulmus*
Subgenus: *U.* subg. *Ulmus*
Section: *U.* sect. *Ulmus*
Species: **U. rubra**

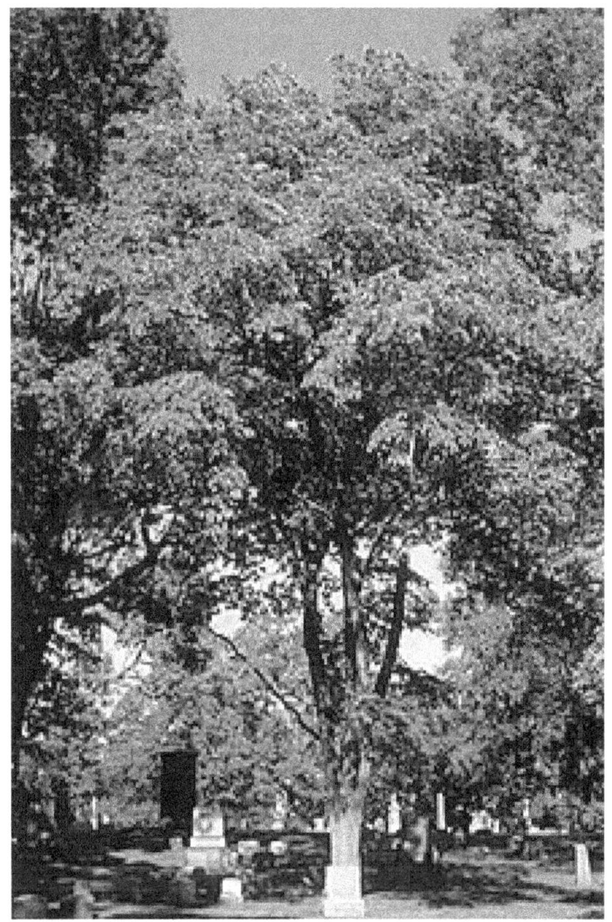

Ulmus rubra, the **slippery elm**, is a species of elm native to eastern North America, ranging from southeast North Dakota, east to Maine and southern Quebec, south to northernmost Florida, and west to eastern Texas, where it thrives in moist uplands, although it will also grow in dry, intermediate soils. Other common names include red elm, gray elm, soft elm, moose elm, and Indian elm. The tree was first named as part of *Ulmus americana* in 1753, but identified as a separate species, *Ulmus rubra*, in 1793 by Pennsylvania botanist Gotthilf Muhlenberg. The slightly later name *U. fulva*, published by French botanist André Michaux in 1803,[6] is still widely used in dietary-supplement and alternative-medicine information.

The species superficially resembles American elm (*U. americana*), but is more closely related to the European wych elm (*U. glabra*), which has a very similar flower structure, though lacks the pubescence over the seed. *U. rubra* was introduced to Europe in 1830

Medicinal

Ulmus rubra has various traditional medicinal uses. The mucilaginous inner bark of the tree is edible has long been used as a demulcent, and is still produced commercially for this purpose in the United States with approval for sale as an over-the-counter demulcent by the U.S. Food and Drug Administration. Sometimes leaves are dried and ground into a powder, then made into a tea.

Uses For Slippery Elm:

Due to its demulcent properties, slippery elm can be used for coughs, sore throat, and colic when added to lozenges or teas. The Food and Drug Administration (FDA) recognizes slippery elm bark as an effective option for these symptoms.

Slippery elm preparations cause an increase in mucus secretion in the gastrointestinal tract that may be useful in the management of gastrointestinal disorders such as stomach and duodenal ulcers, gastroesophageal reflux disease (GERD), irritable bowl syndrome (IBS) and inflammatory bowel disease, although supportive research evidence is lacking. Slippery elm may also promote the expulsion of tapeworms.

When used topically, slippery elm bark can be used to help heal burns and inflammatory skin disorders such as psoriasis, minor wounds, and gout.

Slippery Elm Dosages:

Adults

Slippery elm lozenges as needed for a sore throat or mouth sores.

Powders can be used to make gruels, teas and external skin salves.

Gruel: Mix one teaspoon of the powder with one teaspoon of sugar and add two cups of boiling water, mixing well. Flavor with cinnamon, if desired. Drink one or two cups, twice a day. Good for infants, those who have chronic illnesses or stomach upset.

Tea: Steep two tablespoons of powdered bark for 3-5 minutes in two cups of boiling water. Drink three times a day.

Topical: For skin irritation, mix course slippery elm powder with boiling water to make a poultice. Allow it to cool and then apply it to minor burns, itchy skin, and uncomplicated wounds. Do not apply to open wounds or sores.

Capsules: As directed

Extracts: Slippery elm extract usually comes in a 1:1 concentration, so read the label carefully for directions.

For Children

Same as above. Slippery elm gruel is especially good for infants.

1. Helps Improve Digestive Function

Is slippery elm a laxative? Although it works differently than some other laxatives, it seems to improve symptoms of constipation, IBD and IBS, including in both adults and children. The fresh inner bark can be used in place of, or along with, other natural laxatives.

In one study, the effects of two different formulas on digestive function were compared, both of which included SE in addition to other herbs.

Formula one was associated with a small but significant increase in bowel movement frequency, as well as reductions in straining, abdominal pain, bloated stomach and IBS symptoms. Subjects who took formula two experienced a 20 percent increase in bowel movement frequency and significant reductions in straining, abdominal pain, bloating and global IBS symptom severity, as well as improvements in stool consistency. Ultimately, both formulas led to improvements.

SE has also been shown in certain studies to treat diarrhea and diverticulitis. Additionally, it may help protect against ulcers and excess acidity in the GI tract because it causes reflux stimulation of nerve endings, and that reaction leads to increased mucus secretion. Not only does this help most people, but it can actually give much relief to your dog too.

2. May Aid in Weight Loss (When Combined With a Low-Calorie Diet)

Since SE has the ability to improve digestion, this may aid in weight loss.

A study performed at New York Chiropractic College used normal participants from the faculty, staff, students and community members to participate in a 21-day weight loss program. Nutritional supplements containing digestive enzymes that were intended to facilitate digestion, reduce cholesterol levels, increase metabolic rate and mediate inflammatory processes were consumed 30 minutes before each meal.

The regimented supplementation program included daily supplementation with a one green drink, as well as a "cleanse supplementation" containing slippery elm plus other herbs and minerals. The cleansing mixture was taken before each meal during week two of the study. During week three, the cleanse supplementation was replaced with prebiotic and probiotic supplementation.

At the end of the study researchers found that participants experienced clinically meaningful reductions in weight and low-density lipoprotein cholesterol. It was concluded that "Weight loss and improvements in total cholesterol and low-density lipoprotein cholesterol levels occurred after a low-energy-density dietary intervention plus regimented supplementation program."

3. Can Help Reduce Oxidative Stress

Because it contains compounds called phenolics, SE may act as a natural free radical scavenger and fighter of oxidative stress.

Phenolics are antioxidants that have been shown to elicit cellular responses that counter oxidant stress, which contributes to aging and many chronic diseases. Plant phenolics also seem to help protect against pathogens due to their natural antifungal effects.

4. May Help Prevent Breast Cancer

SE was first promoted as an option to help treat breast cancer, including DCIS, in the 1920s. The inner bark of SE has become an herbal remedy used by some to help support cancer recovery for prevention, and for improving quality of life and side effects among those undergoing conventional breast cancer treatments.

Though more studies need to be conducted, slippery elm — when combined with certain herbs such as burdock root, Indian rhubarb and sheep sorrel (which together form the supplement called Essiac) — may improve conditions for women with breast cancer and improve depression, anxiety and fatigue.

Because it has immune-boosting benefits and anti-inflammatory effects, it may help relieve pain associated with breast cancer.

5. May Reduce Severity of Symptoms of Psoriasis

SE has been shown in certain studies help patients with psoriasis, a condition that currently has no cure.

In one study, five case studies were evaluated of patients with psoriasis following a specific dietary regimen. The subjects were asked to follow a dietary protocol that included a diet of fresh fruits and vegetables, small amounts of protein from fish and fowl, fiber supplements, olive oil, and avoidance of red meat, processed foods and refined carbohydrates. They were also asked to consume saffron tea and slippery elm bark water daily.

The five psoriasis cases, ranging from mild to severe at the study onset, improved on all measured outcomes over a six-month period, demonstrating that SE makes a great addition to any psoriasis diet treatment.

Slippery Elm Interesting Facts

Slippery elm trees, identified by their "slippery" inner bark, may live to be 200 years old. Sometimes called red elm, gray elm or soft elm, this tree grows best on moist, rich soils of lower slopes and flood plains, although it may also grow on dry hillsides with limestone soils.

Although SE trees are abundant and associated with many other hardwood trees, they are not important lumber trees; instead they have been used mostly for medicinal purposes throughout history.

In the U.S., SE trees are uncommon in much of the South, but grow abundantly in the southern part of the lake states and in the corn belt of the Midwest. They can be found growing from Maine west to New York, extreme southern Quebec, southern Ontario, northern Michigan, central Minnesota and in certain other areas.

As described above, there are many medicinal uses for slippery elm. Some Native American tribes believed SE could make childbirth easier. It was also consumed as a tea and was used to treat sore throats. The Iroquois were known to scrape the bark of the slippery elm tree to treat infections, swollen glands and conditions affecting the eyes.

However health-related purposes were not the only use of SE. The bark supplied material for the sides of winter houses and roofs of the Meskwaki. The inner bark was used by many tribes by boiling the bark to make fiber bags, large storage baskets, ropes and cords, making slippery elm one of the most versatile trees on the planet.

How to Use

SE bark can typically be found at your local health food store in a variety of forms — including tea, lozenges, capsules and tablets, poultice, and extract. If possible, speak with an herbalist or nutritionist for help finding what works for you.

Here are some of the most common uses and forms:

- Diarrhea (in humans and pets): treatment by ingestion of capsules, tablets, tea, tincture and extracts
- Cough (humans and cats): treatment by lozenges, tea, tincture, and extracts
- Acid reflux: treatment by tea, and extracts
- Constipation (pets, especially cats): treatment by powder or extract added to food
- External skin conditions (humans and pets): treatment by shampoo or topical cream infused with extract.

Dosage Recommendations:

Dosage is usually dependent on weight.

If making SE tea at home (see below) use about 2–3 teaspoons of powder per one-cup serving. You can consume the tea 1–2 times daily.

A general recommendation in capsule/tablet form is a dosage of about 1,600 milligrams daily, taken in 2–3 divided doses. Because the concentration of SE varies depending on the specific supplement, always read the product's dosage recommendations carefully.

Recipes

There are many ways you can incorporate SE into your diet. Here are a few recipes to try:

Slippery Elm Tea

INGREDIENTS:

- 1 tablespoon slippery elm bark powder
- 1 cup boiling water
- 1 teaspoon local honey (optional)
- 3 ounces almond or coconut milk
- 1/2 teaspoon of cacao
- Sprinkle of cinnamon

DIRECTIONS:

1. Add boiling water to cup.
2. Add the slippery elm bark powder and stir well.
3. Then add the honey, almond or coconut milk.
4. Stir again.
5. Top of with a sprinkle of cinnamon.

STINGING NETTLE

Stinging Nettle herb and leaf

LATIN NAME Urtica dioica

Kingdom: Plantae
Clade: Tracheophytes
Clade: Angiosperms
Clade: Eudicots
Clade: Rosids
Order: Rosales
Family: Urticaceae
Genus: *Urtica*
Species: **U.dioica**

Urticae herba/-folium
Brennesselkraut/Brennesselbltter

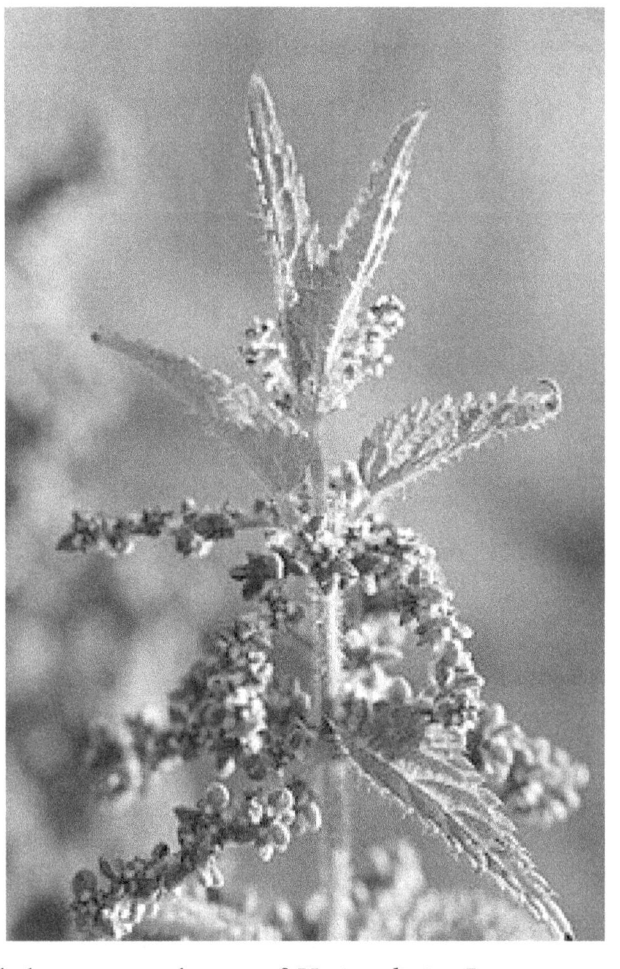

Name of Drug

Urticae herba, stinging nettle herb.
Urticae folium, stinging nettle leaf.

Composition of Drug

Stinging nettle herb consists of fresh or dried above-ground parts of *Urtica dioica* L., *U.urens* L.[Fam.Urticaceae], and/or hybrids of these species, collected during flowering season, as well as their preparations in effective dosage.

Stinging nettle leaf consists of fresh or dried leaves of *U.dioica* L., *U.urens* L.and/or hybrids of these species, gathered during flowering season, as well as their preparations in effective dosage.

Stinging nettle leaf and herb contain mineral salts, mainly calcium and potassium salts, and silicic acid.

Uses
Internal and external application:

- As supportive therapy for rheumatic ailments.

Internal:

- As irrigation therapy for inflammatory diseases of the lower urinary tract and prevention and treatment of kidney gravel.

Contraindications
None known.

Note: No irrigation therapy if edema exists due to impaired heart or kidney function.

Side Effects
None known.

Interactions with Other Drugs

None known.

Dosage

Unless otherwise prescribed:

Average daily dosage:

- 8 - 12 g of drug;
- equivalent preparations.

Mode of Administration

Comminuted herb for teas and other galenical preparations for internal use, as stinging nettle spirit for external application.

HISTORY

Stinging nettle is considered by many to be a bothersome pest, but the nettle has been used since ancient times as a source of food, fiber, and medicinal preparations. In Denmark, burial shrouds made of nettle fabrics have been discovered that date back to the Bronze Age (3000-2000 BC). Europeans and Native Americans used the fibers from stinging nettle to make sailcloth, sacking, cordage, and fishing nets. These fibers have also been used to produce cloth similar in feel and appearance to silky linen. During World War I, the German Empire, plagued by textile shortages, used nettles as a substitute for cotton. Captured German uniforms were found to be 85% nettle fiber.

Stinging nettle is one of the richest sources of chlorophyll in the vegetable kingdom. A decoction of the plant has been used to produce a green dye for clothing for centuries. At the beginning of the Second World War, a request by the British government was made for the collection of 100 tons of nettles, which were used for the extraction of this green dye for camouflage. This property has also been used commercially in Germany as a food coloring agent for canned vegetables.

In ancient Egypt reports are found of the use of nettle infusion for the relief of arthritis and lumbago pains. A standard practice of flogging oneself with the fresh nettle plant, called urtification, was prescribed to treat such illnesses as chronic rheumatism, lethargy, coma, paralysis, and even typhus, and cholera. This practice of urtification is known to many cultures and has been used for thousands of years. The Roman soldiers are said to have brought their own nettle to the British Isles to treat their tired, painful legs on long marches in the cold and wet climate by urtification, thus stimulating the circulation. Documentation or anecdotal reports of its use in this way have been found among the Ecuador Indians, ancient Romans, and Canadian and American native tribes.

Hippocrates (460-377 B.C.) and his followers reported 61 remedies using nettle. In the second century A.D., Galen, the Greek physician, recommended nettle in his book *De Simplicibus* as "a diuretic and laxative, for dog bites, gangrenous wounds, swellings, nose bleeding, excessive menstruation, spleen-related illness, pleurisy, pneumonia, asthma, tinea, and mouth sores." Two hundred years after Galen, Apuleius Platonicus (circa 400 A.D.), in his book *Herbarium of Apuleius,* added nettle combined with hemp or cannabis to "treat symptoms of feeling cold after being burnt (shocked)", and nettle by itself for "cold injury". Throughout the Dark Ages (fifth to tenth centuries) uses of nettle were expanded to include treatment of shingles, constipation, and "dry disease", which probably meant problems with the sinuses or lungs, mucous membranes, and skin.

The 16th century herbalist John Gerard used stinging nettle as an antidote for poison. In the seventeenth century, Culpeper, the astrologer-physician, recommended a nettle and honey extract as a gargle for throat and mouth infections, and claimed that nettles were helpful for "bladder stones or gravel, worms in children, an antiseptic for wounds and skin infections, gout, sciatica, joint aches, and as an antidote to venomous stings from animals". In the nineteenth century, Phelps Brown suggested nettle internally as a diuretic and tonic. He hailed it as a remedy for dysentery, hemorrhoids, bladder and kidney stones, and used the seeds and flowers in wine for fevers. It was also employed in cases of infant diarrhea and eczema.

Stinging nettle has always been recognized for its tonic and nutritional value. It is rich in vitamins and minerals and has traditionally been used primarily in the spring time to stimulate slow winter blood. Its reputation for restorative powers for the sick has been particularly appreciated in poor and rural areas, especially since it is freely available from the fields and ditches. There are reports of the Romans eating nettles as food and using it in the boiling of meat to tenderize it. It is used as a pot plant, in a soup, a tea, and as an ale or beer. Nettle is a traditional remedy for scurvy, anemia, and lack of energy. This is due to its high level of iron, vitamin C, magnesium, and other nutrients. The English poet, Campbell, complained of the little attention paid to the nettle in England. He says, "In Scotland, I have eaten nettles, I have slept in nettle sheets, and I have dined off a nettle tablecloth. The young and tender nettle is an excellent potherb. The stalks of the old nettle are as good as flax for making cloth. I have heard my mother say that she thought nettle cloth more durable than any other species of linen."

The infusion was found to be helpful in increasing milk production, both in humans and in cows. It has been used freely as a gynecological aid by women of the North American aboriginal nations. The juice is taken by pregnant women who are overdue to promote labor. The tips of the plant were chewed during childbirth, as well as the infusion being drunk to relax the muscles.

Stinging nettle has been used throughout history as animal fodder, as vegetarian rennet in cheese making, and is still included in the Passover herbs. The juice was used as a hair rinse and to stimulate hair growth. The leaf was used as a snuff powder or as a local application for nosebleeds, excessive menstruation, and internal bleeding. It is applied to burns and taken in syrup or tincture form to treat urticaria, or nettle rash. It is, in fact, its own remedy. Other uses have included the stems and leaves soaked in water and the water used as an organic pesticide, being applied to plants with mites or aphids. The plant enlivens and conditions the soil, speeding decomposition in compost heaps, and improves the health and vigor of plants.

Modern medicinal uses of nettle are not much different than that of the past. People today still practice urtification, and clinical studies have investigated its use in treating many medical conditions, including allergic rhinitis, rheumatic complaints, eczema, anemia, bleeding (both internally and externally), and acute arthritis. It is in demand as a treatment for benign prostate hyperplasia (BPH), high blood pressure, and urinary tract infections. It is used in treating skin eruptions and freeze-dried as a treatment for hay fever and allergies. It is also being promoted as a textile product once again.

CHEMICAL CONSTITUENTS

Numerous analyses of nettle have revealed the presence of more than fifty different chemical constituents. The roots of stinging nettle have been studied extensively and found to contain starch, gum, albumen, sugar, and two resins. Histamine, acetylcholine, choline, and serotonin are also present. In addition, oleanol acid, sterols and steryl glycosides (including 3-beta-sitosterin), scopoletin (a coumarin), secoisolariciresinol, and neo-olivil (both lignans), and homovanillyl alcohol have been found. An immunologically active polysaccharide fraction was isolated which yielded neutral sugar, protein, and uronic acid. Methalonic extract of the roots were investigated for their inhibitory effect in aromatase, a key enzyme in steroid hormone metabolism. Many active constituents such as phytosterols, pentacyclin triterpenes, coumarins, ceramides, and hydroxyl fatty acids have been isolated from the lipophilic fraction, the compounds having an affiliation for lipids. Six isolectins, collectively referred to as *U. dioica* agglutinin (UDA), and some polysaccharides were isolated from the hydrophilic fraction (compounds that dissolve or mix with water), and are considered to be very important pharmacological findings.

Fresh nettle leaves contain a similar range of constituents, with smaller amounts of plant sterols, but proportionally higher levels of flavonol glycosides such as quercitin, and carbonic and formic acid. Many carotenoids have been found such as beta-carotene, violaxanthin, xanthophylls, zeaxanthin, luteoxanthin, and lutein epoxide. In a study done by Kavalali and Akcasu in 1983, an anti-coagulant was isolated from nettle leaves. Terpene diols, terpene diol glucosides, and alpha-tocopherol were also detected. Five new monoterpenoid components were found, as well as 18 phenolic compounds and eight lignans, some of which were previously unknown. In relatively recent studies done by Weglarz and Roslon in 2000 and 2001, the content of polyphenolic acids both in the leaves and rhizomes was found to be higher in the male form of the plant than the female form, but the chemical composition of the female polyphenolic acids were much more complex. An acetylcholine synthesizing enzyme, choline acetyl-transferase, was found, and it appears that Urtica dioica is the only plant to have this enzyme.

Stinging nettle is a powerhouse of nutrients. It contains on average 22% protein, 4% fats, 37% non-nitrogen extracts, 9-21% fiber, and 19-29% ash. The leaves contain about 4.8 mg chlorophyll per gram of dry leaves, depending on whether the plant was grown in the sun or shade. Surprisingly, more chlorophyll and carotenoids are found in plants that have been grown in the shade. The dried leaf of nettle contains 40% protein. They are one of the highest known sources of protein in a leafy green, and of superior quality than many other green leafy vegetables, The fresh leaves contain vitamins A, C, D, E, F, K, P, and b-complexes as well as thiamin, riboflavin, niacin, and vitamin B-6, all of which were found in high levels, and act as antioxidants.   The leaves are also noted for their particularly high content of the metals selenium, zinc, iron, and magnesium. They contain boron, sodium, iodine, chromium, copper, and sulfur. They also contain tannic and gallic acids, gum, and wax. Sixteen free amino acids have been found in the leaves, as well as high silicon levels in the leaves, stems and roots. Amino acids in dehydrated nettle meal are nutritionally superior to those of alfalfa meal.

Samples of dried flowers have been analyzed for nutrient content. They were found to be rich in alpha-tocopherol, riboflavin, iron, zinc, calcium, phosphorous, and potassium. However, the analyses indicated that as a result of the drying and storage process, total loss of vitamin C and a substantial loss of beta-carotene had been incurred.

The hairs contain an acrid fluid. The active principles of this fluid are thought to be acetylcholine, histamine, and formic acid. Formic acid is the same acid that ants have in their saliva glands. Other chemicals found in the hairs are silica, serotonin, and 5-hydroxy tryptamine. Many of these chemicals are smooth muscle stimulants. *U. dioica* contains a high level of UDA acetylcholine in both the fresh hairs and leaves.

There are few studies of the seeds, but those that have been done have found linoleic acid and linolenic acid as well as vitamins C, E, and B6, thiamin, riboflavin, niacin, iron, zinc, copper, calcium, phosphorous, magnesium, manganese, sodium, potassium, and selenium.

UDA, the six isolectins previously mentioned, are found in the rhizomes, roots, and seeds, but not in the leaves and stems. These lectins differ from all the other plant lectins due to its molecular structure. It was shown to possess both antifungal and insecticidal activity and to act synergistically with chitinase in inhibiting fungal growth. It was also shown to directly inhibit cell proliferation and block the binding of epidermal growth factor to its receptor on a tumor cell line.   It is a potent and selective inhibitor of the HIV virus and shows anti-prostatic activity by interfering with sex-hormone binding globulin (SHBG). Nettle influences hormones through its wealth of lipids including triglycerides, fatty acids, tocopherols, sterols, and galactosyldiglycerides.

MEDICINAL QUALITIES

Stinging nettle is an astringent, diuretic, tonic, anodyne, pectoral, rubefacient, styptic, anthelmintic, nutritive, alterative, hemetic, anti-rheumatic, anti-allergenic, anti-lithic/lithotriptic, haemostatic, stimulant, decongestant, herpatic, febrifuge, kidney depurative/nephritic, galactagogue, hypoglycemic, expectorant, anti-spasmodic, and anti-histamine.

Nettle leaf is among the most valuable herbal remedies. Because of its many nutrients, stinging nettle is traditionally used as a spring tonic. It is a slow-acting nutritive herb that gently cleanses the body of metabolic wastes. It is one of the safest alteratives, especially in the treatment of chronic disorders that require long-term treatment. It has a gentle, stimulating effect on the lymphatic system, enhancing the excretion of wastes through the kidneys.

Nettle's iron content makes it a wonderful blood builder, and the presence of vitamin C aids in the iron absorption. As a hemetic (an herb rich in iron), this is an excellent herb for anemia and fatigue, especially in women. It "promotes the process of protein transanimation in the liver, effectively utilizing digested proteins, while simultaneously preventing them from being discharged through the body as waste products."

Stinging nettle is beneficial during pregnancy due to its rich mineral value and vitamin K, which guards against excessive bleeding. It is also a good supplement to strengthen the fetus. It is used during labor to ease the pains, and will increase milk production in lactating women. Stinging nettle is often recommended for pre-menstrual syndrome because of its toxin-ridding activity. When the liver is sluggish, it processes estrogen slowly, contributing to the high levels that cause or aggravate PMS. It acts as a restorative remedy during menopause, and the astringency of the herb helps in excessive menstrual flow.

As a diuretic, stinging nettle increases the secretion and flow of urine. This makes it invaluable in cases of fluid retention and bladder infections. It is also anti-lithic and nephridic, breaking down stones in the kidneys and gravel in the bladder.

The leaves of the fresh nettle plant are stimulating, thus making it a powerful rubefacient. Arthritis, bursitis, rheumatism, gout, and tendonitis have all been treated successfully with urtification. In a group of eighteen patients with joint pain treated with the topical use of the nettle sting, all except one respondent were sure that the therapy had been very helpful, and several considered themselves cured. However, there are other, less painful ways of treating arthritic diseases using stinging nettle. Boron is a trace mineral essential for healthy bones. James A. Duke states in his book *The Green Pharmacy*, "The recommended beneficial dose of boron is 2-3 milligrams daily. An analysis of stinging nettle provided to me [James Duke] by the USDA scientists shows that it contains 47 parts per million of the mineral boron, figured on a dry-weight basis. That means that a 100-gram serving of stinging nettle, prepared by steaming several ounces of young, tender leaves, could easily contain more than the 2-3 milligram recommendations. According to the Rheumatoid Disease Foundation, boron is effective because it plays a role in helping bones retain calcium. It also has a beneficial influence on the body's endocrine (hormonal) system, and hormones play a role in helping the body maintain healthy bones and joints."

Stinging nettle acts similarly to dandelion leaf, promoting the elimination of uric acid from joints with an alkalizing diuretic activity. In an open multi-clinical trial of 219 patients with arthritis, nettle leaf was compared with non-steroidal anti-inflammatory drug (NSAID) therapy, demonstrating a similar reduction in pain and immobility, with excellent tolerability. In an article by Rob McCaleb in 1998 it states, "In an open randomized study, singing nettle given in combination with a sub-therapeutic dose of an anti-inflammatory drug was as effective as a full dose of the drug alone for arthritis pain relief. Forty patients experiencing acute arthritis took part in the study, with half taking the full 200 mg standard dose of the prescription drug diclofenac. The other subjects took 50 mg of diclofenac along with 50 g of stewed nettle leaf. All subjects ate the same foods during the study and only those with uncomplicated medical histories were included, based on very specific criteria. Researchers used both objective and subjective tests to measure effectiveness. The results were impressive: a combination of 50 g nettle leaf with one-quarter of the normal dose of diclofenac was just as effective in relieving pain as the full dose of the drug alone. The authors noted '50 mg diclofenac is unlikely to produce such a profound effect.' Previous research has shown that doses of 75 mg diclofenac are inadequate for arthritis pain relief."

A study conducted by the National College of Naturopathic Medicine in Portland, Oregon found positive evidence of freeze-dried nettle leaf for treating hay fever, asthma, seasonal allergies, and hives. Australians have been using nettle for years as a treatment for asthma, but Americans didn't catch on to this until about 1990. "In a double-blind placebo-controlled randomized study of 98 patients with allergic rhinitis the effect of a freeze-dried preparation of Urtica dioica was compared against placebo. Based on daily symptom diaries and the global response recorded at the follow-up visit after one week of therapy, *U. dioica* was rated higher than placebo in relieving symptoms."

In an open 14-day clinical study, 32 patients diagnosed with myocardial or chronic venous insufficiency were treated with 15 ml of nettle herb juice three times daily. "A significant increase in the daily volume of urine was observed throughout the treatment, the volume in day two being 9.2% higher than the baseline amount in patients with myocardial insufficiency and 23.9% higher in those with chronic venous insufficiency. Minor decreases in body weights and systolic blood pressure were also observed."

As a styptic (an arrestor of local bleeding), stinging nettle is an effective remedy for nose bleeds. It can be applied locally or sniffed. The astringency of stinging nettle proves its usefulness in hemorrhoids, diarrhea, and bleeding in the urinary organs. It also treats mouth and throat infections. Nettle leaf is useful to correct symptoms of gastrointestinal excess, such as gas, nausea, and mucus colitis. It is also used as an anodyne to relieve the pain of burns and scalds.

Numerous studies conducted mostly in Germany have shown the root to have a beneficial effect on enlarged prostate glands. There have been several clinical trials that have demonstrated the efficacy of stinging nettle in treating benign prostatic hyperplasia (BPH) stages I and II. A combination of nettle root and saw palmetto berries was found to be equal to the generic prescription drug finasteride, without side effects. These studies suggest that the root extract may inhibit interaction between a growth factor and its receptor in the prostate. However, it has been observed that the herb does not reduce the size of the already enlarged prostate. "In a randomized, reference-controlled, multi-center, double-blind clinical trial 543 patients with stage I and II BPH compared therapeutic equivalence between finasteride and a combination nettle root/saw palmetto fruit extract. For 48 weeks, patients were given 2 capsules of the herb combination or 1 capsule of finasteride per day. The primary variable was the change of the maximum urinary flow after 24 weeks of therapy. Urodynamic parameters such as average urinary flow, micturition (nighttime urination) flow, and micturition time were monitored as secondary variables. An increase in urinary flow rate was observed in both treatment groups. The average urinary flow increased, whereas the micturition time decreased in both groups to a similar extent. The International Prostate Symptom Score decreased from 11.3 to 8.2 after 24 weeks and 6.5 at week 48 for the herbal group, and from 11.8 to 8.0 and to 6.2 at week 48 for the finasteride group. Fewer adverse reactions were reported from the nettle root/saw palmetto treatment group than the finasteride group".

A decoction of nettle is valuable in diarrhea and dysentery, with profuse discharges, and in hemorrhoids, various hemorrhages, and scorbutic affections. It has been recommended in febrile affections, gravel, and other nephritic complaints. The fresh leaves were found to show anti-tumoural activity in animal studies and strong anti-mutagenic activity. Nettle leaves are high in antioxidants with vitamin activities and have high potassium to sodium ratio. All this indicates it as an excellent natural source for protection against neoplastic diseases (tumors), cardiovascular disorders, and immune deficiency.

"A combined analysis of stinging nettle's traditional uses and demonstrated activities in clinical trials suggests that the root is a good pelvic decongestant, justifying its use in any condition that is affected by such a state, including passive menorrhagia, fibroids, and dysmenorrhea." Applied externally and taken internally, stinging nettle tea is helpful for acne and eczema. Warts rubbed with the freshly expressed juice disappear without any pain being produced. Stinging nettle has been found to treat Alzheimer's disease. It contains considerable amounts of the mineral boron which can double levels of the hormone estrogen circulating in the body. Estrogen has been found in several studies to help improve short-term memory and elevate the moods.

In the respiratory system nettles help clear catarrhal congestion. The seeds are an excellent lung astringent, particularly useful for bronchitis, tuberculosis, and consumption. They are recommended as a remedy for goiter and to reduce body weight. They are also considered anthelmintic, expelling worms and other parasites.

The stimulating effect of stinging nettle is used as a rinse for the hair. This will regenerate hair growth and restore original hair color. It is used by the personal hair care industry in anti-dandruff products and scalp conditioners. Clairol uses more than 40 tons of nettles a year as a hair conditioner. In addition, Russian studies show that nettle tea has anti-bacterial activity. Mouthwashes and toothpastes containing nettle can reduce plaque and gingivitis. Many oral health care products in health food stores contain nettle.

The following is a concise reference of the ailments stinging nettle treats:

*Congestion
  Coughs
  Tuberculosis
  Bronchitis
  Lung congestion
  Laryngitis
  Consumption

*Joints/muscles
  Arthritis
  Rheumatism
  Gout
  Bursitis
  Tendonitis
  Loss of muscular power

Paralysis

*Allergies
  Hay fever
  Seasonal allergies
  Asthma
  Hives

*Neurological disorders
  Sciatica
  Neuralgia
  MS

*Spring tonic

*Circulation

*Hair
  Loss of
  Restores color
  Scalp Conditioner
  Dandruff

*Stones
  Gravel from bladder
  Kidney stones
  Increase urine output

*Internal bleeding
  Excessive menstruation
  Hemorrhoids
  Ulcers
  Lungs/stomach
  Bleeding piles
  Diarrhea/dysentery

*External bleeding
  Nose bleeds

Other

*Skin complaints
  Eczema
  Acne
  Insect bites
  Chicken pox

*Urinary Tract Infection
  Bladder infection

*Women's complaints
  Increase lactation
  PMS
  Menopause
  Prenatal/eases labor

*Anemia/fatigue

*Burns and scalds

*Enlarged prostate

*Pelvic decongestant

*Parasites

*Goiter/scrofula

*Debility

*Blood purifier/builder

*Metabolic disorders

*Fever/cold

*Ague

*Lupus

*Bladder infections

*Lowers blood sugar

*Raises blood pressure

*Gingivitis

*Scurvy

*Celiac disease

*Weight loss

DOSAGES

To use as an infusion (tea): Pour one cup boiling water over 2-3 tablespoons leaves or plant and steep for 10-20 minutes or until desired temperature. Drink 1-3 cups daily.

To use a tincture (alcohol extract): Put 15-20 drops (0.25-0.3 ml) in a small amount of water and take 2 times daily of the herb, or 30 drops (0.5 ml) 2-3 times daily of the root.

To use the juice: Mix with an equal amount of water and take 1 teaspoon at a time.

To use as a decoction: Take 2-4 fluid ounces as needed.

Encapsulated form: Take 2 capsules of 600 mg 2-3 times daily of the herb, or a total of 320 to 1,200 mg daily of the root.

To help prevent seasonal allergies or hay fever, two 300 mg nettle leaf capsules or tablets, or a 2-4 ml tincture, three times per day can be taken during allergy season. For acute attacks, the freeze-dried encapsulated herb can be taken two capsules every five minutes until symptoms have diminished. For hives, 1-2 capsules can be taken every 2-4 hours as needed.

An infusion, tincture, powder, or the fresh juice can be applied externally to cuts and wounds, hemorrhoids, to nostrils for nosebleeds, insect bites or stings, and to soothe and heal burns and scalds. An ointment can also be applied, especially to hemorrhoids.

An infusion of the aerial parts can be taken to stimulate the circulation and to cleanse the system in arthritis, rheumatism, gout, and eczema. Drink 1-3 cups a day. A compress (a soaked cloth in the tea or tincture) can also be applied to painful arthritic joints, gout, neuralgia, sprains, tendonitis, and sciatica.

For prostate problems or BPH, 240 mg per day of the root extract in capsules or tablets can be taken. If this is purchased from a commercial source, it will most likely be combined with saw palmetto or pygeum extracts.

A tincture of the seeds can be used to raise thyroid function and reduce goiter, for skin problems, and in heavy uterine bleeding. The regular seeds, in doses of 14 or 16, and repeated three times daily, are highly recommended as a remedy for goiter.

The juice can be obtained by liquidizing the whole fresh plant to make a good tonic for debilitating conditions, anemia, and to soothe nettle stings. This is also prescribed for cardiac insufficiency with edema. For warts, rub with the freshly expressed juice 3 or 4 times a day, continuing for 10-12 days. To help prevent balding, a tincture or infusion of nettle leaf can be taken. As a rinse for dandruff, falling hair, and as a general conditioner, an infusion or decoction of the root can be taken. The juice of the roots and leaves mixed with honey can relieve bronchitis. An infusion can be taken to increase lactation in nursing mothers and for post-menopausal health. Drink 1-3 cups a day.

THUNDER GOD ROOT LEI GONG TENG

LATIN NAME Tripterygium wilfordii

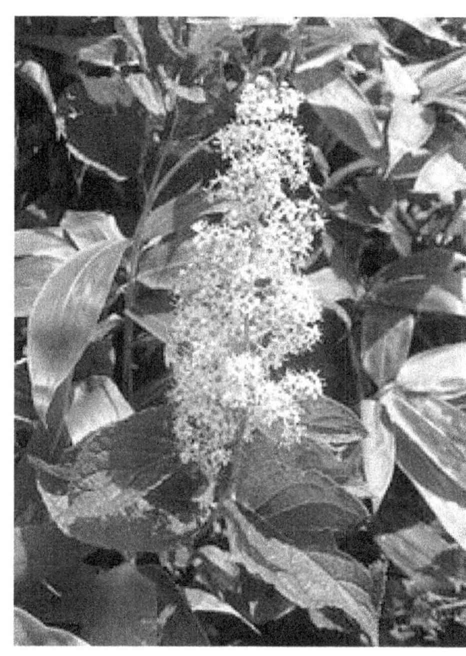

Kingdom: Plantae
Clade: Tracheophytes
Clade: Angiosperms
Clade: Eudicots
Clade: Rosids
Order: Celastrales
Family: Celastraceae
Genus: *Tripterygium*
Species: **T. wilfordii**

Pinyin name: Lei Gong Teng
Literal name: "thunder vine"
Original source: Zhong Guo Yao Ci Dian
(Journal of Chinese Medicinal Plants)
English name: tripterygium, common broad lily root
Botanical name: Tripterygium Wilfordii Hook F.
Pharmaceutical name: Radix Tripterygii Wilfordii
Properties: bitter, acrid, cool
Channels entered: Liver
Safety index: toxic

Background Lei gong teng (radix tripterygii wilfordii) is a native plant that grows in many parts of China and Burma. It is a deciduous climbing vine that grows up to 12 meters in length. The twigs are brown, angular and downy. The leaves are light green, smooth on top, and pale gray with light hairs underneath. The flowers are hermaphroditic, and usually bloom in September. The fruits are threewinged and brownish red, about 1.5 centimeters long. The root is the medicinal part of the plant, and is generally collected in autumn. Traditional Chinese Medicine Traditionally, lei gong teng dispels wind and dampness, and is usually used to treat bi zheng (painful obstruction syndrome). Lei gong teng relieves pain and reduces swelling in patients who have swollen joints and difficulty moving. It can be used alone or with other antirheumatic herbs. This herb is also known as qi bu si, literally, "seven steps to death," implying that it is extremely toxic. Because of its toxicity, the daily dose should be kept between five and 12 grams, with a maximum of 15 grams. Classic texts specifically instructed users to peel and discard the root bark of this herb before decocting. In addition, lei gong teng should be cooked for at least 60 minutes before the addition of other herbs, then cooked for another 15 minutes.

Prolonged decoction (between one and two hours) is recommended to decrease its toxicity. Side-effects are minimal when this herb is prescribed following the proper dosage and preparation. Lei gong teng is contraindicated in pregnancy. It should be used with caution in geriatric and pediatric patients. It should also be used with caution for patients with heart, stomach and spleen disorders. Finally, lei gong teng is toxic, and should not be used by patients who have compromised hepatic functions.1 Clinical Studies and Research There have been many studies published on the potential use of this herb for treatment of arthritis. These in vitro and in vivo studies confirm the therapeutic benefits of this Chinese herb. According to in vitro studies, administration of an extract of lei gong teng once daily for 14 days exhibited a marked effect to suppress the development of arthritis, antibody production and delayedtype hypersensitivity to type II collagen.

On the other hand, therapeutic administration of the herbal extract did not affect the clinical course of the disease.2 In research from the University of Texas and the National Institute of Health, it was reported that the use of a lei gong teng preparation showed that the herb has anti-inflammatory and immunosuppressive effect comparable to prednisone.3 According to one randomized, double-blind trial involving 70 patients with rheumatoid arthritis, the study reported approximately 90 percent of the patients treated experienced significant improvement.4 According to another study, the combination of lei gong teng and fen fang ji (radix stephaniae tetandrae) was found to have a powerful suppressive effect on human immune responses for treatment of rheumatoid arthritis. The mechanisms of action included inhibition of prostaglandin E2 secretion from monocytes, and inhibited IL-1, IL-6, IL-8, and tumor necrosis factor-alpha.5

According to a double-blind, placebo-controlled study, use of a lei gong teng extract for 20 weeks showed therapeutic benefit in patients with rheumatoid arthritis refractory to standard Western drug treatment. Efficacy was defined as 20 percent improvement in disease activity according to the American College of Rheumatology criteria.6 Overdosage The entire tripterygium plant is toxic. The toxicity of the root and bark is greater than that of other parts of the plant. The fresh form is more toxic than the dried form which has been stored for at least a year. Toxic signs include local irritation of the gastrointestinal tract, damage to the central nervous system, internal bleeding and necrosis of the organs.

In severe cases, gross overdose of lei gong teng may cause bleeding in the stomach, intestines, liver and lungs. Other symptoms include dizziness, dry mouth, palpitations, necrosis of mucous membranes and irregular menstruation. Any adverse reactions generally occur within two to three hours after ingestion of the herb. Early reaction is characterized by headache, dizziness, palpitation, fatigue, severe vomiting (sometimes with blood), chills, fever (up to 40° C), continuous abdominal pain, diarrhea (with dark watery stools), generalized aches and pain, tachycardia and irregular heart rhythms. In some cases, patients may present with frequent urination with urgency, and feelings of stabbing pain during urination.

Other patients may exhibit delayed symptoms after two to three days, such as low back pain, hair loss, facial edema, decreased or increased urinary output, and in severe cases, low blood pressure, low body temperature, altered consciousness, convulsions, difficult respiration and purple lips. Hematological disorders have also been noted following chronic use of the herb, with decreased white blood cell and platelet counts due to bone marrow suppression.7 Treatment of Overdosage Early-stage overdose (within four hours of ingestion) should be treated with emetic methods or gastric lavage to eliminate the offending agent from the body. Successful cases of detoxification have been reported using gastric lavage, even with gross overdose.8 Systemic reaction to the herb is generally treated with feng wei cao (herba pteris) or san qi (radix notoginseng) given as decoction (Hu Nan Yi Yao Za Zhi [Hunan Journal of Medicine and Herbology] 1977;5:3). While this herb is toxic to humans, it has no toxicity for goats and rabbits. It was found that goats or rabbits that consume lei gong teng regularly have developed resistance and antibodies to the toxicity of the herb.

VALERIAN

Valerian root

LATIN NAME Valeriana *officinalis*

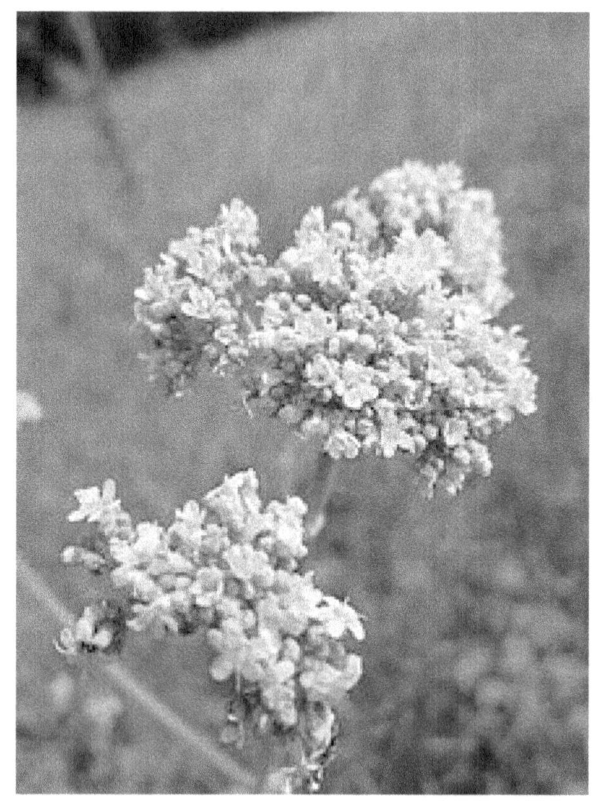

Kingdom: Plantae
Clade: Tracheophytes
Clade: Angiosperms
Clade: Eudicots
Clade: Asterids
Order: Dipsacales
Family: Caprifoliaceae
Genus: *Valeriana*
Species: **V. officinalis**

Valerianae radix
Baldrianwurzel

Name of Drug

Valerianae radix, valerian root.

Composition of Drug

Valerian root, consisting of fresh underground plant parts, or parts carefully dried below 40° C, of the species *Valeriana officinalis* L.[Fam.Valerianaceae], and its preparations in effective dosage.

The roots contain essential oil with monoterpenes and sesquiterpenes (valerenic acids). Preparations of valerian used therapeutically (infusion, extract, fluidextract, tincture) no longer contain the thermolabile and chemically unstable valepotriates.

Uses
Restlessness, sleeping disorders based on nervous conditions.

Contraindications
None known.

Side Effects
None known.

Interactions with Other Drugs

None known.

Dosage

Unless otherwise prescribed:

Infusions:

- 2 - 3 g of drug per cup, once to several times per day.

Tincture:

- - 1 teaspoon (1 - 3 ml), once to several times per day.

Extracts:

- Amount equivalent to 2 - 3 g of drug, once to several times per day.

External Use:

- 100 g for one full bath;
- equivalent preparations.

Mode of Administration

Internal:

- As expressed juice from fresh plants, tincture, extracts, and other galenical preparations.

External:

- As a bath additive.

Actions

Sedative
Sleep-promoting

HISTORY OF VALERIAN

Anxiety, depression, and insomnia are just a few of the countless disorders that are the consequences of a stressful lifestyle. Anyone suffering one of these illnesses knows of the negative results that usually accumulate from the stress. Nerves are tested to the point where relationships are challenged and personal well-being is sacrificed.

Countless amounts of money is being spent in the research and development of the pharmaceutical drugs that are meant to aid in such conditions. These drugs are most often prescribed by physicians to their patients. These patients suffer a broad range of symptoms ranging in intensity. Many people find that taking these drugs may cause severe side-effects and lead to physical and psychological dependence. Often, these patients are discovering that the medications that they have been prescribed do not fix their complaints.

People are becoming so fed up with their physicians and these pharmaceutical companies that they are turning their back on these allopathic medications. More and more people are discovering that nature provides the best healing tools, edible plants or herbs. Fantastic results are produced from using herbal remedies and by making lifestyle modifications and improvements. There are several herbs that produce promising results when used to aid nerve conditions. The powerful herb Valerian has had great success treating such anxiety disorders.

Valerian is an herb that has been documented for hundreds of years for having sedating medicinal qualities. The root of the plant is most commonly used for it's medicinal value. The strong smell of the root makes it easy identifiable. Historic texts dating back to 460 B.C. refer to the unpleasant smell as phu. Variations of the word phu, have been referenced in medical vocabulary from the fifteenth century. These texts gave directions to harvest Valerian in August. Common in use since the age of Hippocrates, Valerian was used by Greeks for several common ailments. Dioscorides, the Greek physician, used Valerian for conditions with the liver, the urinary tract, and the digestive tract. Arab physicians even advocated the use of the herb to patients.

In addition to using the herb chiefly for medicinal purposes, Valerian has even been used by Eastern countries as a scent for one's bath water and as a perfume. Some people used the root to give scent to their clothing. It's hard to believe that anyone would care to use such a foul smelling root for pleasant aromatic purposes but there were and still are several species of Valerian whose roots smelled more appealing.

Before the herb was named Valerian, it was referred to as nard. The origin of Valerian's name is debated. Some say that it is derived from the Latin word meaning good health, valere. Others insist that the herb was named after it was used treating medical conditions by Valerius. Centuries ago Valerian was referred to as Amantilla and has consistently been referred to as "all-heal."

Throughout history Valerian was used as a spice. A recipe from the 1500's containing Valerian stated, "Men who begin to fight and when you wish to stop them, give to them the juice of Amantilla and peace will be made immediately." [i] Anglo-Saxton recipes containing Valerian have also been found and it was often consumed in salads. People in many parts of Europe used the root as additive to stews. It continues to be added to edible dishes around the world.

Valerian has been used in folklore for spiritual purposes. Historically, it has been found as an ingredient in love spells and to bring fighting couples back together. Utilizing Valerian for these purposes was not nearly as common because it was used more effectively for it's medicinal qualities.

Use of medicinal herbs in old English folk medicine was vital. Valerian was effective and people continued to be use it during a time when blood letting was the most popular "healing" method in use. Though it was popular with the country people, physicians also used the herb because of it's effective healing ability.

Valerian is used across the world for the sedating and soothing medicinal qualities that it provides, especially for the nerves. People are not the only beneficiaries of Valerians properties, animals are recipients too. It is not unusual to see a cat instantly attracted to any Valerian plant with bruised leaves or stems. Their reaction is similar to the way they act when they encounter catnip. It is known that many of the historic apothecaries judged the quality of the Valerian they used by the way a cat reacted to it. Many have experienced success in catching rats with a Valerian laced trap. These vermin are enticed by the Valerian plant. It has even been suggested that the rat charmer, the Pied Piper scented his body with the herb.

Gardener's may find that soil containing Valerian will contain greater amounts of earthworms. The herb will increase phosphorus levels and help to provide the soil with additional minerals. The presence of Valerian in a garden may keep animals away from other well loved plants because of their appeal to the strong smelling herb.

Valerian has long been cultivated across the world for the sedating medicinal qualities that it provides. French pharmacists maintained an inventory of herbs that was as impressive as the amount of drugs that were stocked. Phamacuetical companies in the mid-Nineteenth century found their drugs produced a higher quality of results when they added Valerian as an ingredient. Native Americans were known to use chewed Valerian in their ears to provide relief from earaches.

Despite the popularity of allopathic medicine in the early twentieth century, Valerian was still being sought after by many in the medical community in America. Herbal use was even accepted for treating soldiers in World War I. Europeans continued to use the herb during Word War II to help ease the stress of the active air raids that their country was experiencing. Valerian was accepted in the United States medical field for over a hundred years in the U.S. Pharmopoeia until 1942. It was also published in the National Formulary through the mid-twentieth century.

There are at least eighty, yes eighty, over-the-counter sleep medications that include Valerian as an ingredient. The herb is quite popular in Europe and many of these medications are manufactured there. Several countries still cultivate the herb to meet the demand for market use. These countries include: England, Belgium, Holland, India, China, and the United States. The Chinese continue to use it in Traditional Chinese Medicine and Valerian remains an active herb in Ayurvedic practice. The herb remains of the Food and Drug Administration's list of edible foods and even the World Health Organization recognizes the use of Valerian for relaxing the nerves.

It has been suggested that the prescription drug Valium may have derived it's name from Valerian. Perhaps there could be some truth to that...somewhere but the two are not chemically the same. The drug Valium does not contain Valerian. The herb, Valerian is much more safe to use the Valium.

CHEMICAL CONSTITUENTS

One of the foremost active properties of the Valerian is the oil which is only found under the top layer of the root. Concerning the oil of Valerian, Grieve's book, <u>A Modern Herbal</u>, explains that, "It is of complex composition containing valerenic, formic and acetic acids, the alcohol known as borneol, and pinene." The valerenic acid in Valerian is the constituent that has scientifically been proven to give Valerian it's foul smell.

Valeprotriates are chemical constituents that are known for producing a strong sedating effect. In <u>A Green Pharmacy</u>, James A. Duke discusses how bornyl esters were mostly credited for the herbs sedative qualities but an Italian study discovered otherwise. Valeprotriates were once thought to be carcinogenic but further research has indicated that is false and that these constituents are not harmful. This particular study found that the chemicals valeranone and kessyl esters were also components which contributed to Valerian's relaxing qualities. These components cannot be isolated and used to reproduce the same soothing effect. Working as a group is the only way that these constituents are able create the calming effects that Valerian provides. Since the Valerian herb also acts as a stimulant about twenty percent of users will react to these chemicals in such a manner.

Also found in Valerian are anti-arrhythmic compounds that can help to regulate the heart by slowing any palpitations of concern. Valerian contains compounds called sesquiterpenes that also produce sedating effects. Other constituents that are contained in Valerian include the alkaloid, Chatarine, formic acid, glucoside, gums, phosphorous, resins, and silica.

MEDICINAL QUALITIES

Valerian is widely known for its powerful effectiveness as a nervine herb. Nervine herbs can be either stimulating or calming. They work as a tonic to tone the nerves. Our nerves are put to the test every day and sometimes we have no idea how much stress we are experiencing until we hit our breaking point. Instead of modifying stressful habits and other factors that are daily influences, many people are using addictive prescription medication in order to provide relief. The original cause of the affliction is completely over looked while new conditions arise. Using herbs like Valerian can help to provide relief and eliminate the need for prescription medications.

Valerian has proven to be a mild sedative and is popular for treating sleep conditions. When used before sleep it has been quickly effective for anyone suffering from insomnia or restlessness. This herb is great for anyone unable to sleep throughout the entire night because it will help to provide a solid night of sleep. Any nocturnal anxiety, nightmares, and panic attacks can be alleviated by Valerian use. Anyone using Valerian should awaken alert, unlike waking after the use of many sleep aides that create morning-after side effects.

Many studies have been conducted that provide evidence that using Valerian is effective in inducing sleep, but that results may not be obtained unless two to three weeks of use is completed. One such study was conducted with twenty Hispanic volunteers that complained of having trouble sleeping. Upon completion of the trial, eighty percent claimed to have moderate to significant improvement in sleep quality.

It has shown to be especially helpful for women suffering sleeplessness caused by menopause. Valerian can also provide relief for women not yet experiencing the effects of menopause. Women nationwide suffering from PMS and menstrual cramping should push aside the Midol bottles and give Valerian a try. The use of hot Valerian can stimulate a woman's menstrual cycle.

Physical pain is one reason many people seek out alleviation from over-the-counter drugs, prescription medications, and even illegal narcotics. Valerian has been known for centuries as a reliable pain reliever and relaxant. Many over-the-counter pain medications are sold constantly to provide relief from pain caused from ailments such as headaches and joint pain . It may also help to ease the severe pain caused by migraines. Valerian can decrease the feeling of mild to intense pain.

Pharmaceutical companies make billions of dollars in profits annually from their sales of medication to aid in depression. Once again, addictions to medications are created by use of these prescription drugs. There are many herbs that can be used for depression instead of turning to these prescriptions. Valerian is one of them.

The rate of Attention Deficit Disorder (ADD) has skyrocketed in the United States over the last couple of decades. People diagnosed with this disorder are prescribed medication in order to be able to concentrate. In many scenarios, the medication itself has caused severe psychological damage. People that have trouble focusing and are hyperactive are successful with taking Valerian as a way to help control these conditions. These patients found that using the herb allowed them to be able to concentrate for longer amounts of time. Their nerves were stimulated to allow them to focus with better coordination.[i]

The use of Valerian has also been found to be useful for lowering blood pressure. It is well known that high levels of stress can cause an elevation in blood pressure. Taking Valerian can provide relief to the stress and can in turn lower blood pressure. Valerenic acid contains an enzyme that prevents the breakdown of gamma-amino butyric acid, which is known for its ability to regulate blood pressure.[ii]

Valerian is calming and soothing to the digestive muscles. Its ability to relax the digestive system makes Valerian useful in certain cases of upset stomach and constipation. It has even displayed success in healing stomach ulcers. The constituent valerenic acid is so soothing to irritated muscles that it has been used with success to provide relief for people suffering from Irritable Bowel Syndrome.
Recently in Iowa there were outbreaks of measles and the whooping cough amongst vaccinated children in the state. All children are at risk from these diseases, so a little awareness can provide a great deal of relief for these little ones. Valerian can be given to small children that are having trouble sleeping due to an illness and can be directed for

use in the occurrence of measles. This herb can provide relief for anyone suffering from the whooping cough because of its ability to relax internal muscles.

In addition to other afflictions, the ancient Greeks used Valerian for urinary tract disorders and as a decongestant. I assume that Valerians ability to relax muscles could allow kidney stones to pass easier, and for phlegm to break apart for ejection. This herbs success in calming muscle spasms has even made it a choice herb to help people suffering from epilepsy. It became widely known to be used for epilepsy in 1592, when Fabius Calumna cured himself of the condition by using Valerian. [iii]

The use of Valerian to aid in treatment of the optic nerves to increase eyesight has also been documented. Herbalists praise that external use of Valerian. It has provided great results for people suffering from skin conditions like bruises, sores, and acne. People suffering from the pain of rheumatoid arthritis may want to try a topical application of an infusion of Valerian to provide some relief. This herb has also had great results in easing the itching and appearance of hives. Historical references called for spinal fomentations of Valerian to provide stimulation for the nerves.

There have been animal studies that have confirmed Valerian is successful in lowering blood pressure and protecting the liver. The World Health Organization sponsored studies in Bulgaria for traditional herbs known for their healing properties on the cardiovascular system.[iv] Results from Valerian use were highly promising. Current studies are being conducted to obtain results for a possible link between the anti-tumor properties of Valerian in treating cancer. Germans have also released evidence supporting Valerians corrective role in several studies. These studies confirmed the herb is useful in lowering blood pressure, relaxing nerve conditions, and ceasing muscle spasms. Italian researchers have also provided evidence that Valerian is one of the best herbs to support the digestive tract.

DOSAGES

Anyone who is just beginning to take Valerian should begin with small doses and increase the amount of herb used as needed. This is because Valerian is very powerful, so a little care with administration of this herb will ensure safe and effective results. Valerian is known for its effectiveness as a sedative and should be used responsibly. Anyone using Valerian should not attempt to do tasks that require full alertness, such as drive. Alcohol and narcotics should not be taken when using Valerian. There is only one known severe overdose of Valerian. On this occasion, a woman took twenty times the recommended dosage and attempted suicide. This does not by any means make Valerian accountable, and the herb remains on the Food & Drug Administration's list of safe foods. This instance only confirms the importance of following dosage instructions and using the herb with care. One can benefit from the great healing properties of Valerian by using several different methods of application.

Preparing a cup of Valerian tea is a common but stinky way to obtain medicinal results. The strong tasting tea is tolerable and can be a relaxing method of using Valerian before bedtime. An infusion of Valerian should be used as opposed to a decoction. A decoction should be avoided since the root of this herb should not be boiled so that vital essential oils are not lost. Infusions of Valerian are used for external applications. Dr. Christopher recommended using two ounces of this infusion before meals and again before bedtime. Otherwise, a cup of tea steeped with two teaspoons of the dried herb may be used before retiring for the night.

Using a tincture form of Valerian is great for those who find the smell of the herb unpleasant. In addition, a tincture of Valerian will maintain it's medicinal value for several years. The recommended dosage for a tincture of Valerian is one to two teaspoons daily.

Using Valerian in a powdered or capsule form is an easy way to take Valerian but a little extra attention is required. The dosage for the powdered form of Valerian is between three hundred milligrams to one gram. If purchasing a marketed form of Valerian, careful examination of the label will provide the amount of herb and how many capsules to take. Typical dosage, depending on content, is about two capsules. Filling individual capsules with powdered Valerian would require great care to assure that dosage instructions are safe and accurate.

Another recommended form of use is an elixir of Valerian. Elixirs contain high concentrations of the herb and need to be used in small doses. Generally, a half a teaspoon to one full teaspoon are taken. Only five to fifteen drops is advised if a fluid extract is being used. For solid extracts the dosage instructions would be between three hundred to six hundred milligrams.

As mentioned earlier, commercial formulas may contain additional herbs besides Valerian. Therefore, dosage instructions should be followed as they will vary depending what the formula consists of. The average amount of volatile oil from Valerian in commercial preparations is about .05 percent. With this in mind, a preparation that contains a higher percentage of the oil will not require as high of a dosage. Also one should to keep in consideration that the precious qualities contained in the root may vary in potency.

WILLOW

White Willow bark

LATIN NAME Salix alba

Kingdom: Plantae
Clade: Tracheophytes
Clade: Angiosperms
Clade: Eudicots
Clade: Rosids
Order: Malpighiales
Family: Salicaceae
Genus: *Salix*
Species: **S. alba**

Salicis cortex
Weidenrinde

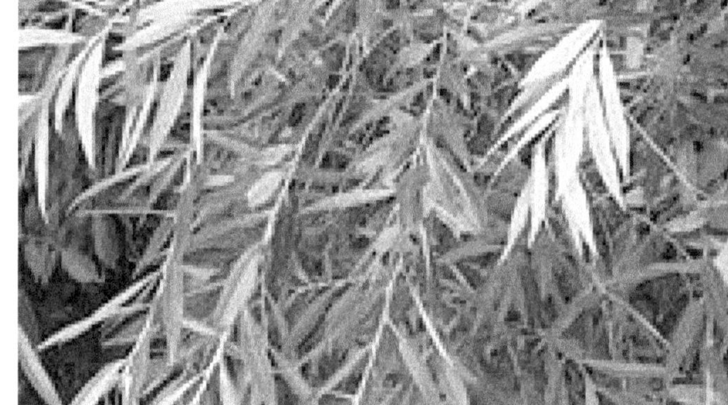

Name of Drug

Salicis cortex, white willow bark.

Composition of Drug

White willow bark consists of the bark of the young, 2- to 3-year-old branches harvested during early spring of *Salix alba* L., *S.purpurea* L., *S.fragilis* L.and other comparable *Salix* species [Salicaceae], as well as their preparations in effective dosage.The bark contains at least 1 percent total salicin derivatives, calculated as salicin ($C_{13}H_{18}O_7$, MW 286.3) and related to the dried herb.

Uses
Diseases accompanied by fever, rheumatic ailments, headaches.

Contraindications
See Interactions with Other Drugs

Side Effects
See Interactions with Other Drugs

Interactions with Other Drugs

Because of white willow bark's active constituents, interactions like those encountered with salicylates may arise. However, in reviewing the scientific literature available so far, there are no definite indications for this.

Dosage

Unless otherwise prescribed:

- Average daily dosage corresponding to 60 - 120 mg total salicin.

Mode of Administration

Liquid and solid preparations for internal use.

Note: Combinations with diaphoretic drugs could be considered.

Actions

Antipyretic
Antiphlogistic
Analgesic

Relieves Pain

Due to its rich blend of antioxidants and organic compounds, willow bark functions as a very successful analgesic. For thousands of years, it has been traditionally used to relieve pain from injuries and illness, with great success. More than 2,500 years ago, the earliest recorded use of an herb was of willow bark, in Chinese traditional medicine. Although it was mentioned in older texts dating back to the Egyptians, this was the first documented use of willow bark for pain relief!

Anti-inflammatory Properties

Inflammation takes on many different forms within our bodies. If you are looking to eliminate the inflammation in your respiratory tracts, gastrointestinal system, or joints, then willow bark can quickly soothe your symptoms. If you prepare a decoction or a tea of this bark, you will feel the inflammation and topical pain from arthritis, irritable bowel syndrome (IBS), gout, and other conditions disappear.

Reduces Fever

One of the most important anti-inflammatory properties of willow bark is in the reduction of fevers. Fevers are a symptom of an infection in the body, but reducing a fever or breaking it is important to speed up the healing process and get the organs working normally again. It has been used to treat fevers for thousands of years.

Eases Menstruation

For many women who suffer from abnormally heavy periods or severe menstrual symptoms, taking a small glass of willow bark can do wonders for everything from period pains and cramping to mood swings and unnecessary stress hormones in the body. Its relaxing characteristics are particularly good in these circumstances, as they can help re-balance hormones in a woman's body.

Soothes Stomach Disorders

The high content of tannins can help soothe the stomach and prevent gastrointestinal distress during other illnesses or periods of a weakened immune system. Willow bark can be slow-acting, its effects can be long-lasting, making it an effective herbal remedy to occasionally add to your health regimen, but it should not be consumed daily unless advised by a doctor or trained herbalist.

Weight Loss

Many people turn to willow bark to enhance their weight loss efforts, namely because the herb combines so well with other fat-burning and metabolism-boosting substances. It can intensify the effects of these herbs healthily, thereby increasing their efficacy and improving your results even further.

Skin Care

The appearance of the skin is very important for many people, and the high content of antioxidant compounds found in willow bark can have a major impact on the health of the skin. Whether applied topically or consumed, willow bark can increase blood flow to the skin due to its antioxidants, while also reducing the appearance of wrinkles and age marks. Furthermore, it can eliminate inflammation in the skin and ease the pain of insect bites and irritation.

Eliminates Migraines

If you suffer from chronic headaches and migraines, you might be able to benefit significantly from the pain-relieving qualities of willow bark. It can help eliminate migraines by lowering the blood pressure in the small capillaries and blood vessels in the head, easing pressure and relieving those painful, debilitating symptoms. It can also be used as a preventive method for regular headaches.

YARROW

LATIN Achillea millefolium

Kingdom: Plantae
Clade: Tracheophytes
Clade: Angiosperms
Clade: Eudicots
Clade: Asterids
Order: Asterales
Family: Asteraceae
Genus: *Achillea*
Species: **A. millefolium**

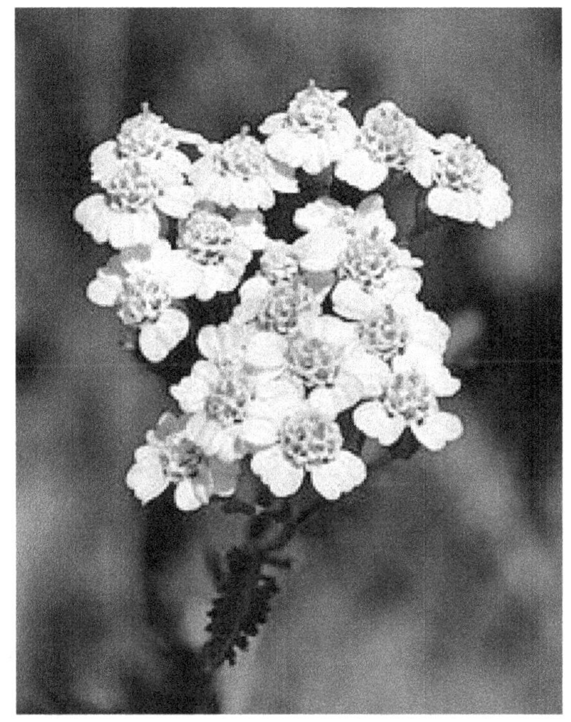

Achillea millefolium, commonly known as **yarrow** /ˈjæroʊ/ or **common yarrow**, is a flowering plant in the family Asteraceae. It is native to temperate regions of the Northern Hemisphere in Asia and Europe and North America.[2] It has been introduced as a feed for livestock in New Zealand[3] and Australia, where it is a common weed of both wet and dry areas, such as roadsides, meadows, fields and coastal places.[3]

In New Mexico and southern Colorado, it is called *plumajillo* (Spanish for 'little feather') from its leaf shape and texture. In antiquity, yarrow was known as *herbal militaris*, for its use in stanching the flow of blood from wounds.[4] Other common names for this species include gordaldo, nosebleed plant, old man's pepper, devil's nettle, sanguinary, milfoil, soldier's woundwort, thousand-leaf, and thousand-seal

Description

Clusters of 15 to 40 tiny disk flowers surrounded by three to eight white to pink ray flowers are, in turn, arranged in a flat-topped inflorescence (Wenatchee Mountains, Washington).

Achillea millefolium is an erect, herbaceous, perennial plant that produces one to several stems 0.2–1 m (0.66–3.28 ft) in height, and has a spreading rhizomatous growth form. Leaves are evenly distributed along the stem, with the leaves near the middle and bottom of the stem being the largest. The leaves have varying degrees of hairiness (pubescence).

The leaves are 5–20 cm (2.0–7.9 in) long, bipinnate or tripinnate, almost feathery, and arranged spirally on the stems. The leaves are cauline, and more or less clasping.

The inflorescence has 4 to 9 phyllaries and contains ray and disk flowers which are white to pink. The generally 3 to 8 ray flowers are ovate to round. Disk flowers range from 15 to 40. The inflorescence is produced in a flat-topped capitulum cluster and the inflorescences are visited by many insects, featuring a generalized pollination system.The small achene-like fruits are called cypsela.

The plant has a strong, sweet scent, similar to that of chrysanthemums

Folklore

The English name yarrow comes its Saxon (Old English) name *gearwe*, which is related to both the Dutch word *gerw* (alternately *yerw*) and the Old High German word *garawa*. In the eastern counties it may be called yarroway.

The genus name *Achillea* is derived from mythical Greek character, Achilles, who reportedly carried it with his army to treat battle wounds.The specific name *millefolium* as well as the common names milfoil and thousand weed come from the featherlike leaves which appear to be divided into a thousand.

For its historical use in wound healing particularly in the military it was called bloodwort, herbe militaris, knight's milfoil, staunchweed, and, from its use in the US Civil War, soldier's woundwort. Its use in either starting or stopping nosebleeds led to the common name nosebleed. For its association with the Evil One it was called bad man's plaything, devil's nettle, and devil's plaything. It was called old man's pepper due to its pungent flavor, while the name field hop came from its use in beer making in Sweden.

Other traditional names for *A. millefolium* include arrowroot, carpenter's weed, death flower, eerie, hundred leaved grass, knyghten, old man's mustard, sanguinary, seven-year's love, snake's grass, soldier, and thousand seal.

Overview

Yarrow is a chemically polymorphic perennial herb from a genus of complex taxonomy, native to Europe, Asia, and North America, now distributed in the temperate zone worldwide. Many species, subspecies, and microspecies have been recognized and named (Bruneton, 1995; Budavari, 1996; Leung and Foster, 1996; Wichtl and Bisset, 1994). Yarrow adapts itself to new surroundings and can change its morphology and chemical composition significantly, depending on its environment. New subspecies evolve by polyploidy (changes in chromosome number). The subspecies can be differentiated by their chromosome numbers, determined by microscopic examination (Bradley, 1992; Zeylstra, 1997). The material of commerce comes mostlyfrom southeastern and eastern European countries and the United Kingdom (BHP, 1996;Wichtl and Bisset, 1994).In Germany, a small amount of yarrow is cultivated (Lange and Schippmann, 1997). The material used in Ayurvedic medicine grows wild in the Himalayan mountains from Kashmir to Kumaon (Nadkarni, 1976).

Yarrow has been used as medicine by many cultures for hundreds of years (Budavari, 1996; Zeylstra, 1997). Its English common name is a corruption of the Anglo-Saxon name *gearwe*; the Dutch, *yerw*. The genus name *Achillea* may have been derived from the *Achilles* of Greek mythology, who was fabled to have had his wounds treated by topical use of the herb. The species name *millefolium* is derived from the many segments of its foliage. The ancient Europeans called it *Herba Militaris,* the military herban ointment made from it was used as a vulnerary drug on battle wounds (Grieve, 1967).Yarrow flower was formerly official in the *United States Pharmacopeia.* Today, it is official in the national pharmacopeias ofAustria, the Czech Republic,France, Germany,Hungary,Switzerland, and Romania. Additionally, it is listed in the Indian *Ayurvedic Pharmacopoeia* for fevers and wound healing (Karnick, 1994).

Its uses in North American aboriginal medicine are well documented. Yarrow tea is used by healers of the Micmac nation as a diaphoretic remedy to treat fevers and colds. The stalks are also pounded into a pulp and applied topically to bruises, sprains, and swellings(Lacey, 1993).Yarrow has been the subject of an ongoing study of herbal drugs used by people of the Micmac and Malecite nations of the Canadian Maritime provinces. The study began with an examination of the observations and writings of early European settlers and missionaries. Modern phytochemical studies, using techniques including nuclear magnetic resonance spectroscopy and combined gas chromatography-mass spectrometry, have identified a range of phytosterols and triterpenes occurring in yarrow, which may help explain its successful therapeutic applications in Micmac and Malecite medicines (Chandler et al., 1979; Chandler et al., 1982; Chandler and Hooper, 1982; Chandler, 1983; Hooper and Chandler, 1984). The Abnaki people use yarrow tea as a drug to treat colds, fevers, and grippe (Rousseau, 1947). People of the Algonquin and Quebec nations use it internally to treat colds and other respiratory disorders. The powder is also used as an analgesic snuff for headaches (Black, 1980). Yarrow infusions and decoctions are used as a gastrointestinal aid by the Cherokee, Gosiute, Iroquois, and Mohegan nations (Chamberlin, 1911; Hamel and Chiltoskey, 1975; Herrick, 1977; Tantaquidgeon, 1928, 1972).

In Germany,yarrow flower is licensed as a standard medicinal tea. It is also used as a cholagogue component in numerous preparedbiliary and/or gastrointestinal medicines. It is also used externally as a sitz bath to treat vegetative pelvipathia (Bradley, 1992; Braun et al., 1997; Wichtl and Bisset, 1994).In the United States, yarow is used as adiaphoretic or febrifuge component of traditional cold and flu/fever compounds marketed asdietary supplement products, often used in combination with echinacea herb, elder flower, ginger rhizome, and peppermint leaf. It is also used as a component of topical styptic preparations.

The approved modern therapeutic applications for yarrow flower are supportable based on its long history of use in well established systems of traditional medicine,on phytochemical investigations,and on pharmacological studies in animals.

German pharmacopeial gradeyarrow flower must be composed of the dried aerial parts (capitulums with maximum 5% stems) harvested during the flowering period, containing not less than0.2% (v/m)volatile oils with minimum 0.02% proazulene, calculated as chamazulene on a dry-weight basis. It must have a bitter value of maximum 5000. Botanical identity must be confirmed by thin-layer chromatograhy (TLC) as well as macroscopic and microscopic examinations (DAB, 1997; DAC, 1986; Wichtl and Bisset, 1994).The *Swiss Pharmacopoeia* also requires not less than 0.2% volatile oils, though not more than 10% peduncles of inflorescences (Ph.Helv.VII, 1987; Wichtl and Bisset, 1994). The *British Herbal Pharmacopoeia* requires not less than 15% water-soluble extractive, among other quantitative standards and identity tests (BHP, 1996).

Both the *Austrian Pharmacopoeia* and the *French Pharmacopoeia* require >0.3% volatile oil and the characterization of azulenes (Bruneton, 1995; AB, 1981; Ph.Fr.X, 1990; Wichtl and Bisset, 1994).According to Bruneton, these requirements can only be fulfilled by the pink flower subspecies (*sudetica,* from mountain areas), or by other species entirely (e.g., *A. collina*),becausethe official species at best contains only traces of azulenes(Bruneton, 1995). The most widespread species [*Achillea millefolium* L. ssp. *millefolium*] is hexaploid and the volatile oil contains no chamazulene (Bradley, 1992).

Description

Yarrow herb consists of the fresh or dried aboveground parts of *A. millefolium* L. [Fam. Asteraceae], harvested at flowering season, and its preparations in effective dosage. Yarrow flower consists of the dried inflorescence of *A. millefolium* L. *s.l.* [Fam. Asteraceae] and its preparations in effective dosage. The preparation contains essential oil and proazulene.

Chemistry and Pharmacology

Yarrow contains 34% condensed and hydrolysable tannins; 0.31.4% volatile oils, mostly linalool, borneol, camphor, *b*-caryophyllene, 1,8-cineole, and sesquiterpene lactones composed of guaianolides, mainly achillicin (a proazulene), achillin, leucodin, and germacranolides (dihydroparthenolide, achillifolin, millefin); flavonoids (apigenin, luteolin, isorhamnetin, rutin); amino acids (alanine, histidine, leucine, lysine); fatty acids (linoleic, palmitic, oleic); phenolic acids (caffeic, salicylic); vitamins (ascorbic acid, folic acid); alkaloids and bases (achiceine, achilleine, betaine, choline); alkanes (tricosane); polyacetylenes; saponins; sterols (*b*-sitosterol); sugars (dextrose, glucose, mannitol, sucrose); and coumarins (Bradley, 1992; Bruneton, 1995; Leung and Foster, 1996; Newall et al., 1996; Wichtl and Bisset, 1994).

The Commission E reported choleretic, antibacterial, astringent, and antispasmodic activities.

The *British Herbal Compendium* reported diaphoretic, antipyretic, anti-inflammatory, spasmolytic, aromatic bitter, hemostatic, hypotensive, and emmenagogic activities (Bradley, 1992). Anti-inflammatory activity was reported in laboratory mice and rats with an aqueous extract of yarrow flower heads (Leung and Foster, 1996; Newall et al., 1996). It is possible that its anti-inflammatory and antispasmodic properties are due to its flavonoids content (Bruneton, 1995). Choleretic activity has been confirmed in animal experiments. Antimicrobial activity against a range of bacteria has been reported for aqueous and ether extracts of yarrow (Wichtl and Bisset, 1994).

Uses

The Commission E approved the internal use of yarrow flower for loss of appetite and dyspeptic ailments, such as mild, spastic discomforts of the gastrointestinal tract, and externally as a sitz bath for painful, cramp-like conditions of psychosomatic origin in the lower part of the female pelvis.

The *British Herbal Compendium* lists its internal use for feverish conditions, common cold, and digestive complaints; and its topical use for slow-healing wounds and skin inflammations (Bradley, 1992). The German Standard License for yarrow tea indicates its use for mild cramp-like or spasmodic gastrointestinal-bilious complaints, for gastric catarrh, and for appetite stimulation (Bradley, 1992; Wichtl and Bisset, 1994).

Contraindications

Allergy to yarrow and other composites.

Side Effects

None known.

None known.

Dosage and Administration

Internal:

Unless otherwise prescribed: 4.5 g per day of cut herb, or 3 g of cut flower for teas and other galenical preparations; pressed juice of fresh plants.

Infusion: 1-2 g in 150 ml boiled water for 10 to 15 minutes, three times daily between meals.

Succus (pressed juice from fresh herb): 5 ml (1 teaspoon), three times daily between meals.

Fluidextract 1:1 (g/ml): 1-2 ml, three times daily between meals.

Tincture 1:5 (g/ml): 5 ml, three times daily between meals.

External:

Unless otherwise prescribed: Sitz baths.

Sitz bath: 100 g yarrow per 20 liters (5 gallons) of warm or hot water, just enough to cover the hips with the knees up; wrap upper body in towels; soak 10 to 20 minutes, rinse.

About The Author

Dr. Earendil M. Spindelilus D.N.M., M.H., C.R. -
Traditional Naturopath, Holistic Practitioner,
Clinical Master Herbalist, Certified Nutritionist,
Certified Reflexology, Member of Plant Savers of
America, Member of American Botanical
Council.

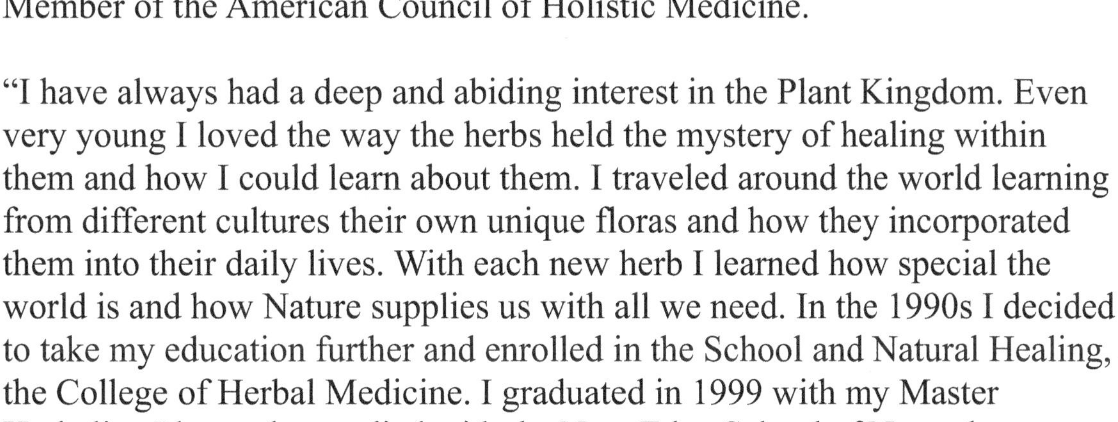

He holds a Doctorate degree in Natural Medicine.
I have also been a lecturer since 1999. Board
Certified Diplomate of Natural Medicine.
Member of the American Council of Holistic Medicine.

"I have always had a deep and abiding interest in the Plant Kingdom. Even
very young I loved the way the herbs held the mystery of healing within
them and how I could learn about them. I traveled around the world learning
from different cultures their own unique floras and how they incorporated
them into their daily lives. With each new herb I learned how special the
world is and how Nature supplies us with all we need. In the 1990s I decided
to take my education further and enrolled in the School and Natural Healing,
the College of Herbal Medicine. I graduated in 1999 with my Master
Herbalist. I have also studied with the New Eden School of Natural
Medicine where I completed my Doctorate in Natural Medicine."

To date, my wife have run two medical centers for natural healing. It has
always been a great joy meeting with our patients. We are all meant to live a
happy, healthy life and when we allow our body to perform it's innate ability
to heal itself then this can happen. I am also a past board member of the
Reflexology Association of California as well as a published author/writer of
numerous holistic books and articles. I am also a past host of a holistic radio
show.

**OTHER BOOK BY DR. EARENDIL SPINDELILUS
IN THE HEALING NATURALLY SERIES**

A Holistic Approach To Healing Lyme Disease

Healing Lyme Disease Naturally

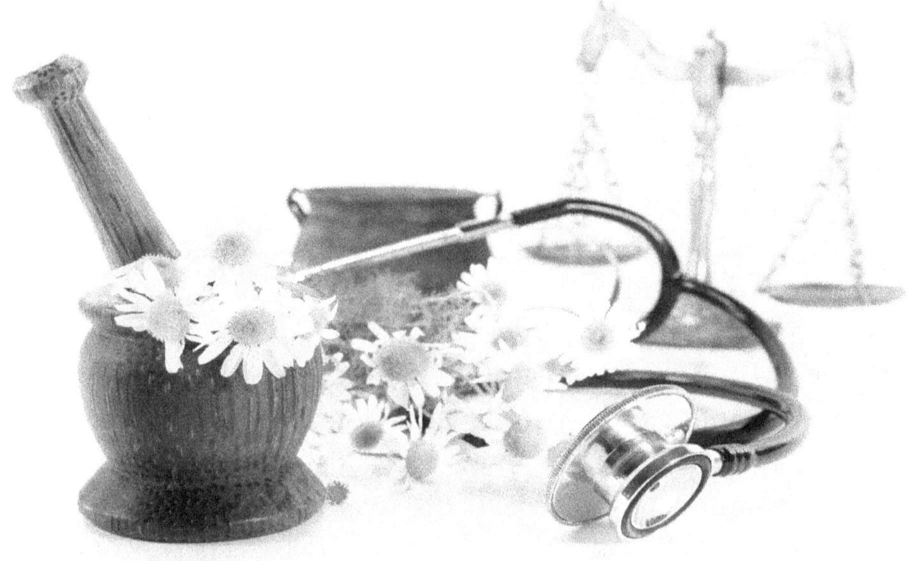

Dr. Earendil M. Spindelilus
D.N.M., M.H., C.R., PSc.D

Case Histories From A Successful Naturopathic Clinic

Healing Chronic Disease Naturally

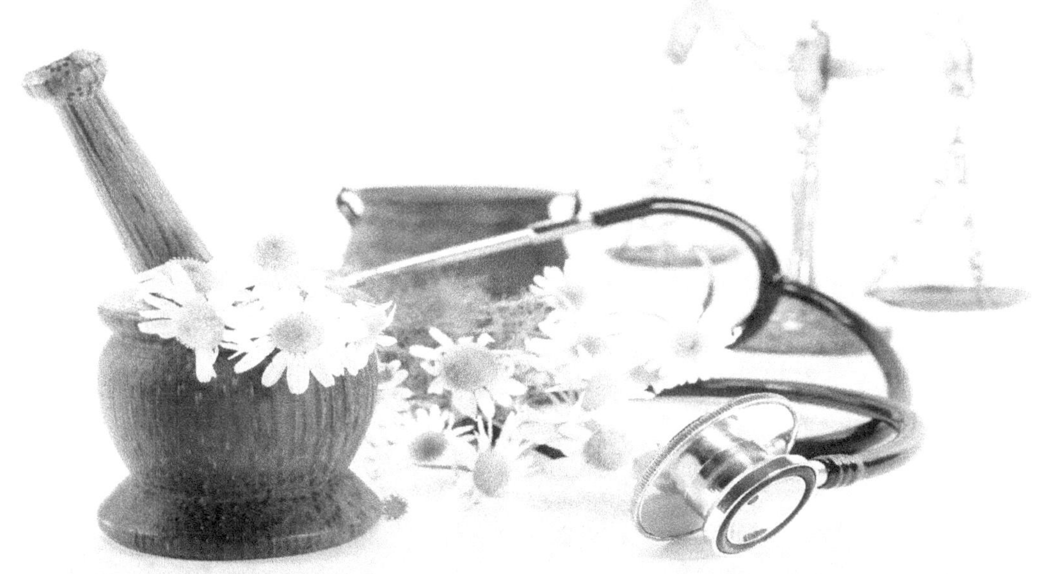

Dr. Earendil M. Spindelilus
D.N.M., M.H., C.R., PSc.D

A Complete Body Repair

Healing Candida, Parasites and Heavy Metal Toxicity Naturally

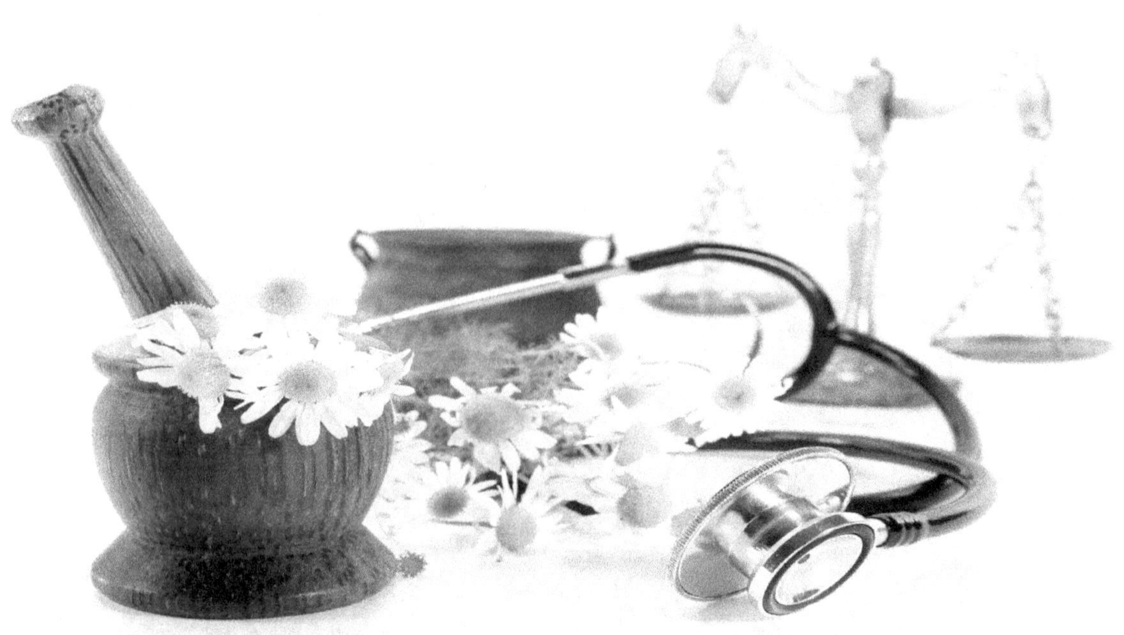

Dr. Earendil M. Spindelilus
D.N.M., M.H., C.R., PSc.D

Holistic First ✚ Aid

Healing Emergencies Naturally

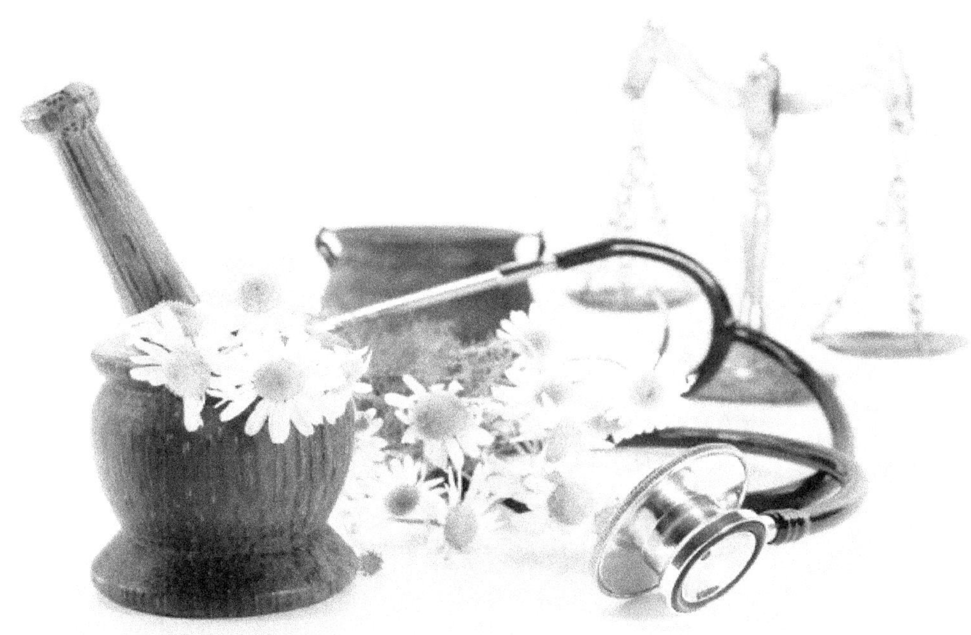

Dr. Earendil M. Spindelilus
D.N.M., M.H., C.R., PSc.D

The Handbook Of Holistic Healing

Healing The Body Naturally

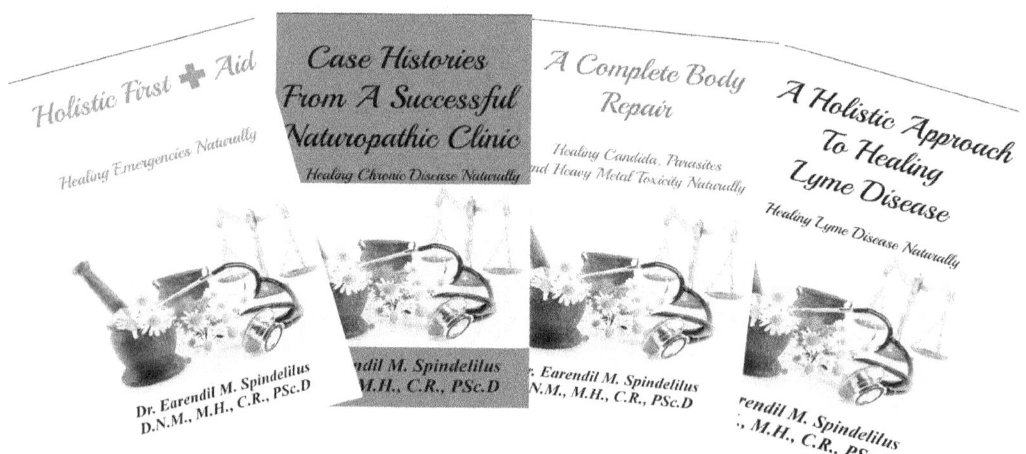

**The Complete Healing Naturally Series
By Dr. Earendil Spindelilus
Plus A Bonus Section For Treating Your
Companion Animals!**

Dr. Earendil M. Spindelilus
D.N.M., M.H., C.R., PSc.D

Curing Chronic Disease With A Raw Vegan Diet

Healing With A Raw Vegan Diet Naturally

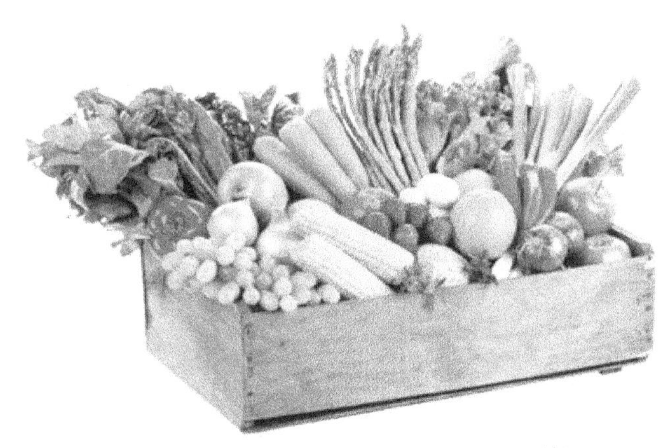

Dr. Earendil M. Spindelilus
D.N.M., M.H., C.R., PSc.D

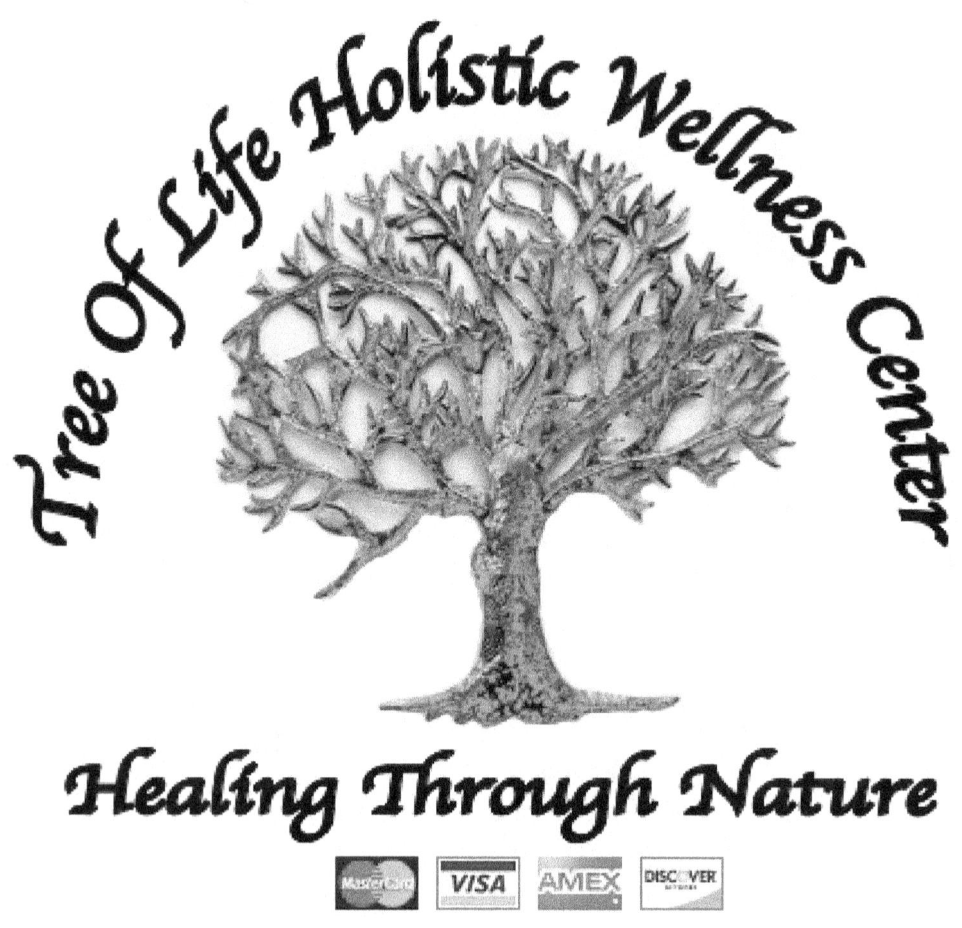

Tree Of Life Holistic Wellness Center also also online classes in Herbalism and Nutrition. If you are interested please feel free to check out our school and website at:

http://www.treeoflifehwc.com/ Practice website

http://www.treeoflifehwc.com/online-holistic-classes.html Classes Description

https://tree-of-life-holistic-studies.thinkific.com/ School Site

www.ingramcontent.com/pod-product-compliance
Lightning Source LLC
Chambersburg PA
CBHW080858160726
48000CB00009B/2769